Endometriosis

Endometriosis

An Enigma

Edited by
Seema Chopra

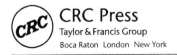

CRC Press
Taylor & Francis Group
Boca Raton London New York

CRC Press is an imprint of the
Taylor & Francis Group, an **informa** business

CRC Press
Taylor & Francis Group
6000 Broken Sound Parkway NW, Suite 300
Boca Raton, FL 33487-2742

First issued in paperback 2021

© 2020 by Taylor & Francis Group, LLC
CRC Press is an imprint of Taylor & Francis Group, an Informa business

No claim to original U.S. Government works

ISBN-13: 978-1-138-32796-2 (hbk)
ISBN-13: 978-1-03-217328-3 (pbk)
DOI: 10.1201/9780429448980

Publisher's Note

Library of Congress Cataloging-in-Publication Data

Names: Chopra, Seema, editor.
Title: Endometriosis : an enigma / edited by Seema Chopra.
Other titles: Endometriosis (Chopra)
Description: Boca Raton : CRC Press, [2020] | Includes bibliographical references and index. |
Summary: "Endometriosis is a complex gynecological disorder with multifactorial etiology. It is an estrogen-dependent disorder that occurs in 6-10% of women in the general population and in 35-50% of women with pain and/or infertility. This book aims to discuss different aspects from basic to advanced levels, in turn exploring this benign but chronic disease"-- Provided by publisher.
Identifiers: LCCN 2020002845 (print) | LCCN 2020002846 (ebook) | ISBN 9781138327962 (hardback) | ISBN 9780429448980 (ebook)
Subjects: MESH: Endometriosis--therapy | Endometriosis--complications | Infertility, Female--etiology
Classification: LCC RG483.E53 (print) | LCC RG483.E53 (ebook) | NLM WP 390 | DDC 618.1--dc23
LC record available at https://lccn.loc.gov/2020002845
LC ebook record available at https://lccn.loc.gov/2020002846

Visit the Taylor & Francis Web site at
http://www.taylorandfrancis.com

and the CRC Press Web site at
http://www.crcpress.com

Contents

Preface

Knowledge and practice in the field of gynecology is constantly changing. With ongoing research, changes in treatment modalities become necessary, as well as appropriate.

Endometriosis is a complex gynecological disorder that can affect women from menarche until menopause. It is a benign, estrogen-dependent disorder with multifactorial etiology. Endometriosis is characterized by the presence of functional endometrial glands and stroma outside the uterine cavity, resulting in chronic pelvic pain, dysmenorrhea, dyspareunia, and infertility, thus affecting the quality of life.

Several theories have been put forth to explain the etiopathogenesis of this disease. There is increasing evidence to suggest that endometriosis is at least partially a genetic disease.

At the time of diagnosis, most patients with endometriosis have had the disease for an unknown period, making it difficult to initiate any clinical experiments that would definitively determine the etiology or progression of the disease. As of now, the gold standard for diagnosis is laparoscopic visualization of endometriotic lesions. The use of biomarkers, such as CA-125, is not sensitive enough to detect the disease in the early stages.

Peripheral biomarkers show promise as diagnostic aids, but further research is necessary before these can be recommended in routine clinical care. Panels of markers may allow increased sensitivity and specificity of any diagnostic tests.

Management is both medical and surgical, depending upon age, fertility preservation, symptomatic relief, and whether or not the disease is extra pelvic/deep endometriosis. The disease is notorious for recurrence and requires long-term management.

Availability of new drugs, alternative medicines, and lifestyle modifications are helpful for the women inflicted with the disease. Therefore, this book aims to help the readers get a concise knowledge in the field of endometriosis as a valued resource, with evidence based from literature and recent guidelines.

The support of the publisher, CRC Press/Taylor & Francis, for completion of this book is highly appreciated.

Seema Chopra

Acknowledgments

This book is dedicated to all the courageous women living with endometriosis who have helped us understand this entity.

I thank my family and friends for their constant support and encouragement in successful completion of this responsibility.

I sincerely hope that the resource material will be able to answer the queries in the minds of readers of this book.

Editor

Seema Chopra, MBBS, MD, is a consultant (additional professor) in the Department of Obstetrics and Gynecology at the Postgraduate Institute of Medical Education and Research (PGIMER), Chandigarh, a well-established and reputed tertiary care institute in North India. She has more than 70 publications to her credit in international as well as national journals and as an author of book chapters. She is an active participant in national and international conferences and research projects. Conducting seminars, teaching postgraduate students, and administrative responsibilities are part of her curriculum. She is also designated nodal in-charge of sexually transmitted infections (STI)/reproductive tract infections (RTI) of the state chapter under the National AIDS Control Organization (NACO), as well as nodal officer for the STI reference laboratory in her institute in collaboration with the Department of Microbiology. She has been invited for lectures at various scientific meetings, public forums, and panel discussions, as well as for conducting drills in continuing medical education (CME) and other workshops. She has attended/organized live surgical workshops and has a special inclination toward minimally invasive surgery. She has been involved in the management of gynecological as well as obstetrical emergencies for more than 25 years in her career. Her areas of interest are related to endometriosis: early diagnosis and medical, surgical management of this entity to help these women for relief of symptoms, as well as part of infertility treatment. She is actively conducting research on the recurrence of endometriosis after conservative laparoscopic surgery and suppression with medical therapy as part of a postgraduate thesis.

Contributors

Neelam Aggarwal
Department of Obstetrics and Gynecology
PGIMER
Chandigarh, India

Neha Aggarwal
Department of Obstetrics and Gynecology
Maulana Azad Medical College
Delhi, India

Aashima Arora
Department of Obstetrics and Gynecology
PGIMER
Chandigarh, India

Rashmi Bagga
Department of Obstetrics and Gynecology
PGIMER
Chandigarh, India

Girdhar Singh Bora
PGIMER
Chandigarh, India

Rinnie Brar
Department of Obstetrics and Gynecology
PGIMER
Chandigarh, India

Seema Chopra
Department of Obstetrics and Gynecology
PGIMER
Chandigarh, India

Shalini Gainder
Department of Obstetrics and Gynecology
PGIMER
Chandigarh, India

Nalini Gupta
Department of Cytology and Gynecological
  Pathology
PGIMER
Chandigarh, India

Parikshaa Gupta
Department of Cytology and Gynecological
  Pathology
PGIMER
Chandigarh, India

Rajesh Gupta
Department of General Surgery
PGIMER
Chandigarh, India

Bharti Joshi
Department of Obstetrics and Gynecology
PGIMER
Chandigarh, India

Japleen Kaur
Fellowship Reproductive Endocrinology
PGIMER
Chandigarh, India

Aditya Kulkarni
Department of General Surgery
PGIMER
Chandigarh, India

Neethi Mala Mekala
PGIMER
Chandigarh, India

Rakhi Rai
Department of Obstetrics and Gynecology
AIIMS
Delhi, India

Minakshi Rohilla
Department of Obstetrics and Gynecology
PGIMER
Chandigarh, India

Nancy Sahni
Department of Dietetics
PGIMER
Chandigarh, India

Indu Saroha
Department of Obstetrics and Gynecology
PGIMER
Chandigarh, India

Aditya Prakash Sharma
Department of Urology
PGIMER
Chandigarh, India

Bharti Sharma
Department of Obstetrics and Gynecology
PGIMER
Chandigarh, India

Pooja Sikka
Department of Obstetrics and Gynecology
PGIMER
Chandigarh, India

Sujata Siwatch
Department of Obstetrics and Gynecology
PGIMER
Chandigarh, India

Arshi Syal
Government Medical College and
  Hospital
Chandigarh, India

Natural history: Basics of endometriosis

ARSHI SYAL AND SEEMA CHOPRA

Endometriosis is a relatively common and potentially debilitating condition affecting women of reproductive age. Symptomatic endometriosis can result in long-term adverse effects on personal relationships, quality of life, and work productivity. As there is no clarity regarding the etiopathogenesis to date, researchers have shown a keen interest in the history of endometriosis over the past few decades.

Although, medical texts older than 4000 years have described this entity [1], Karl von Rokitansky was the first to diagnose endometriosis microscopically in 1860 [2].

As long as 2500 years ago, the disease with symptomatology of chronic pelvic pain was treated as a true organic disorder. As it was difficult to differentiate the menstrual pain from the severe pain due to endometriosis, during the middle ages, there was a shift from organic cause into the belief that women with pelvic pain were malingering or immoral, had female weakness, or were misbehaving. There was development of an attitude of indifference to the patients' true pain. Hence, through the ages, the historical diagnosis of hysteria in women with severe pelvic pain may have indeed been endometriosis, thus leading to delays in a correct diagnosis during the twentieth century.

Hippocratic doctors believed that endometriosis-like symptoms are a result of delaying childbearing, which triggers diseases of the uterus. This may be an indirect pointer toward the existence of the disease in women with dysmenorrhea, as they were encouraged to marry at a young age and produce children so that the ectopic endometrial tissue remained quiescent. This also implies that the disease prevalence rates were higher than the 5%–15% that is often reported nowadays. If it is considered plausible that the existence of endometriosis was so common historically, we will have to reconsider the modern theories that suggest links between endometriosis and environmental toxins such as dioxins, polychlorinated biphenyls (PCBs), and chemicals [1].

ANCIENT DESCRIPTIONS SUGGESTING THE DIAGNOSIS OF ENDOMETRIOSIS

In 1999, Vincent J. Knapp [3] reported a number of old dissertations as old as the eighteenth and even the seventeenth centuries; this started a new discussion revolving around the history of endometriosis, thus focusing our attention to the exploration of women's diseases that had onset during the eighteenth century. On evaluation of these texts, no description of macroscopic features of endometriosis could be found. Also, it was not possible in those early times even to predict the presence of endometrial (or even epithelial) tissue in the lesions described by those authors without a microscope. Therefore, substantiating the presence of the specific features of endometriosis during the seventeenth and eighteenth centuries seems nearly impossible.

The Barker hypothesis [4] proposes that early exposures, including those arising from unhealthy lifestyles of parents, during sensitive windows of human development, such as pregnancy, may permanently reprogram the developing embryo or fetus for extra-uterine life. Thus, this theory generated considerable interest in the potential early origins of health and disease. This reprogramming is speculated to occur largely through epigenetic mechanisms [5].

In an attempt to verify the early origins of health and disease hypothesis, many investigators have assessed in utero exposures with diagnosis of endometriosis in adult women. It was demonstrated that in utero diethylstilbestrol (DES) was associated with higher odds of an endometriosis diagnosis in these women and a lesser chance of having this diagnosis with in utero exposure to cigarette smoking and increasing birth weight [6].

There has been research to document the possible role for endocrine disrupting chemicals (EDCs), defined as exogenous chemicals that can interfere with hormonal milieu in the body, including alterations in estrogen signaling [7]. The Endocrine Society published a statement on EDCs citing strong evidence of adverse reproductive outcomes following exposure, including the possibility of epigenetic changes and transgenerational effects with early exposure to these agents [8].

While speculative, this finding may suggest a role for in utero environmental tobacco smoke and endometriosis that has not been previously reported. Irrespective of route of exposure, active smoking, or passive exposure from environmental sources, the biologic dose of tobacco chemicals and metabolites may be the relevant exposure [6].

The ENDO Study was carried out with the specific aim to assess the relation between persistent environment chemicals and endometriosis [9]. There were positive associations between endometriosis and select organochlorine pesticides such as aromatic fungicides and hexachlorocyclohexane [10], polychlorinated biphenyls [11], perfluorochemicals, and dioxins. Its etiology remains unknown despite investigating a number of probable mechanisms for the same. Bisphenol A (BPA) has the ability to interact with estrogen receptors and stimulate estrogen production, being similar to endogenous estrogens, and therefore can alter gonadotropin hormone secretion [12]. Similar observations between these chemicals and endometriosis have not been substantiated by many authors in the literature, underscoring remaining critical data gaps.

Another environmental toxin widely used in plastics to increase its resilience, namely phthalate, produces anti-androgenic effects largely through the reduction in testosterone production and, possibly, reduced estrogen production at high doses [13].

It was observed that mEHP was the only phthalate consistently associated with endometriosis across cohorts, though significance was only achieved when disease was restricted to comparison women with a normal pelvis in the operative cohort. Also of note is the observation that three of the phthalate metabolites (mono (2-ethyl-5-carboxyphentyl) phthalate [mECPP], mono (2-ethyl-5-hydroxyhexyl) phthalate [mEHHP], mono (2-ethyl-5-oxohexyl) phthalate [mEOHP]) associated with endometriosis are derived from the parent compound di-(2-ethylhexyl)-phthalate (DEHP), which is the most widely used phthalate and is present in cosmetics and other personal care products that are a source of continuous human exposure [14]. Despite their relatively short half-lives, ubiquitous occurrence of BPA and phthalates may produce prolonged exposures for users, thus causing toxic levels and the related effects.

While going through the evolution of this entity, an important question often asked is, "Who identified endometriosis?" To have a plausible answer, two non-complementary methods were used: searching for ancient descriptions of similar symptoms associated with endometriosis or, as an alternative evidence, identifying researchers who mentioned various pathological features associated with the different phenotypes of endometriosis. Rokitansky, in the middle of the nineteenth century, suggested the presence of endometrial glands and stroma in neoplasias of the ovary and the uterus. However, Cullen was the first scientist to delineate peritoneal endometriosis and named it "adenomyoma" using histological parameters of endometrial structure and activity. On the other hand, Rokitansky was the first to describe an adenomatous polyp, a form of adenomyosis. The description of an "ovary containing uterine mucosa" was first published in 1899 by Russel [15].

What is the natural course of endometriosis?

As there are no set diagnostic criteria for endometriosis without invasive testing for the presumptive diagnosis of this pathology for chronic pelvic pain as seen in almost all adolescent girls who report painful periods, the natural course of symptomatic endometriosis is difficult to delineate. Also, it is not possible to exclude a diagnosis of endometriosis clinically; hence, follow-up is not stringent so as to know the natural evolution of endometriosis [16].

The definition of the expression "discovering endometriosis" is the starting point for our historical journey. The word "discovery" may imply imagining its existence in the susceptible group, naming it as endometriosis, giving details clinical symptoms, sometimes describing it as a separate pathophysiological entity, or confirming it on histological examination. In the early days, the term "adenomyoma" was used to describe peritoneal, extraperitoneal (scar), and deep-infiltrating endometriosis, ovarian endometrioma, and adenomyosis, as all these varieties were considered together. In the 1920s, these two entities were described as separate entities [17,18].

OVARIAN ENDOMETRIOSIS

The work of Carl Rokitansky was not recognized initially as endometriosis, probably because he had described these lesions as sarcomas [19]. It was realized later, as reported by Batt, that Rokitansky had utilized a "personal" definition of these tumors as described in his opus magnum *A Manual of Pathological Anatomy*.

Further, in 1920, cases of "ovarian hematomas" described by Smith [20] could have been endometriosis, as one such case, in particular, had all the characteristics of ovarian endometriosis; clinically the patient had severe dysmenorrhea, which was markedly relieved after its surgical removal.

Similarly, Sampson described 23 cases of ovarian hematomas of endometrial type in his publication "Perforating Hemorrhagic (Chocolate) Cysts of the Ovary" [21]. Finally, the term "perforating hemorrhagic cyst" was omitted and, instead, "ovarian endometrioma" was coined, which included hematomas or hemorrhagic cysts of endometrial (Müllerian) type. While rupture of the endometrial cyst was considered as the cause of peritoneal endometriosis by Sampson [22], several authors proposed that endometriotic lesions on the cortex invaded the ovary, or lymphatic spread of endometrial cells led to endometriosis [23]. Finally, it was histological evidence given by Hughesdon in 1957, demonstrated on a surgical specimen of 27 ovaries with chocolate cyst in situ that ovarian cortex formed the wall of the cyst in 90% of the cases. This also confirmed the findings of Sampson's original article "Perforating Hemorrhagic Cysts of the Ovary" [21] or Halban's [23] hypothesis of lymphatic theory that the presence of an inner cortex in the cyst is indicative that relation of the cyst to the surface is primary. This was further confirmed objectively on endoscopy by Brosens et al. [24]. They showed that chocolate cysts were lined by the ovarian cortex, which was partially covered by a thin lining of endometrial tissue.

IDENTIFICATION OF ADENOMYOMA

Initially, Rokitansky, in the middle of the nineteenth century [19], described three cases of fibrous polyps of the uterus with additional glandular tubes in some of them. These also contained a smooth muscle component in addition to the usual features of endometrial polyps. On histological examination, they were composed of "endometrial glands intimately mixed with smooth muscle and thick-walled blood vessels." Later on, the term "adenomyoma" was coined by both Cullen and Von Recklinghausen [25], followed by Pick and Rolly around the end of the nineteenth century.

ADENOMYOSIS AND ENDOMETRIOSIS—THE DIFFERENTIATION

With ongoing research, Sampson, in 1925 [26], postulated that endometrial tissue that sloughs into uterine veins, the theory of retrograde menstruation, could be the cause of adenomyosis and spread of disease beyond the pelvis in menstruating women. In an attempt to redefine the terminology, Sampson first introduced the term "endometriosis" interchangeably with the term "implantation adenomyoma." It was the exact description of the anatomical picture for the mucosal invasion of the myometrium by the endometrial glands by Frankl [18] as "adenomyosis uteri." He also enumerated the criteria to differentiate it from endometriosis, stating, "In an adenomyoma the glands originate independently within the myoma as an autochthonous (indigenous) growth, while in adenomyosis, even when localized, the direct connection of the endometrium with the islands of mucosa located in the musculature can be established in serial sections. In the majority of cases of genuine adenomyoma, which are extremely rare, the glands are not accompanied by stroma." Thus, at this point, "adenomyoma" was subdivided into two separate entities, endometriosis and adenomyosis.

REFERENCES

1. Nezhat C, Nezhat F, Nezhat C. Endometriosis: Ancient disease, ancient treatments. *Fertil Steril* 2012;98(6 Suppl):S1–62.
2. Batt RE. *A History of Endometriosis*. London: Springer; 2011, pp. 13–38.
3. Knapp VJ. How old is endometriosis? Late 17th- and 18th-century European descriptions of the disease. *Fertil Steril* 1999;72:10–4.
4. Barker DJ. The fetal and infant origins of adult disease. *BMJ* 1990;301(6761):1111. Comment in The effects of preterm birth and its antecedents on the cardiovascular system. [*Acta Obstet Gynecol Scand.* 2016].
5. Daxinger L, Whitelaw E. Understanding transgenerational epigenetic inheritance via the gametes in mammals. *Nat Rev Genet* 2012;13(3):153–62.
6. Wolff EF, Sun L, Hediger ML, Sundaram R, Peterson CM, Chen Z, Buck Louis GM. In utero exposures and endometriosis: The Endometriosis, Natural History, Disease, Outcome (ENDO) Study. *Fertil Steril* 2013;99(3):790–5, Copyright © 2013.
7. Crews D, McLachlan JA. Epigenetics, evolution, endocrine disruption, health and disease. *Endocrinology* 2006;147:S4–10.
8. Zoeller RT, Brown TR, Doan LL, Gore AC, Skakkebaek NE, Soto AM, Woodruff TJ, Vom Saal FS. Endocrine-disrupting chemicals and public health protection: A statement of principles from The Endocrine Society. *Endocrinology* 2012;153(9):4097–110.
9. Buck Louis GM, Peterson CM, Chen Z et al. Bisphenol A and phthalates and endometriosis: The Endometriosis: Natural History, Diagnosis and Outcomes Study. *Fertil Steril* 2013;100(1):162–9.e2.
10. Buck Louis GM, Chen Z, Peterson CM et al. Persistent lipophilic environmental chemicals and endometriosis: The LIFE Study. *Environ Health Perspect* 2012;120:811–6.
11. Porpora MG, Medda E, Abballe A et al. Endometriosis and organochlorine environmental pollutants: A case control study on Italian women of reproductive age. *Environ Health Perspect* 2009;1117:1070–5.
12. Takeuchi T, Tsutsumi O, Ikezuk Y et al. Elevated serum bisphenol A levels under hyperandrogenic conditions may be caused by decreased UDP-glucuronosyltransferase activity. *Endocrine J* 2006;53:485–91.
13. Okubo T, Suzuki T, Yokoyama Y, Kano K, Kano I. Estimation of estrogenic and anti-estrogenic activities of some phthalate diesters and monoesters by MCF-7 cell proliferation assay in vitro. *Biol Pharm Bull* 2003;26:1219–24.
14. Silva MJ, Barr JA, Reidy NA et al. Urinary levels of seven phthalate metabolites in the U.S. population form the national health and nutritional examination survey (NHANES) 1999–2000. *Environ Health Perspect* 2004;112:331–8.
15. Benagiano G, Brosens I, Lippi D. The history of endometriosis. *Gynecol Obstet Invest* 2014;78:1–9.
16. Hickey M, Ballard K, Farquhar C. Endometriosis. *BMJ* 2014;348:g1752.
17. Benagiano G, Brosens I. Who identified endometriosis? *Fertil Steril* 2011;95:13–6.
18. Frankl O. Adenomyosis uteri. *Am J Obstet Gynecol* 1925;10:680–4.

19. Rokitansky C. *A Manual of Pathological Anatomy (transl by W.E. Swaine).* Philadelphia: Blanchard & Lea, 1855, vol I: General pathological anatomy, pp. 189–190.
20. Smith RR. Hemorrhage into the pelvic cavity other that of ectopic pregnancy. *Am J Obstet Gynaecol* 1920;1:240–2.
21. Sampson JA. Perforating hemorrhagic (chocolate) cysts of the ovary. *Arch Surg* 1921;3: 245–323.
22. Sampson JA. Peritoneal endometriosis due to the menstrual dissemination of endometrial tissue into the peritoneal cavity. *Am J Obstet Gynecol* 1927;14:422–69.
23. Halban J. (The lymphatic origin of the so-called heterotopic adenofibromatosis.) *Arch Gynäkol* 1925;124:457–82.
24. Brosens IA, Puttemans PJ, Deprest J. The endoscopic localization of endometrial implants in the ovarian chocolate cyst. *Fertil Steril* 1994;61:1034–8.
25. Cullen T. Adenomyoma of the round ligament. *Johns Hopkins Hosp Bull* 1896;7:112–3.
26. Sampson JA. Heterotopic or misplaced endometrial tissue. *Am J Obstet Gynecol* 1925;10:649–64.

Epidemiology

POOJA SIKKA AND RINNIE BRAR

Endometriosis remains a disease marred with confusion due to the absence of an easy, noninvasive diagnosis; changing definitions; and the absence of a validated classification system. Endometriosis is one of the most common diagnoses in women with pelvic pain. Prevalence estimates vary from about a 4% occurrence of largely asymptomatic endometriosis found in women undergoing tubal ligation to 50% of teenagers with intractable dysmenorrhea. It is important to clearly distinguish among subtle, typical, cystic, and deep endometriosis and to understand the shifts that have occurred, mainly in the recognition of subtle endometriosis and deep endometriosis. Estimations of subtle endometriosis range from 5% to 50% and from 50% to 80% in asymptomatic or symptomatic women, respectively.

INTRODUCTION

To describe the incidence and prevalence of endometriosis is as difficult as is managing it. Over the past few years, endometriosis has become one of the most common diagnoses in women with pelvic pain. Whether managed medically or surgically, it constitutes a significant burden on the quality of life of women, their families, their healthcare providers, and healthcare facilities. Prevalence estimates of the disease in populations that visit a doctor vary from about a 4% occurrence of largely asymptomatic endometriosis found in women

undergoing tubal ligation to 50% of teenagers with intractable dysmenorrhea. The prevalence of endometriosis is undoubtedly higher in women with infertility. However, there is great variation in the published estimates (as much as 30–40 times). This is primarily because studies on endometriosis focus on women who have a higher probability of having the disease, such as women with pelvic pain and infertility.

EPIDEMIOLOGY

Advances in understanding the epidemiology of endometriosis have lagged behind other diseases because of methodologic problems related to the disease definition. It was first described in 1860. The definition of endometriosis has changed over time, contributing to bias in the literature and clinical practice. Initially in the mid-1980s, nonpigmented or subtle endometriosis was introduced, and later, the recognition of deep endometriosis progressively increased. The concept arose when it was seen that even after surgery, symptomatic relief in pain did not happen. Taken together, the absence of an easy, noninvasive diagnosis; the changing definitions; the absence of a clear understanding of the pathophysiology; and the absence of a validated classification system, endometriosis remains a disease marred with confusion.

Nevertheless, a better picture of the epidemiology of endometriosis has emerged over the past few decades [1,2]. This is because of wider use of computed tomography (CT) scans, magnetic resonance imaging (MRI), and laparoscopy [3]. General awareness among women and gynecologists about the disease has led to using these tests. To correctly define the epidemiology of endometriosis, it is important to clearly distinguish among subtle, typical, cystic, and deep endometriosis and to understand the shifts that have occurred, mainly in the recognition of subtle endometriosis and deep endometriosis. Estimations of subtle endometriosis range from 5% to 50% and from 50% to 80% in asymptomatic or symptomatic women, respectively [4–6]. For typical lesions, estimations are less than half of these figures, but those data were collected before the 1990s. For severe endometriosis, either cystic or deep, estimations in the population range between 1% and 10%.

A poorly addressed problem is the variability of prevalence by region and country. There is a clinical impression that African Americans have lower rates and Asians have higher rates of endometriosis than Caucasians. No systematic studies are available, but it is obvious that the prevalence of very severe deep endometriosis must be higher in Europe, from where this type of lesion is reported. In Arab countries, endometriosis is rare. A variety of personal risk factors for endometriosis have also been described. Women with endometriosis may be taller and thinner. Menstrual factors reported to increase risk include dysmenorrhea, early menarche, and shorter cycle lengths. There is support for the idea that lifestyle exposures that might raise or lower estrogen levels could affect risk, including a decreased risk associated with smoking and exercise and an increased risk associated with caffeine or alcohol use. These risk factors appear to be compatible with the central importance of retrograde menstruation influenced by outflow obstruction that might affect its amount, immune factors that might affect its ability to be cleared, or hormonal stimuli that might affect its growth. In this model, dysmenorrhea could be either a disease symptom or a manifestation of outflow obstruction. There is an established hereditary basis for endometriosis.

The role of nutrition, of lifestyle, of personality traits, of the immune system, of the peritoneal fluid, and other variables is not well understood. Various speculations have been made. For most of these factors, indirect evidence strongly suggests a modulating role. The key question that remains, however, is to find an answer to the question whether endometriosis is a normal endometrial cell or an abnormal endometrial cell. This is important to understanding the prediction, prevention, and management of the disease. The etiopathogenesis of the disease is discussed in Chapter 3.

REFERENCES

1. Parazzini F, Esposito G, Tozzi L et al. Epidemiology of endometriosis and its comorbidities. *Eur J Obstet Gynecol Reprod Biol* 2017;209:3–7.
2. Cramer DW, Missmer SA. The epidemiology of endometriosis. *Ann N Y Acad Sci* 2002;955:11–22.
3. Janssen EB, Rijkers AC, Hoppenbrouwers K et al. Prevalence of endometriosis diagnosed by laparoscopy in adolescents with dysmenorrhea or chronic pelvic pain: A systematic review. *Hum Reprod Update* 2013;19:570–82.
4. Fuldeore MJ, Soliman AM. Prevalence and symptomatic burden of diagnosed endometriosis in the United States: National estimates from a cross-sectional survey of 59,411 women. *Gynecol Obstet Invest* 2017;82:453–61.
5. Mowers EL, Lim CS, Skinner B et al. Prevalence of endometriosis during abdominal or laparoscopic hysterectomy for chronic pelvic pain. *Obstet Gynecol* 2016;127:1045–53.
6. Stuparich MA, Donnellan NM, Sanfilippo JS. Endometriosis in the adolescent patient. *Semin Reprod Med* 2017;35:102–9.

Etiopathogenesis of endometriosis

POOJA SIKKA AND RINNIE BRAR

Endometriosis is a chronic, progressive, and troublesome disease of women in the reproductive age group. It was first described in 1860. The disease is increasingly being diagnosed over the years. Still, it is one of the most underdiagnosed diseases and mean time period from onset of symptoms to definitive diagnosis is around seven to eight years. The incidence of disease is reported to be 10%–15%. However, in women with chronic pelvic pain and infertility, endometriosis can be found in almost 50%. In many women, the disease may not present any symptom, so it may go undiagnosed.

The research today is focused mainly on etiopathogenesis of the disorder so that targeted treatment can be provided to the patients. In the past several decades, significant progress toward exposing the enigma associated with this disorder has been made. Still, many aspects of the disease are unclear. For example, can endometriosis be prevented or predicted? What triggers malignancy in endometriosis?

The answers can only be provided if the mechanism of the disease is understood. A thorough understanding of the etiopathogenesis of endometriosis is essential for the development of newer diagnostic tests and effective treatments of the disease. Maybe it is a disease with several mechanisms of origin, several symptoms, and several treatments.

WHAT IS ENDOMETRIOSIS?

Endometriosis is defined as the presence of functioning glands and stroma of the uterus outside the endometrium. It can manifest in two forms:

- Presence of endometrium in the extra uterine organs
- Presence of endometrium in the uterine wall

WHAT IS THE PATHOLOGY?

An endometriotic lesion has typical histological resemblance to the endometrial glands and stroma. They exhibit cyclical changes characteristic of menstruation and decidualize during pregnancy. The process of endometriosis formation is generally a diffuse one. In the ovary, however, blood and debris get collected, then get encapsulated to form a cyst. With progression of the pathology, absorption of fluid elements causes the blood to become inspissated and give a tarry or chocolate look. As the cyst grows, its endothelial lining becomes thinned, stretched, and ultimately destroyed.

WHAT IS ADENOMYOSIS?

The myometrium is invaded by endometrial glands. The invasion, however, has to be at least one high power field from the basal endometrium to label it as adenomyosis.

Other areas where endometriosis has been reported include urinary bladder, ureter, bowel, episiotomy or cesarean section scars, rectovaginal septum, vulva, cervix, pleura, lungs, and kidneys.

ETIOLOGY

The disease has a few known and many supposed etiological factors. The precise etiopathogenesis of endometriosis is unknown, but several theories regarding the phenomena involved in its development have been proposed. Besides the classic retrograde menstruation theory, lymphatic and vascular metastases, iatrogenic direct implantation, coelomic metaplasia, embryonic remnants, and mesenchymal cell differentiation or induction, the persistence of a form of embryonic endometriosis may also be involved, as well as the theory of the possible role of endometrial stem/ progenitor cells. Genetics also plays a role in the development of endometriosis. Recent studies have highlighted the role of oxidative stress, defined as an imbalance between reactive oxygen species (ROS) and antioxidants, which may be implicated in the pathophysiology of endometriosis causing a general inflammatory response in the peritoneal cavity.

RISK FACTORS

Family history: The risk of developing endometriosis is 10 times higher in women with a family history of the disease in first-degree relatives. No specific gene has been identified and therefore a multifactorial inheritance is suggested.

Early menarche, nulliparity, and polymenorrhea: Endometriosis is an estrogen-dependent disorder. When we compare ectopic endometriotic tissue with eutopic, an increased activity of the aromatase enzyme and decreased activity of 17β-Hydroxysteroid dehydrogenase (17β-HSD) type 2 is found. Increased aromatase activity is the consequence of the higher production of prostaglandin E2 (PGE2), which is stimulated by higher locally bioavailable E2 concentration. These findings support the ability of endometriotic lesions for E2 biosynthesis and confirm treatments which lead to hypoestrogenism.

GENITAL TRACT (MÜLLERIAN ANOMALIES)

Whenever, in medical science, we are unable to precisely decipher the past, present, and future of any disease, we propose several theories. It is because all facts about the disease cannot be explained by one single mechanism. Endometriosis is one such disorder. All proposed mechanisms remain to be conclusively confirmed. Of recent interest are the theories of oxidative stress and immune dysfunction.

Various proposed theories behind the etiopathogenesis of endometriosis are presented here.

Retrograde menstruation theory: The theory of retrograde menstruation was proposed by Sampson. According to this theory: eutopic endometrium is transferred through patent fallopian tubes into the peritoneal cavity during menstruation every month. It must have been proposed as a mechanism when in women with patent tubes undergoing laparoscopy during the perimenstrual time of the cycle, the menstrual blood would have been seen in the pouch of douglas. When the collection of this menstrual blood in the pelvis or, to be more precise, over the ovaries becomes significant, it causes symptoms. This theory is supported by the fact that the prevalence of endometriosis is very high in adolescent girls with congenital obstructed or compromised tracts.

Coelomic metaplasia theory: According to this theory, endometriosis originates from the metaplasia of cells, which are present in the mesothelial lining of the visceral and abdominal peritoneum. Transformation of normal peritoneal cells into endometrium-like cells occurs as a result of either hormonal or immunological triggers.

Theory of abnormal embryogenesis: Ectopic endometrial tissue has also been detected in female fetuses. This theory postulates that residual cells of the Wolffian or Müllerian ducts persist and develop into endometriotic lesions that respond to estrogen. Furthermore, recent theories suggest coelomic metaplasia to be the origin of the adolescent variant of a severe and progressive form of endometriosis. However, endometriotic lesions can also be found in areas outside of the course of Müllerian duct.

Stem cell theory: The stem cells are supposed to exist in the basalis layer of the endometrium since the basalis layer of the endometrium is not shed with the monthly menstrual shedding of the functional layer. Recently, clonogenic cells have been identified and proposed to be involved in the formation of ectopic endometrial lesions. These cells are thought to represent the stem cell population in the human endometrium. Stem cells are pluripotent cells. This means that they have the ability to differentiate into one or several types of specialized cells. The undifferentiated endometrial stem cells may be less responsive to ovarian steroids than the terminally differentiated cells due to a lack of expression of hormone receptors. Retrograde menstruation can lead to the abnormal translocation of normal endometrial basalis, which can result in the involvement of stem cells in the formation of endometriotic deposits. Brosens et al. (2020) postulated that the uterine bleeding in neonatal girls contains a high amount of endometrial progenitor cells and that some of these cells may reside and reactivate in response to ovarian hormones later in life.

Leyendecker et al. (2004) proposed that women with endometriosis abnormally shed the endometrial basalis tissue, which, in combination with retrograde menstruation, initiates endometriotic deposits. The evidence that some of the endometrial stem cells have a bone marrow origin further supports the hematogenous dissemination theory of these cells. On the other hand, aberrant stem cells can relocate from the endometrium to an ectopic site and generate endometrium-like lesions. Endometrial tissue produces several chemokines and angiogenic cytokines so this lesion can reside in the ectopic sites due to neovascularization.

The last possibility of stem cell involvement in endometriosis is the differentiation of the peritoneal, hematopoietic, or ovarian stem cells into endometrium-like tissue. Cytokines flow between the uterine cavity and the peritoneal cavity through the fallopian tubes. This connection may regulate the endometrium-like differentiation of the resident stem cell population in the peritoneal cavity.

Autoimmune disease or immune deficiency theory: Endometriosis can occur when a defective immune response is present. This theory is supported by the fact that autoimmune diseases are found to be more common in women with endometriosis. Women with endometriosis have a higher concentration of activated macrophages, decreased cellular immunity, and a repressed natural killer (NK) cell function. Ectopic endometrial cells in the peritoneum induce an inflammatory response, and macrophages and leukocytes are activated locally. This inflammatory response may have a negative influence, which prevents elimination of ectopic endometrial cells that now can grow in ectopic sites.

Many theories have been suggested but none exclusively explains all facets of the disease. Still, we are unclear about its etiopathogenesis. Given the late stage at time of diagnosis at present, young girls may ask for the availability of screening tests for endometriosis in the coming years. Further research is suggested in the form of biomarkers or other immunological tests for understanding of the mechanism of development of disease. It would be wonderful if we could predict the occurrence of endometriosis in women and young girls and protect them from the morbidity of pain and infertility.

SUGGESTED READING

1. Greene AD, Lang SA, Kendziorski JA et al. Endometriosis: Where are we and where are we going? *Reproduction*, 2016 Sep; 152(3):R63–78. doi: 10.1530/REP-16-0052. [Epub 2016 May 10. Review].
2. Gordts S, Koninckx P, Brosens I et al. Pathogenesis of deep endometriosis. *Fertil Steril* 2017 Dec;108(6):872–85. e1. doi: 10.1016/j.fertnstert.2017.08.036. [Epub 2017 Oct 31. Review].
3. Gargett CE, Schwab KE, Brosens JJ et al. Potential role of endometrial stem/progenitor cells in the pathogenesis of early-onset endometriosis. *Mol Hum Reprod* 2014;20:591–8.
4. Donnez J. Introduction: From pathogenesis to therapy, deep endometriosis remains a source of controversy. *Fertil Steril* 2017;108:869–71.
5. Donnez J, Donnez O, Dolmans MM et al. Introduction: Uterine adenomyosis, another enigmatic disease of our time. *Fertil Steril* 2018;109:369–70.
6. Kvaskoff M, Mu F, Terry KL et al. Endometriosis: A high-risk population for major chronic diseases? *Hum Reprod Update* 2015;21:500–16.
7. Brosens I, Benagiano G. Endometriosis, a modern syndrome. *Indian J Med Res* [serial online 2011] 2020 Jan 1;133:581–93.
8. Leyendecker G, Kunz G, Herbertz M, Beil D, Huppert P, Mall G, Kissler S, Noe M, Wildt L. Uterine peristaltic activity and the development of endometriosis. *Ann N Y Acad Sci.* 2004 Dec;1034:338–55. Review.

4

Molecular basis and biomarkers of disease activity

PARIKSHAA GUPTA AND NALINI GUPTA

Endometriosis refers to non-uterine, ectopic localization of endometrial tissue in any other tissue or organ of the body [1]. Though the exact incidence is not known, it is estimated that the disease affects around 10% of women in the reproductive age group [2]. The clinical symptoms are varied and depend upon the location of the ectopic endometriotic tissue. The most common presenting symptom is chronic pelvic pain with or without infertility. In recent years, with advancements of research in this field, considerable insights have been obtained in terms of pathogenesis of endometriosis; however, advancements in terms of rapid and early diagnosis and therapy are still lagging.

Establishing an early diagnosis of this complex disease is quintessential for prompt management in women with endometriosis. However, more often than not, diagnostic delays occur with the majority of these women having to undergo multiple unnecessary tests and treatments until a definite diagnosis is made. This is because a definite diagnosis of endometriosis cannot be established based on the clinical features alone as these show a significant overlap with those seen in a number of other gynecological conditions. The undue diagnostic delays are associated with a momentous increase in the physical and emotional, as well as psychosocial, stress in these women, simultaneously adding to an ever-increasing socioeconomic burden on society. To date, the standard approach to establish the diagnosis of endometriosis still involves laparoscopic exploration of the abdomen and biopsy of the suspicious lesions for histopathological demonstration of ectopic endometrial glands and stroma [3]. Like for many other diseases, there is a need for identification of effective biomarkers and development of rapid, noninvasive or minimally invasive, biomarker-based tests, which may be of help in early diagnosis of the disease, as well as in predicting disease activity. With the advancements in understanding of pathogenetic mechanisms of endometriosis, several biomarkers have recently been proposed for early and relatively noninvasive diagnosis of endometriosis.

These can be broadly categorized under the following groups:

- Biomarkers in peripheral blood
- Endometrial biomarkers
- Biomarkers in urine

- Biomarkers in body fluids
- Genetic biomarkers
- Molecular and proteomic biomarkers

BIOMARKERS IN PERIPHERAL BLOOD

The ease of obtaining a peripheral blood sample makes it a useful minimally invasive method for testing for various endometriosis-related biomarkers. Several authors have conducted studies exploring the role of multiple biomarkers in detection of endometriosis. However, none of these have been found to be of significant utility in diagnosing endometriosis and hence have not been recommended as an alternative to surgical exploration [4,5].

Markers related to inflammation and oxidative stress

GLYCOPROTEINS

Cancer antigen 125 (CA-125) is the most commonly implicated and studied biomarker for endometriosis. It is basically a marker indicating inflammation in the peritoneum. Multiple studies have evaluated the diagnostic role of CA-125 in patients with endometriosis using several different cutoff values and have found variable sensitivities and specificities with each set of values. In a recent meta-analysis published on the Cochrane database, the authors evaluated all such studies and found that none of the cutoff values had sufficient diagnostic accuracy so as to label this biomarker as either a useful replacement test or a triage test [4]. However, in another recent systematic review and meta-analysis, the authors concluded that a cutoff value of >30 U/mL for CA-125 may be useful as a rule-in test for endometriosis [6]. Based on analysis of various other studies evaluating the role of CA-125, the diagnostic utility of this biomarker seems to be limited, mainly owing to the lower specificity as it is elevated not only in endometriosis but a plethora of other gynecological diseases as well. This is compounded by low sensitivity, as this marker has been seen to be elevated mainly in advanced endometriosis and the elevation is much more inconsistent in the early stages [6,7]. Regardless of its shortcomings, CA-125 is still the most widely used marker in studies evaluating other diagnostic endometriosis biomarkers.

Other glycoprotein biomarkers include galectin-9, glycodelin A, and follistatin. Galectin-9 is basically an immunomodulatory protein. Studies have found its levels to be significantly elevated in endometriosis as compared with normal healthy women. However, the levels were also found to be elevated in females with other gynecological diseases, thereby suggesting that using high levels of galectin-9 may not be of practical utility to diagnose endometriosis [8].

Glycodelin A is a cell proliferation promotor that also promotes neovascularization. It also exhibits immunosuppressive properties and acts via inactivation of T and NK (natural killer) cells. Several studies have previously been conducted to explore the diagnostic utility of this marker for endometriosis; however, they have yielded conflicting results, with some suggesting a significant association of the elevated levels with endometriosis while the others indicating only a limited clinical utility [4,9].

CYTOKINES AND INFLAMMATORY PROTEINS

Endometriosis is known to thrive in inflammatory conditions. Foci of endometriosis, similar to the normal uterine endometrium, undergo cyclical shedding, thereby inducing an ambient inflammatory response [10]. The development of inflammatory response has been known to promulgate the primary endometriotic lesions [11,12]. Based on this knowledge, several researchers have implicated several cytokines and inflammatory proteins as biomarkers for minimally invasive diagnosis of endometriosis. The roles of these mediators as biomarkers for endometriosis in peripheral blood has been explored in multiple studies; however, many of these have yielded inconsistent and rather conflicting results [5].

Of all the cytokines, interleukin-6 (IL-6) is the most widely studied biomarker in the context of endometriosis. The authors of a recent meta-analysis found a sensitivity of 63% and a specificity of 69% for IL-6, when a cutoff value of >1.90–2.00 pg/mL was chosen [5]. IL-35, which is an inhibitory cytokine involved in immune tolerance and produced by regulatory T cells, has been seen to be elevated in cases of endometriosis as compared with others [13]. Other inflammatory cytokines that have been studied in endometriosis include IL-1, IL-8, IL-10, IL-12, IL-17, IL-23, monocyte chemoattractant protein-1 (MCP-1), tumor necrosis factor alpha (TNF-α), interferon gamma (IFN-γ), and many others. Although some studies in the literature have shown some of these markers to be significantly elevated in women with endometriosis, there are other studies that have suggested against or have shown a limited role of cytokine measurements in diagnosing endometriosis [14–16]. This is mainly because cytokine measurements, rather than being simple, are complex owing to variability with circadian rhythms, methods of sample collection, short half-lives, and methods of assessment [17].

MARKERS OF OXIDATIVE STRESS

The cyclical bleeding, besides eliciting inflammation, also leads to increased oxidative stress in the tissues by causing increased accumulation of iron from the damaged and ruptured red blood corpuscles. It has been demonstrated by several authors that the levels of proteins related to oxidative stress are elevated in patients with endometriosis. Levels of active as well as total myeloperoxidase have been found to be elevated in association with endometriosis as compared to women with other gynecological diseases [18]. Researchers have also found significant reduction in serum levels of superoxide dismutase, paraoxonase (PON1), and high-density lipoproteins in women with endometriosis [14].

AUTOIMMUNE MARKERS

Abnormalities in the numbers and/or functions of immune cells have been implicated in the development and also the progression of endometriosis. These abnormalities include increased number of activated macrophages, increased polyclonal activation of B cells, defective natural killer (NK) cell and regulatory T-cell functions, and increased levels of cytokines involved in regulating autoimmunity including IL-27, IL-6, and transforming growth factor beta (TGF-β). Some researchers have found increased levels of autoantibodies in patients with endometriosis. In a recent meta-analysis, the authors found the detection of autoantibodies in the sera of these patients to be a useful biomarker; however, this test can neither be used as a replacement to the gold standard nor does it qualify to be a triage test [4]. Recently, some authors attempted to study the diagnostic utility of an immunomarker panel comprising anti-tropomodulin 3b, anti-tropomodulin 3c, anti-tropomodulin 3d, anti-tropomyosin

3a, anti-tropomyosin 3c, and anti-tropomyosin 3d autoantibodies for endometriosis [19]. They found a higher sensitivity of detecting endometriosis using this panel of six immunomarkers in comparison with some previously used biomarkers, including CA-125. However, validation of these results by further studies is needed before large-scale diagnostic application.

Markers related to cell survival, adhesion, and migration

As per the retrograde menstruation theory, after shedding from the endometrium, the endometrial cells enter the peritoneal cavity. In the peritoneal cavity, the endometrial cells, before attaching onto the peritoneum, need to survive the new environment by evading apoptosis. Thereafter, the survival depends on the establishment of new vasculature. Some researchers have demonstrated elevated levels of FAS/CD95 in the sera of patients with endometriosis, thereby providing evidence to the apoptosis-evasion hypothesis [20]. The authors also found elevated levels of an angiogenic factor, hypoxia-inducible factor 1 alpha (HIF-1α). A few studies have also demonstrated upregulation of the mRNA of factors such as survivin, vascular endothelial growth factor (VEGF), and vascular cell adhesion molecule 1 (VCAM-1) in cases of endometriosis compared with controls [21,22]. Studies comparing the diagnostic utility of biomarker panels comprising apoptotic and angiogenic markers with panels comprising inflammatory markers have also been conducted, and the authors have found relatively higher utility of the former than the latter [23].

CIRCULATING ENDOMETRIAL CELLS

Circulating endometrial cells have previously been identified as circulating cells, which are vimentin positive (stromal cells), pan-cytokeratin positive (epithelial cells), ER/PR (estrogen or progesterone receptor) positive, and leucocyte common antigen (CD45) negative. Researchers have found elevated numbers of circulating endometrial cells in cases of endometriosis as compared to controls [24].

CIRCULATING CELL-FREE DNA (cfDNA)

A few studies have found elevated levels of circulating cfDNA in cases of endometriosis compared with controls, thereby indicating a potential role for cfDNA in the diagnosis of endometriosis [25]. However, this needs to be validated in further large-scale studies.

Markers related to pain

Pain is one of the most common symptoms in women with endometriosis. Several studies focusing on the pain pathways have been conducted. A literature review shows that many authors have demonstrated elevated levels of brain-derived neurotropic factor (BDNF) in the plasma of these patients compared with controls. However, the role is limited in diagnosis of peritoneal endometriosis and deeply infiltrative endometriosis [26].

ENDOMETRIAL BIOMARKERS

Many previous studies have evaluated the role of various endometrial biomarkers in rapid, noninvasive, or minimally invasive diagnosis of endometriosis. A recent systematic review published in the literature included 54 studies on the role of endometrial markers. In all, more than 90 endometrial biomarkers were assessed in these studies; however, around 77 were not found to be associated with endometriosis. Of the remaining 22, only 2 markers, namely, CYP19 and PGP9.5, could be evaluated in the review as only these had been assessed in sufficient numbers. However, the authors found that neither of these can be recommended as a diagnostic test that can be used for endometriosis [27].

It has been seen that the levels of glycodelin and EWI-2 (EWI-2 is also referred to as immunoglobulin superfamily member 8 [IGSF8].) are significantly lower in uterine endometrium of cases of endometriosis and endometriomas compared with normal controls [28,29].

BIOMARKERS IN URINE

Urine has been recognized as one of the most useful and easily available samples to be tested for an early, noninvasive diagnosis of endometriosis. Detection of proteins associated with endometriosis is relatively easy in urine samples owing to higher concentrations of plasma proteins in urine due to selective glomerular filtration, and hence, urine samples are preferred for proteomics [30]. However, care needs to be taken while evaluating these results as there are several factors that might influence the concentrations, as well as expression of urinary proteins such as intake of certain medications like diuretics or dehydration. Various methods that can be used to study urinary proteins include electrophoresis, Western blotting, enzyme-linked immunosorbent assay (ELISA), matrix-assisted laser desorption/ionization–time of flight (MALDI-TOF), mass spectrometry, and liquid chromatography tandem mass spectrometry (LQ-MS/MS) [31]. There are a few studies in the literature wherein the authors have evaluated certain urinary biomarkers of endometriosis. Some of the commonly implicated urinary biomarkers have been described below.

Soluble feline McDonough sarcoma (fms)-like tyrosine kinase-1 (sFlt-1), an anti-angiogenic factor, downregulates VEGF and hence VEGF-mediated neovascularization. The overexpression of sFlt-1 leading to pathological neovascularization in breast and colonic cancers has been reported. Some researchers have shown significantly high urinary levels of sFlt-1 in patients with confirmed endometriosis, corrected for creatinine, compared with controls [32]. They also observed a much higher elevation during the secretory phase of the menstrual cycle in the patients, in contrast to the controls in whom the levels did not fluctuate significantly during the menstrual cycle. The elevated urinary levels also correlated with the stage of the disease, which means that the levels were elevated significantly in initial stages of the disease but not in the advanced stage. An important observation in the study was that though the urinary levels were significantly elevated in endometriosis patients, the serum levels did not show any significant variation.

Matrix metalloproteinases (MMPs) are endopeptidases that play a role in degradation and remodeling of the extracellular matrix, thereby facilitating cellular migration. Three MMPs, including MMP-2, MMP-9, and MMP-9/NGAL, have been found to be significantly elevated in urine in the cases of endometriosis when compared with controls [33]. Additionally, increased expression of MMP-2 and MMP-9 has been seen in the uterine as well as ectopic endometrial tissue in these patients [34].

Vitamin D–binding protein (VDBP) plays a role in chemotaxis and migration of monocytes, neutrophils, and fibroblasts. The urinary levels of VDBP, corrected for creatinine, are significantly elevated in cases of endometriosis, thereby supporting the association of inflammation with endometriosis [35]. However, serum levels do not show any significant elevation in these patients compared with the controls.

Cytokeratin-19 (CK-19), a cytoskeletal protein, has been found to be elevated in urine, but not serum, in cases of endometriosis, as opposed to controls [36]. However, more recent studies have not shown any significance of urinary levels of CK-19 in cases of endometriosis [37].

BIOMARKERS IN SALIVA

Like urine, saliva is also a convenient, noninvasive, easily available sample that can be tested for biomarkers of endometriosis. Some researchers have used saliva for studying hormonal variations and identifying various genetic aberrations in patients with endometriosis. An important prerequisite to biomarker testing in saliva is proper sample collection.

In order to ensure uniformity in this process, guidelines have been framed by the World Endometriosis Research Foundation–Endometriosis Phenome and Biobanking Harmonization project (WERF-EPHECT), highlighting the use of properly validated collection kits as well as appropriate sample storage conditions so that the specimen quality is not compromised.

Hormones

Hormonal levels, including progesterone and cortisol, have been estimated in patients with endometriosis, and some studies have found significant differences in the hormonal levels in patients of endometriosis compared with controls. Some authors have found significant morning hypocortisolism in these patients [38].

Cell-cycle regulatory factors

WNT4 is an important cell-cycle regulatory protein. Some researchers have conducted genome-wide association studies (GWAS) using salivary samples alone and have shown an association of endometriosis with WNT4 in patients with confirmed endometriosis [39]. p27 (the cyclin-dependent kinase inhibitor 1B), is an enzyme inhibitor, which is encoded by the *CDKN1B* gene. A study using buccal swabs has shown a significantly higher prevalence of a V109G substitution in the *p27* gene in patients of endometriosis [40].

BIOMARKERS IN PERITONEAL FLUID

Peritoneal fluid (PF) contains many cells, such as mesothelial cells, macrophages, and lymphocytes. When activated, the resident macrophages, as well as the mesothelial cells, can produce cytokines. Peritoneal fluid cytokines play a pivotal role in the etiopathogenesis. Peritoneal fluid thus serves as a useful potential sample for diagnostics as well as disease monitoring. The major disadvantage associated with PF testing is the fact that it has to be collected at the time of surgery, thereby making the entire procedure more invasive than other samples such as urine and peripheral blood. As is the case with other biomarkers, although many markers have been evaluated in the PF, to date there is no single reliable biomarker or biomarker panel that can replace the gold standard. Some of the important peritoneal fluid biomarkers that have been extensively studied for their potential role in endometriosis have been listed in Table 4.1 [31].

PROTEOMIC BIOMARKERS

Several previous studies in the literature have evaluated expression in the endometrial cells among patients with endometriosis. Researchers have shown at least 72 dysregulated genes in women with endometriosis by sequencing mRNA from the secretory phase endometrial samples. Of these, 4 upregulated proteins including MMP-11, Fos proto-oncogene, dual specificity phosphatase and serpin family E member 1, and adenosine deaminase 2 were validated using quantitative polymerase chain reaction (PCR). Similarly, several acyl carnitines were found to be elevated while trimethylamine-N-oxide was decreased in the cases of endometriosis using mass spectrometry methods. Studies using nuclear magnetic resonance spectrometry have revealed that metabolites containing valine, fucose, and choline, amino acids lysine/arginine, and lipoproteins were upregulated, while creatinine was downregulated in patients with late stages of the disease [41].

GENETIC BIOMARKERS

Endometriosis is a complex disorder having a multifactorial etiopathogenesis. The disease is not only regulated by several environmental factors but

Table 4.1 Commonly studied biomarkers of endometriosis in peritoneal fluid

Biomarkers	Basic action	Role in endometriosis
Tumor necrosis factor-α	• Activates helper T cells and other cytokines • Proinflammatory • Promotes angiogenesis	Significantly elevated PF levels in patients with endometriosis
RANTES	• Regulates inflammation by recruiting NK cells, histiocytes, and granulocytes	Elevated PF levels correlate with disease severity
Interferon-γ	• Induces expression of MHC class II molecules • Proinflammatory • Macrophage activation	Controversial, decreased PF levels have been seen in patients with endometriosis
Interleukin-6	• Anti-inflammatory • Stimulates of antibody production • Development of effector T cells	Significantly elevated levels in moderate to severe endometriosis, no significance in mild disease
Interleukin-8	• Neutrophil chemotactic factor • Proinflammatory • Promotes angiogenesis	Controversial, significantly elevated PF levels in mainly early stages of the disease
Interleukin-10	• Human cytokine synthesis inhibitory factor • Anti-inflammatory	Significantly elevated PF levels in all stages of the disease
Interleukin-13	• Anti-inflammatory • Inhibits macrophage and lymphocyte activation	Significantly reduced PF levels in endometriosis
Interleukin-18	• Stimulates Th1 and Th2 immune responses • Induces the production of interferon-γ, IL-4, TNF-α, IL-5, and IL-13	Controversial, some studies showing significantly higher PF levels in endometriosis while others demonstrating lower PF levels in these patients compared with controls
TGF-β-1	• Inhibits natural killer cells • Regulates cell proliferation and angiogenesis • Inhibits macrophages	Significantly higher PF levels in endometriosis, correlating with disease severity
FAS ligand	• Regulates apoptosis • Stimulates secretion of IL-8	Significantly higher PF levels in moderate to severe endometriosis, no significance in early disease
Leptin	• Hormone of energy expenditure • Anti-inflammatory • Regulates angiogenesis	Significantly elevated PF levels in early-stage endometriosis compared with late-stage disease

Abbreviations: PF, peritoneal fluid; MHC, major histocompatibility complex; TGF, transforming growth factor; RANTES, regulated on activation, normal T cell expressed and secreted.

multiple genetic factors as well. This is supported by the fact that the relatives of these patients carry a much higher risk for the disease as compared to general population. Moreover, several twin studies have also demonstrated an increased concordance in monozygotic twins as compared to dizygotic twins [31,42]. Several researchers have tried to identify the genes associated with endometriosis using linkage and GWAS. However, the success rates have been low, probably because the disease is regulated by interplay of multiple genes.

GWAS have identified several candidate genes associated with endometriosis. Some studies have shown an association of the disease with a single nucleotide polymorphism (SNP) *PvuII* in the estrogen receptor 1 gene; however, the same could not be validated by subsequent studies. A study evaluating the association of ten estrogen-metabolizing SNPs in cases of endometriosis showed significant association of vIV A→C variant in the hydroxysteroid (17-β) dehydrogenase 1 (*HSD17B1*) gene with endometriosis [43]. Similarly, *PROGINS* polymorphism in the progesterone receptor gene has also been found to be positively associated with endometriosis; however, the association has not been found to be statistically significant [42].

Given the role of cytokines, including TNF-α and various interleukins and their receptors in the etiopathogenesis of the disease, roles of polymorphisms in their respective genes have also been explored by researchers in several studies. The results, however, have been inconsistent, with some studies showing a positive association with some cytokine polymorphisms with others failing to do so.

GWAS has shown a positive association of endometriosis with the SNP *rs1096523*, which is located in the cyclin-dependent kinase inhibitor 2B antisense RNA (*CDKN2BAS*) gene on chromosome 9p21. *CDKN2BAS* regulates the expression of *CDKN2A*, which controls proliferation of endometrium and is implicated in etiopathogenesis of endometriosis [44]. Additionally, a similar association has been observed with *rs16826658m* in the linkage disequilibrium block which also includes the gene *WNT4* on chromosome 1p36 [44]. *WNT4* signaling plays a role in the development of ovarian follicles, fallopian tubes, and the uterus from the Müllerian ducts. An association of endometriosis has also been found with the locus 9p21 that is also associated with other diseases, including malignant melanoma, basal cell carcinoma, coronary artery disease, type 2 diabetes, glioma, and nevi [42]. A few other loci that have been linked to increased susceptibility for endometriosis include 7p15.2 (a region between NFE2L3 and HOXA10) and 10q26. However, the clinical significance of these genetic variants in predicting the risk of the disease is still unclear. Recently, some researchers have demonstrated an increased prevalence of an inherited polymorphism of a *let-7* miRNA-binding site in the *KRAS* gene in patients with endometriosis as the first described genetic marker for endometriosis risk and also a potential therapeutic target [45].

CONCLUSION

Advances in research have led to identification of a number of noninvasive and/or minimally invasive biomarkers for early diagnosis of endometriosis. However, despite a large number of biomarkers being available, promising results are sparse, and to date, no single biomarker is capable of accurately diagnosing endometriosis and replacing histopathological diagnosis. The major reason for this is the complex etiopathogenesis of the disease. To conclude, endometriosis can most likely be diagnosed using a panel of biomarkers rather than a single biomarker alone.

REFERENCES

1. Giudice LC. Clinical practice. Endometriosis. *N Engl J Med* 2010;362(25):2389–98.
2. Eisenberg VH, Weil C, Chodick G, Shalev V. Epidemiology of endometriosis: A large population-based database study from a healthcare provider with 2 million members. *BJOG* 2018;125(1):55–62.
3. Kennedy S, Bergqvist A, Chapron C et al. ESHRE guideline for the diagnosis and treatment of endometriosis. *Hum Reprod* 2005;20:2698–704.
4. Nisenblat V, Bossuyt PM, Shaikh R, Farquhar C, Jordan V, Scheffers CS, Mol BW, Johnson N, Hull ML. Blood biomarkers for the non-invasive diagnosis of endometriosis. *Cochrane Database Syst Rev* 2016;(5):CD012179.
5. May KE, Conduit-Hulbert SA, Villar J, Kirtley S, Kennedy SH, Becker CM. Peripheral biomarkers of endometriosis: a systematic review. *Hum Reprod Update* 2010;16(6):651–74.

6. Hirsch M, Duffy J, Davis CJ, Nieves Plana M, Khan KS; International Collaboration to Harmonise Outcomes and Measures for Endometriosis. Diagnostic accuracy of cancer antigen 125 for endometriosis: A systematic review and meta-analysis. *BJOG* 2016;123(11):1761–8.

7. Mol BW, Bayram N, Lijmer JG, Wiegerinck MA, Bongers MY, van der Veen F, Bossuyt PM. The performance of CA-125 measurement in the detection of endometriosis: A meta-analysis. *Fertil Steril* 1998;70(6):1101–8.

8. Brubel R, Bokor A, Pohl A, Schilli GK, Szereday L, Bacher-Szamuel R, Rigo J Jr, Polgar B. Serum galectin-9 as a noninvasive biomarker for the detection of endometriosis and pelvic pain or infertility-related gynecologic disorders. *Fertil Steril* 2017;108(6):1016–25.e2.

9. Vodolazkaia A, El-Aalamat Y, Popovic D et al. Evaluation of a panel of 28 biomarkers for the non-invasive diagnosis of endometriosis. *Hum Reprod* 2012;27(9):2698–711.

10. Sourial S, Tempest N, Hapangama DK. Theories on the pathogenesis of endometriosis. *Int J Reprod Med* 2014;2014:179515.

11. Ekarattanawong S, Tanprasertkul C, Somprasit C, Chamod P, Tiengtip R, Bhamarapravatana K, Suwannarurk K. Possibility of using superoxide dismutase and glutathione peroxidase as endometriosis biomarkers. *Int J Womens Health* 2017;9:711–6.

12. Scutiero G, Iannone P, Bernardi G, Bonaccorsi G, Spadaro S, Volta CA, Greco P, Nappi L. Oxidative stress and endometriosis: A systematic review of the literature. *Oxid Med Cell Longev* 2017;2017:7265238.

13. Zhang C, Peng Z, Ban D, Zhang Y. Upregulation of interleukin 35 in patients with endometriosis stimulates cell proliferation. *Reprod Sci* 2018;25(3):443–51.

14. Fassbender A, Burney RO, O DF, D'Hooghe T, Giudice L. Update on biomarkers for the detection of endometriosis. *Biomed Res Int* 2015;2015:130854.

15. Rocha AL, Vieira EL, Maia LM, Teixeira AL, Reis FM. Prospective evaluation of a panel of plasma cytokines and chemokines as potential markers of pelvic endometriosis in symptomatic women. *Gynecol Obstet Invest* 2016;81(6):512–7.

16. Pateisky P, Pils D, Kuessel L, Szabo L, Walch K, Obwegeser R, Wenzl R, Yotova I. The serum levels of the soluble factors sCD40L and CXCL1 are not indicative of endometriosis. *Biomed Res Int* 2016;2016:2857161.

17. O DF, Aalamat YE, Waelkens E, Moor BD, D'Hooghe T, Fassbender A. Multiplex immunoassays in endometriosis: an array of possibilities. *Front Biosci (Landmark Ed)* 2017;22:479–92.

18. O DF, Waelkens E, Peterse DP et al. Evaluation of total, active, and specific myeloperoxidase levels in women with and without endometriosis. *Gynecol Obstet Invest* 2018;83(2):133–9.

19. Gajbhiye R, Bendigeri T, Ghuge A et al. Panel of autoimmune markers for noninvasive diagnosis of minimal-mild endometriosis. *Reprod Sci.* 2017;24(3):413–20.

20. Karakus S, Sancakdar E, Akkar O, Yildiz C, Demirpence O, Cetin A. Elevated Serum CD95/FAS and HIF-1α levels, but not Tie-2 levels, may be biomarkers in patients with severe endometriosis: A preliminary report. *J Minim Invasive Gynecol* 2016;23(4):573–7.

21. Kuessel L, Wenzl R, Proestling K, Balendran S, Pateisky P, Yotova 1st, Yerlikaya G, Streubel B, Husslein H. Soluble VCAM-1/soluble ICAM-1 ratio is a promising biomarker for diagnosing endometriosis. *Hum Reprod* 2017;32(4):770–9.

22. Acimovic M, Vidakovic S, Milic N, Jeremic K, Markovic M, Milosevic-Djeric A, Lazovic-Radonjic G. Survivin and VEGF as novel biomarkers in diagnosis of endometriosis. *J Med Biochem* 2016;35(1):63–8.

23. Vodolazkaia A, El-Aalamat Y, Popovic D et al. Evaluation of a panel of 28 biomarkers for the non-invasive diagnosis of endometriosis. *Hum Reprod* 2012;27(9):2698–711.

24. Chen Y, Zhu HL, Tang ZW et al. Evaluation of circulating endometrial cells as a biomarker for endometriosis. *Chin Med J (Engl)* 2017;130(19):2339–45.

25. Zachariah R, Schmid S, Radpour R, Buerki N, Fan AX, Hahn S, Holzgreve W, Zhong XY. Circulating cell-free DNA as a potential biomarker for minimal and mild endometriosis. *Reprod Biomed Online* 2009;18(3):407–11.

26. Rocha AL, Vieira EL, Ferreira MC, Maia LM, Teixeira AL, Reis FM. Plasma brain-derived neurotrophic factor in women with pelvic pain: A potential biomarker for endometriosis? *Biomark Med* 2017;11(4):313–7.

27. Gupta D, Hull ML, Fraser I, Miller L, Bossuyt PM, Johnson N, Nisenblat V. Endometrial biomarkers for the non-invasive diagnosis of endometriosis. *Cochrane Database Syst Rev* 2016;4:CD012165.

28. Zheng T, Yang J. Differential expression of EWI-2 in endometriosis, its functional role and underlying molecular mechanisms. *J Obstet Gynaecol Res* 2017;43(7):1180–8.

29. Focarelli R, Luddi A, De Leo V, Capaldo A, Stendardi A, Pavone V, Benincasa L, Belmonte G, Petraglia F, Piomboni P. Dysregulation of GdA expression in endometrium of women with endometriosis: Implication for endometrial receptivity. *Reprod Sci* 2018;25(4):579–86.

30. Hortin GL, Sviridov D. Diagnostic potential for urinary proteomics. *Pharmacogenomics* 2007;8:237–55.

31. D'Hooghe T. Biomarkers for endometriosis. In: D'Hooghe T, editor. *State of the Art.* Switzerland: Springer International Publishing AG; 2017.

32. Cho SH, Oh YJ, Nam A et al. Evaluation of serum and urinary angiogenic factors in patients with endometriosis. *Am J Reprod Immunol* 2007;58:497–504.

33. Becker CM, Louis G, Exarhopoulos A, Mechsner S, Ebert AD, Zurakowski D, Moses MA. Matrix metalloproteinases are elevated in the urine of patients with endometriosis. *Fertil Steril* 2010;94(6):2343–6.

34. Chung HW, Wen Y, Chun SH, Nezhat C, Woo BH, Lake Polan M. Matrix metalloproteinase-9 and tissue inhibitor of metalloproteinase-3 mRNA expression in ectopic and eutopic endometrium in women with endometriosis: a rationale for endometriotic invasiveness. *Fertil Steril* 2001;75:152–9.

35. Cho S, Choi YS, Yim SY, Yang HI, Jeon YE, Lee KE, Kim HY, Seo SK, Lee BS. Urinary vitamin D-binding protein is elevated in patients with endometriosis. *Hum Reprod* 2012;27(2):515–22.

36. Tokushige N, Markham R, Crossett B, Ahn SB, Nelaturi V, Khan A, Fraser IS. Discovery of a novel biomarker in the urine of women with endometriosis. *Fertil Steril* 2011;95:46–9.

37. Kuessel L, Jaeger-Lansky A, Pateisky P, Rossberg N, Schulz A, Schmitz AA, Staudigl C, Wenzl R. Cytokeratin-19 as a biomarker in urine and in serum for the diagnosis of endometriosis—a prospective study. *Gynecol Endocrinol* 2014;30(1):38–41.

38. Petrelluzzi KF, Garcia MC, Petta CA, Grassi-Kassisse DM, Spadari-Bratfisch R. Salivary cortisol concentrations and quality of life in women with endometriosis and chronic pelvic pain. *Stress* 2008;11(5):390–7.

39. Bischoff FZ, Simpson JL. Heritability and molecular genetic studies of endometriosis. *Hum Reprod Update* 2000;6(1):37–44.

40. Camargo-Kosugi CM, da Silva ID, Sato H, D'Amora P, Carvalho CV, Nogueira-de-Souza NC, Girão MJ, Schor E. The V109G polymorphism in the p27 gene is associated with endometriosis. *Eur J Obstet Gynecol* 2009;145(2):180–3.

41. O DF, Flores I, Waelkens E, D'Hooghe T. Noninvasive diagnosis of Endometriosis: Review of current peripheral blood and endometrial markers. *Best Practice Res Clin Obstetrics Gynaecol* 2018;50:72–83.

42. Dun EC, Taylor RN, Wieser F. Advances in the genetics of endometriosis. *Genome Med* 2010;2:75.

43. Huber A, Keck CC, Hefler LA, Schneeberger C, Huber JC, Bentz EK, Tempfer CB. Ten estrogen-related polymorphisms and endometriosis: a study of multiple gene-gene interactions. *Obstet Gynecol* 2005;106:1025–31.

44. Uno S, Zembutsu H, Hirasawa A, Takahashi A, Kubo M, Akahane T, Aoki D, Kamatani N, Hirata K, Nakamura Y. A genome-wide association study identifies genetic variants in the CDKN2BAS locus associated with endometriosis in Japanese. *Nat Genet* 2010;42:707–10.

45. Grechukhina O, Petracco R, Popkhadze S et al. A polymorphism in a let-7 microRNA binding site of KRAS in women with endometriosis. *EMBO Mol Med* 2012;4:206–17.

5

Diagnostic evaluation

NEHA AGGARWAL, SEEMA CHOPRA, AND ARSHI SYAL

Endometriosis may have different clinical presentations depending on the primary location. Pelvic pain and infertility are the two most common symptoms associated with it.

PAIN

Dysmenorrhea typically developing after years of pain-free menstrual cycles is suggestive of endometriosis. The pain most often begins 48 hours prior to the onset of menses and persists throughout the menstrual period. The pain may be unilateral or bilateral and is perceived as a sensation of swelling of the internal organs or pelvic heaviness [1]. Endometriosis-associated pain tends to be more severe and responds to a lesser degree to conventional treatment with nonsteroidal anti-inflammatory agents and combined oral contraceptive pills [2,3]. Cyclical pain soon progresses to noncyclical, chronic pelvic pain severe enough to cause functional disability and compromise day-to-day activities [4].

There are primarily three main mechanisms for the underlying cause of pain in endometriosis:

- Focal bleeding from the endometriotic implants.
- Macrophages present in the peritoneal fluid of the women with endometriosis produce various cytokines, growth factors, and prostaglandins, which in turn promote pain and expansion of the ectopic endometrium [5].
- Infiltration or invasion of the nerves by the endometriotic implants [6,7]. The inflammatory mediators further sensitize the nociceptors, which in turn initiate the central neurons [8].

Infiltration of the uterosacral ligament, rectovaginal septum, and posterior cul-de-sac result in dyspareunia. Dyspareunia is present due to traction of fixed uterosacral ligaments during intercourse. There are mixed opinions regarding the correlation between the extent of the endometriotic implants and intensity of the pain.

There are various methods of grading the pain experienced by patients suffering from endometriosis. Though not used much in clinical practice, below are some examples for quantifying the pain:

- Visual Analogue Scale (VAS): Rating the pain from none to worst imaginable [9]
- Numerical Rating Scale: Grading the pain at a score from 1 to 10
- McGill Pain Questionnaire [10]

Although endometriosis usually presents as chronic pain, in some instances, the ovarian endometrioma might rupture and give a clinical picture very similar to that of a ruptured hemorrhagic cyst.

INFERTILITY

The overall incidence of endometriosis is greater in infertile women (13%–33%) than in fertile women (4%–8%) [11,12]. The fecundity rate of women with endometriosis is quite similar to the fecundity rate caused by unexplained infertility (i.e., 0.02–0.10) [13]. In addition, there is increased prevalence of infertility with severe forms of endometriosis when compared with women with mild endometriosis [14–16].

No definite mechanism has yet been identified to establish an association between endometriosis and infertility; however, several biological mechanisms have been suggested. We have briefly discussed these mechanisms below.

Distorted adnexal anatomy

Adhesions as a result of endometriosis can hinder the normal ovum pickup after ovulation and transport by the uterine tubes [17].

Altered peritoneal fluid volume and composition

Women with endometriosis have increased peritoneal fluid volume and high levels of prostaglandin production (PGE2). This induces a classic inflammatory response characterized by increased production of cytokines, such as IL-1, IL-6, and TNF-α. Angiogenic cytokines, such as VEGF and IL-8, production by macrophages is also increased in the peritoneal fluid [18,19]. These inflammatory mediators together contribute in peritoneal adhesion formation and subsequent local angiogenesis. Studies have shown that the inflammatory milieu present in the peritoneal fluid of patients with endometriosis contributes to fragmentation of DNA of sperm [20]. The oxidative stress induced by this chronic inflammation may interfere with sperm–oocyte interaction, impairs the development of embryo, and makes implantation difficult [21].

Impaired implantation

Decreased expression of the cell adhesion molecule $\alpha v\beta 3$ integrin has been held responsible for the implantation failure in endometriosis [22].

Decreased endometrial receptivity

For the transition of endometrium from proliferative to luteal phase, progesterone is required. However, in women with endometriosis, there will be increased activation of steroidogenic factor 1 (SF1) and aromatase activity leading to increased production of estradiol. Highly potent estradiol downregulates the expression of progesterone receptors leading to progesterone resistance and further increasing the level of estradiol by lowering the activity of 17β-hydroxysteroid dehydrogenase (17β-HSD) [23].

SYMPTOMS FROM SPECIFIC SITES

Rectosigmoid lesions

Chronic or cyclical constipation, diarrhea, or hematochezia may arise due to inflammation of the rectal wall or adherence of the rectum to the adjacent structures [24]. Deep infiltrating endometriosis (DIE) is defined as endometriotic lesions penetrating into the retroperitoneal space or the wall of the pelvic organs to a depth of at least 5 mm. DIE complicates around 5%–12% of cases of endometriosis and commonly involves the rectosigmoid colon and, to a lesser extent, the ileum, the appendix, and the sigmoid colon. Lesions usually involve the serosa and muscularis propria but in rare cases can induce transmural inflammation leading to intestinal obstruction. Endometriosis of the ileum could result in partial bowel obstruction, typically during menses; however, endometriosis of the colon rarely results in obstruction owing to the colon's larger diameter.

Urinary tract lesions

Superficial endometriotic lesions involving bladder peritoneum are not symptomatic. DIE involving the urinary tract have been found in 2.6% of the cases [25]. Endometriotic nodules involving the uterosacral ligaments can cause irritation of the pelvic plexus, leading to voiding symptoms, urgency, and dysuria. Cyclical hematuria is an uncommon finding because the non-involvement of the bladder mucosa.

Ureteral endometriosis can result in hydronephrosis, flank pain, and decline of renal function.

Anterior abdominal wall lesions

Scar endometriosis is a very rare entity reported in patients who have undergone any previous abdominal or pelvic surgery. The symptoms are usually of cyclical pain and increase in the size of the endometriotic implants during menses.

Thoracic–diaphragmatic endometriosis

Endometriotic implants, when they involve the thoracic cavity, can lead to cyclical chest or shoulder pain with right-sided predominance, hemoptysis, and pneumothorax.

DIAGNOSTIC EVALUATION

Physical examination

In the majority of the cases, the endometriosis remains confined to the pelvic cavity except the few exceptions of scar and thoracic endometriosis. In the order of decreasing frequency, the primary location of endometriosis are as follows: ovaries, uterine ligaments, pouch of Douglas, and peritoneal surfaces.

On pelvic examination, external genitalia is typically normal. The exception may be the rare cases of episiotomy scars.

On per speculum examination, blue-colored implants or red powder burn lesions are seen on the cervix and the posterior vaginal fornix. These lesions are usually tender and bleed on contact.

On bimanual examination, there may be lateral displacement of the cervix due to unilateral involvement of the uterosacral ligaments. The uterus may be retroverted and exhibit tenderness, decreased mobility, or fixation. Ovarian endometriomas can present as fixed, immobile, and tender adnexal masses. Ovarian endometriomas are bilateral in 30%–50% of cases [26]. Tender nodules can be palpated along the uterosacral ligaments or posterior cul-de-sac, especially if done before the onset of menses.

Digital rectal examination reveals the nodularity and tenderness of the rectovaginal septum.

Serum markers of endometriosis

CA-125 is a transmembrane glycoprotein and is synthesized and secreted by the coelomic epithelium derivatives. Its utility in monitoring the disease remission and recurrence has been well established in epithelial ovarian cancer. Chronic inflammation in endometriosis can cause irritation of the peritoneum, leading to increased production of CA-125 [27]. A study was done by Mol et al. to assess the utility of CA-125 as a noninvasive diagnostic marker for endometriosis. The assay seems to be a poor marker for stage I/II endometriosis but has a better sensitivity in diagnosing stage III/IV disease. Despite having limited utility in diagnosing endometriosis, Mol continued to advocate for the routine measurements of CA-125 in patients who present with infertility, as this could identify the subgroup of patients who will benefit from early laparoscopy [28].

Serum CA-125 may have a role in differentiating endometriomas from other benign cysts, especially when coupled with the transvaginal ultrasonography.

A recent study done by Othman and colleagues has found elevated levels of IL-6 in the serum of the patients with endometriosis when compared with infertile patients with no evidence of endometriosis [29]. The discovery of new biomarkers may be of particular advantage in diagnosing endometriosis.

Diagnostic imaging

ULTRASONOGRAPHY

Transvaginal ultrasonography (TVS) is simple, widely available, and cost effective, and hence, it is the first imaging modality in evaluation for endometriosis. Ovaries are the most common site of endometriotic implants. The classical finding of an ovarian endometrioma on ultrasound is the presence of a "chocolate cyst" caused by the presence of thick, degenerated blood products that result from cyclical bleeding during the menses; it is a homogenous hypoechoic lesion with the ovary, with low to medium echoes (ground glass appearance), and no internal vascularity [30–34]. Occasionally, endometriomas may have thickened walls, a fluid–fluid level, an avascular mural nodule (a retracting clot), and solid masses (due to the presence of older product and fibrosis). A thick, dense fibrous capsule is invariably present at the periphery of the endometrioma. Traditionally, endometriomas are uniloculated but up to 4 thin septations can be found. Use of power Doppler may show only pericystic vascularity with absence of blood flow within it.

Endometriosis, when it involves both the ovaries, the ovaries adhere to one another in the midline, giving the appearance of "kissing ovaries." Ovarian endometriosis is usually present in association with advanced endometriosis.

TVS has 88% sensitivity in differentiating endometriomas from other masses and a specificity of 90% [35].

TVS should be performed during menses or at the time of maximum pain as during this time endometrial implants grow and are easily visualized.

Bladder endometriosis can be accurately diagnosed using transvaginal ultrasonography. The endometriotic implants appear as solid hypoechoic nodules that adhere to the posterior aspect of the bladder dome.

To diagnose rectal endometriosis in ultrasonography, paramount experience is required. So, if the patient presents with symptoms suggesting rectal endometriosis, transvaginal ultrasound can be done to diagnose or rule it out [36].

TVS is a powerful tool for diagnosing ovarian endometrioma and endometriosis of the bladder, but its value in evaluating the superficial peritoneal lesions and deep infiltrating lesions is questionable [35,37].

MAGNETIC RESONANCE IMAGING (MRI)

The use of MRI comes into the play when ultrasonography is inconclusive. MRI can be used as an adjunct to differentiate endometriomas from hemorrhagic cysts or dermoid cysts. Endometriomas are hyperintense on T1-weighted images and show gradual loss of signal with low signal intensity on T2-weighted images. This decrease in signal intensity has been termed as "shading sign" [38]. It reflects the presence of blood products of varying age within the cyst. Another typical finding is the presence of the black peripheral rim containing accumulated hemosiderin-laden macrophages as a result of cyclical bleeding [39].

Hemorrhagic cysts are often confused with endometriomas. The hemorrhagic cysts appear uniloculated and do not exhibit shading sign on T2-weighted images.

Fat-saturated, T1-weighted sequences show persistence of high signal intensity on T1-weighted images in cases of endometriomas. There is loss of signal intensity on fat-saturated images in cases of dermoid cysts [40].

MRI confers benefits in the evaluation of deep infiltrating endometriosis and cul-de-sac obliteration, which are often difficult to visualize laparoscopically. In these cases, MRI may help in preoperative planning. According to one study, the sensitivity and specificity of diagnosing endometriosis is 69% and 75%, respectively [41]. DIE involving the rectosigmoid colon may need resection. MRI can give valuable information on number and location of lesions, depth of infiltration, and distance between the inferior margin of the nodule and the anal border [42].

OTHER MODALITIES

- *Computed tomography (CT)*: CT offers limited value in the evaluation of endometriosis. It may reveal endometriomas as nonspecific masses and does not offer diagnostic images as provided by TVS or MRI. This is because of the fact that CT has poor sensitivity for small implants and plaques.

  Thoracic lesions of endometriosis can be detected by chest CT. Also, their role has been defined in bowel and ureteral endometriosis [43].
- *Cystoscopy*: Cystoscopy may aid in diagnosing the bladder endometriosis and in providing a tissue sample for histological confirmation.
- *Double-contrast barium enema*: It is used to make a diagnosis of endometriosis and also allows the evaluation of length and degree of bowel occlusion. It is an important presurgical imaging tool.

  Clinical symptoms when combined with characteristic imaging features can facilitate in making a diagnosis of endometriosis by use of noninvasive techniques.

Stepwise algorithm for the diagnosis of endometriosis

Suspect endometriosis if the following symptoms are reported:

- Secondary dysmenorrhea
- Chronic pelvic pain
- Dyspareunia
- Chronic/cyclical bowel symptoms
- Chronic/cyclical bladder symptoms
- Infertility

Physical examination:

- Blue-colored/red powder burn lesion on cervix/posterior fornix
- Lateral displacement of cervix
- Uterus retroverted, fixed, tender
- Immobile, tender adnexal mass
- Nodules palpable on posterior cul-de-sac

Presumptive diagnosis of endometriosis

REFERENCES

1. Bieber E. *Clinical Gynaecology*, 2nd ed. Cambridge: Cambridge University Press; 2015.
2. Opoku-Anane J, Lauer MR. Prevalence of endometriosis in adolescent girls with chronic pelvic pain not responding to conventional therapy. Have we underestimated? *J Pediatr Adolesc Gynecol* 2012;25(2):e50.
3. Allen C, Hopewell S, Prentice A et al. Nonsteroidal anti-inflammatory drugs or pain in women with endometriosis. *Cochrane Database Syst Rev* 209;2:CD004753.
4. American College of Obstetricians and Gynecologists: Chronic pelvic pain. Practice Bulletin No. 51, March 2004, Reaffirmed May 2010.
5. Bulun SE. Endometriosis. *N Engl J Med* 2009;360(3):268.
6. Barcena de Arellano ML, Arnold J, Vercellino F et al. Overexpression of nerve growth factor in peritoneal fluid from women with endometriosis may promote neurite outgrowth in endometriotic lesions. *Fertil Steril* 2011;95(3):1123.
7. McKinnon B, Bersinger NA, Wotzkow C et al. Endometriosis-associated nerve fibers, peritoneal fluid cytokine concentrations, and pain in endometriotic lesions from different locations. *Fertil Steril* 2012;97(2):373.
8. Evans S, Moalem-Taylor G, Tracey DJ. Pain and endometriosis. *Pain* 2007;132(Suppl 1):S22–5.
9. Jensen MP, Karoly P. Self-report scales and procedures for assessing pain in adults. In: Turk DC, Malzack R, editors. *Handbook of Pain Assessment*. New York: Guilford Press; 1992, p. 135.
10. Melzack R. The McGill Pain Questionaire: Major properties and Scoring methods. *Pain* 1975;1:277.
11. D'Hooghe M, Debrock S, Hill JA et al. Endometriosis and subfertility: Is the relationship resolved? *Semin Reprod Med* 2003;21:243.
12. Strathy JH, Molgaard CA, Coulam CB et al. Endometriosis and Infertility: A laparoscopic study of endometriosis among fertile and infertile women. *Fertil Steril* 1982;38:667.
13. Hughes EG, Fedorkow DM, Collins JA. A quantitative overview of controlled trials in endometriosis associated infertility. *Fertil Steril* 1993;59:963–70.
14. Matorras R, Rodriguez F, Pijoan JI et al. Women who are not exposed to spermatozoa and infertile women have similar rates of stage I endometriosis. *Fertil Steril* 2001;76:923.
15. D'Hooghe M, Bambra CS, Raeymaekers BM et al. The cycle pregnancy rate is normal in baboons with stage I endometriosis but decreased in primates with stage II and stage III–IV disease. *Fertil Steril* 1996;66:809.
16. Schenken RS, Asch RH. Surgical induction of endometriosis in the rabbit: Effects on fertility and concentrations of

peritoneal fluid prostaglandins. *Fertil Steril* 1980;34:581.

17. Practice Committee of the ASRM. Endometriosis & infertility. *Fertil Steril* 2006;86(4): S156–60.

18. Bedaiwy MA, Falcone T, Sharma RK et al. Prediction of endometriosis with serum and peritoneal fluid markers: A prospective controlled trial. *Hum Reprod* 2002;17:426–31.

19. Pizzo A, Salmeri FM, Ardita FV, Sofo V, Tripepi M, Marsico S. Behaviour of cytokine levels in serum and peritoneal fluid of women with endometriosis. *Gynecol Obstet Invest* 2002;54:82–7. Switzerland: S. Karger AG, Basel; 2003.

20. Mansour G, Aziz N, Sharma R et al. The impact of peritoneal fluid from healthy women and from women with endometriosis on sperm DNA and its relationship to the sperm deformity index. *Fertil Steril* 2009;92:61–7.

21. Pellicer A, Oliveira N, Ruiz A, Remohi J, Simon C. Exploring the mechanism (s) of endometriosis- related infertility: An analysis of embryo development and implantation in assisted reproduction. *Hum Reprod* 1995;10(Suppl 2):91–7.

22. Lessey BA, Castelbaum AJ, Sawin SW et al. Aberrant integrin expression in the endometrium of women with endometriosis. *J Clin Endocrinol Metab* 1994;79:643–9.

23. Giudice L, Evers JLH, Healy DL. *Endometriosis: Science and Practice*. Chichester, West Sussex: Wiley-Blackwell; 2012.

24. Roman H, Bridoux V, Tuech JJ et al. Bowel dysfunction before and after surgery or endometriosis. *Am J Obstet Gynecol* 2013;209(6):524.

25. Antonelli A, Simeone C, Zani D et al. Clinical aspects and surgical treatment of urinary tract endometriosis: Our experience with 31 cases. *Eur Urol* 2006;49:1093.

26. Carbognin G, Guarise A, Minelli L et al. Pelvic endometriosis: US and MRI features. *Abdom Imaging* 2004;29:609.

27. Barbieri RL, Niloff JM, Bast RC Jr et al. Elevated serum concentration of CA-125 in patients with advanced endometriosis. *Fertil Steril* 1986;45:630–4.

28. Mol BW, Bayram N, Lijmer JG, Wiegerinck MA, Bongers MY, van der Veen F, Bossuyt PM. The performance of CA-125 measurement in the detection of endometriosis: A meta-analysis. *Fertil Steril* 1998;70:1101–8.

29. Othman EE, Hornung D, Salem HT et al. Serum cytokines as biomarkers for nonsurgical prediction of endometriosis. *Eur J Obstet Gynecol Reprod Biol* 2007;137:240–6.

30. Bhatt S, Kocakoc E, Dogra VS. Endometriosis: Sonographic spectrum. *Ultrasound Q* 2006;22:273–80.

31. Asch E, Levine D. Variations in appearance of endometriomas. *J Ultrasound Med* 2007;26:993–1002.

32. Kupfer MC, Schwimmer SR, Lebovic J. Transvaginal sonographic appearance of endometriomata: Spectrum and findings. *J Ultrasound Med* 1992;11:129–33.

33. Patel MD, Feldstein VA, Chen DC et al. Endometriomas: Diagnostic performance of US. *Radiology* 1999;210:739–45.

34. Bennett GL, Slywotzky CM, Cantera M, Hecht EM. Unusual manifestations and complications of endometriosis—spectrum of imaging findings: Pictorial review. *AJR Am J Roentgenol* 2010;194(6 Suppl):WS34–46.

35. Mais V, Guerriero S, Ajossa S, Angiolucci M, Paoletti AM, Melis GB. The efficiency of transvaginal ultrasonography in the diagnosis of endometrioma. *Fertil Steril* 1993;60:776–80.

36. Hudelist G, English J, Thomas AE, Tinelli A, Singer CF, Keckstein J. Diagnostic accuracy of transvaginal ultrasound for non-invasive diagnosis of bowel endometriosis: Systematic review and meta-analysis. *Ultrasound Obstet Gynecol* 2011;37:257–63.

37. Fedele L, Bianchi S, Raffaelli R, Portuese A. Pre-operative assessment of bladder endometriosis. *Hum Reprod* 1997;12:2519–522.

38. Glastonbury CM. The shading sign. *Radiology* 2002;224:199.

39. Outwater E, Schiebler ML, Owen RS et al. Characterization of hemorrhagic adnexal lesions with MR imaging: Blinded reader study. *Radiology* 1993;186:489.

40. Kier R, Smith RC, McCarthy SM. Value of lipid- and water- suppression MR images in distinguishing between blood and lipid within ovarian masses. *AJR Am J Roentgenol* 1992;58:321.

41. Stratton P, Winkel C, Premkumar A et al. Diagnostic accuracy of Laparoscopy, magnetic resonance imaging, and histopathologic examination for the detection of endometriosis. *Fertil Steril* 2003;79(5):1078–85.

42. Chamie LP, Blasbalg R, Pereira RM, Warmbrand G, Serafini PC. Findings of pelvic endometriosis at transvaginal US, MR imaging, and laparoscopy. *Radiographics* 2011;31(4):E77–100.

43. Exacoustos C, Malzoni M, Di Giovanni A et al. Ultrasound mapping system or the surgical management of deep infiltrating endometriosis. *Fertil Steril* 2014a;102(1):143.

Adolescents and endometriosis

AASHIMA ARORA

Endometriosis refers to the presence of endometrial glands and stroma outside the endometrial cavity. These ectopic implants may occur anywhere in the body, but are mostly located in the pelvis. The clinical spectrum may vary from a completely asymptomatic nature to a most debilitating pelvic pain. Endometriosis in adolescents will be discussed in detail in this chapter.

PREVALENCE

The exact prevalence of endometriosis among adolescents is not known. The estimated prevalence depends upon whether a symptomatic or an asymptomatic population is being studied and upon the method used for diagnosis. Around 20%–30% of adolescents with chronic pelvic pain and around half of those undergoing laparoscopy for this pain will be diagnosed to have this condition [1]. However, laparoscopy for the sole purpose of diagnosing endometriosis is not warranted in all adolescents with dysmenorrhea. However, pelvic pain not controlled with nonsteroidal anti-inflammatory drugs (NSAIDs) or combined oral contraceptive pills (OCPs) strongly points toward endometriosis [2,3].

CLINICAL PRESENTATION

The average time taken to diagnose endometriosis from onset of clinical symptoms is 9 years, requiring an average of 4.2 physician visits, and this time is the longest in the adolescent age group [4]. This is mainly because the pelvic pain of endometriosis in adolescents may be noncyclic in comparison with adults, who typically present with more specific complaints such as cyclical pain, dyspareunia, and infertility, making the diagnosis easier [3]. Also, dysmenorrhea in adolescents is more often considered "physiological" and hence rarely evaluated seriously. Bowel symptoms such as rectal pain, constipation, cyclic painful defecation, rectal bleeding, and bladder symptoms (e.g., dysuria, urgency, and hematuria) are also common among adolescents.

It may be difficult to diagnose endometriosis in adolescents with pelvic pain merely on the basis of history as similar symptoms occur in patients evaluated laparoscopically for pelvic pain with and without endometriosis. It must be remembered that cases of histologically proven endometriosis have been documented even prior to menarche in girls who have breast development and in many others soon after menarche. Also, around 60% of adult women with endometriosis report symptoms beginning at 20 years of age or earlier [5]. It is a common misbelief that endometriosis presents only after many years of menstruation. Hence, during evaluation of an adolescent with significant pelvic pain, whether it is cyclic or acyclic, endometriosis must be kept as a differential to avoid delay in diagnosis and management.

DIAGNOSIS

Though the gold standard of diagnosis of endometriosis is histological proof of disease by laparoscopically taken biopsy, detailed history and age-appropriate examination may clinch the diagnosis in most adolescents and save an invasive procedure (Figure 6.1). The history must focus on all characteristics of pain: location (diffuse/localized), onset (sudden/gradual), constant/intermittent, magnitude, quality, duration, radiation, relationship to various activities (such as menstruation and sexual, physiologic, or physical activities). The bowel and bladder symptoms must be asked for, in addition to menstrual, sexual, and contraceptive history. It should be assessed how much pain interferes with daily activities and whether or not any treatment for the same has been taken in the past by the adolescent.

General physical examination and abdominal examination are usually normal and a complete pelvic examination may not be possible in all adolescents. Even if bimanual examination is done, it is rare to appreciate fixed retroverted uterus, pelvic nodularity, or large ovarian endometrioma in adolescents. A thorough attempt must be made, either clinically or with help of imaging in case of suspicion, to rule out Müllerian anomalies, as they predispose girls to severe and early onset endometriosis, which can resolve with timely treatment. Congenital anomalies of the genital tract are found in around 10% of adolescents with endometriosis, and endometriosis is present in more than two-thirds of girls with Müllerian anomalies [6,7].

A complete blood count with erythrocyte sedimentation rate (ESR) and a urine routine and microscopy examination are usually performed to rule out chronic inflammatory process and urinary tract infection (UTI), respectively. Though CA-125 is commonly elevated in endometriosis, it is not recommended as a screening test due to its high false-positive rate. It is commonly used by clinicians to follow the progress of disease in confirmed cases, though follow-up based on clinical symptomatology seems more reliable. Imaging is less useful in adolescents compared with adults since endometriomas rarely occurs in this age group. However, imaging may be useful in excluding other causes of pelvic pain such as ovarian torsion/hemorrhage, Müllerian anomalies, appendicitis, and so on. MRI is not recommended as a first-line imaging test; however, it may be of use to better define an abnormality suspected on ultrasound or when Müllerian anomaly is suspected.

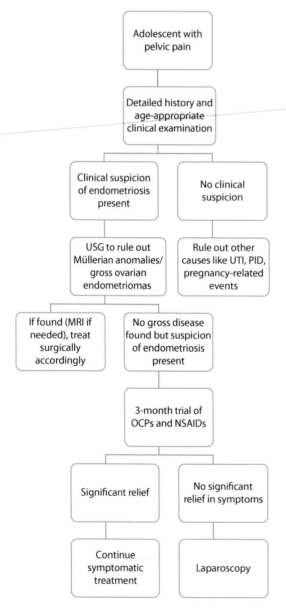

Figure 6.1 Diagnosis of endometriosis.

MANAGEMENT

All adolescents with pelvic pain should not be subjected to invasive diagnosis by laparoscopy.

When initial evaluation suggests endometriosis, a 3-month trial with NSAIDs/OCPs is a reasonable first-line approach [8]. Literature does not suggest benefit of any specific contraceptive pill formulation. Hormonal therapy leads to decidualization and subsequent atrophy of ectopic as well as eutopic endometrial tissue, thereby reducing bleeding and bleeding-related pain. Empirical use of GnRH analogues is not recommended in adolescents due to concern about bone mass accumulation during these years [9,10]. The American College of Obstetricians and Gynecologists (ACOG) also does not recommend use of empirical GnRH therapy for treatment of presumed endometriosis in girls <18 years. However, this may be considered as an option after informed consent in adolescents >18 years of age.

Laparoscopy must be considered if an adolescent with chronic pelvic pain does not respond to NSAIDs/OCPs since endometriosis is present in 35%–70% of these female patients, and definite diagnosis must be made before any further treatment is administered. The initial surgical procedure performed must be both diagnostic and therapeutic. The operating surgeon must be familiar with the appearance of endometriotic implants in adolescents. Studies have reported that red-flame lesions are more common and powder-burn lesions are less common in adolescents compared

with adults [11]. Also, peritoneal defects must be taken to be suggestive of endometriosis. Though controversial, some authors suggest random biopsies, including one from the posterior cul-de-sac, if no evidence of endometriosis is found grossly during laparoscopy.

The revised American Society for Reproductive Medicine (ASRM) classification must be used for staging the disease during laparoscopy. Overall, minimal to mild endometriosis (stage I and II rASRM classification) is most commonly found in adolescents [12]. It should, however, be remembered that the stage of disease or the location of lesions does not correlate with symptoms and, hence, does not dictate further treatment.

As in adults, treatment of stage I and II disease may be excisional or ablative. Electrocautery, endocoagulation, laser ablation, or resection of implants must be done during the initial laparoscopy. Although large endometriomas are rare in this age group, if found, cysts must be removed with as much preservation of ovarian tissue as possible [13]. (See Figure 6.2.)

POSTOPERATIVE TREATMENT

Even though there is no long-term data on the course of adolescents who do not take postoperative therapy after laparoscopic treatment of endometriosis, there is general consensus that after histological confirmation of the disease, adolescents must be started on medical treatment. The basic rationale of medical therapy is decreasing estrogen production from the ovaries and prostaglandin synthesis from the endometriotic implants, thereby causing decidualization and atrophy of ectopic endometrial tissue. The goal of therapy is symptomatic relief and suppression of disease progression which could later impair fertility.

Numerous medical therapeutic options are available for endometriosis, with different benefits, risks, and side effect profiles [9]. The treatment chosen must depend upon the severity of symptoms and compliance. For adolescents <18 years, OCPs are usually the first line while for older adolescents (>16 years or >18 years according to some authors), GnRH analogues and OCPs are both considered first-line options. OCPS may be used cyclically or continuously to retard disease progression and control remaining pain. No particular OCP formulation has been found to be advantageous

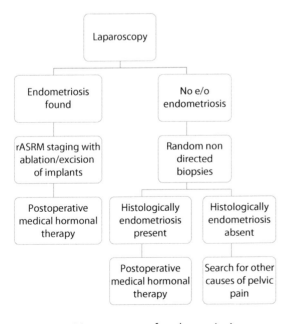

Figure 6.2 Management of endometriosis.

over others. Progestins, by themselves, also relieve symptoms in 80%–100% of patients with endometriosis by not only causing decidualization of endometrial tissue, but by also inhibiting pituitary gonadotropin secretion and ovarian hormone production, finally leading to a hypoestrogenic state. Though usually tolerated well, common side effects include weight gain, bloating, depression, and unscheduled spotting. Oral progestin therapy is preferred over long-term depot intramuscular preparations, which may result in loss of bone density.

GnRH agonists may be prescribed for adults >16–18 years of age with laparoscopy-confirmed disease [5]. This may be in the form of monthly or 3-monthly depot preparations, though the latter are associated with better compliance. Side effects include hot flashes, headache, mood swings, vaginal dryness, and depression. More than 90% of adolescents become amenorrhoeic after 2–3 months of therapy with GnRH and hence have almost complete resolution of symptoms. Initial treatment is usually continued for 6 months, after which either the patient is put on OCPs/progestin therapy or long-term GnRH therapy with add-back therapy with estrogens offered. When on long-term GnRH therapy, baseline bone density must be assessed and followed up every 2 years. Danazol is not commonly used in adolescents because of intolerable side effects, though the efficacy in treating mild-to-moderate disease is equivalent to GnRH.

CONCLUSION

Endometriosis must be considered in every adolescent with secondary dysmenorrhea. As the pain is commonly acyclic and physical examination inconclusive, diagnosis is commonly delayed for many years, leading to progression of disease. Strong clinical suspicion should warrant a trial of hormonal therapy, and early laparoscopy must be done in unresponsive adolescents.

The treating gynecologist must adopt a multi-dimensional approach for the treatment of pain in endometriosis in adolescents in which besides surgery and hormonal therapy, mental health support and complementary and alternative therapies are important components [14,15]. Pain that does not respond to aggressive medical therapy may be due to recurrent disease, pelvic adhesions due to endometriosis or prior surgery, or any different disease process and, hence, should be managed as per the cause.

REFERENCES

1. Goldstein DP, De Cholnoky C, Emansi SJ. Adolescent endometriosis. *J Adolesc Health Care* 1980;1:3741.
2. Harel Z. A contemporary approach to dysmenorrhea in adolescents. *Pediatr Drugs* 2002;4:797–805.
3. Laufer MR, Goietein L, Bush M, Cramer DW, Emans SJ. Prevalence of endometriosis in adolescent girls with chronic pelvic pain not responding to conventional therapy. *J Pediatr Adolesc Gynecol* 1997;10:199–202.
4. Ballweg ML. Big picture of endometriosis helps provide guidance on approach to teens: Comparative historical data show endo starting younger, is more severe. *J Pediatr Adolesc Gynecol* 2003;16(3 Suppl):S21–6.
5. ACOG Committee Opinion: No. 310. Endometriosis in adolescents. *Obstet Gynecol* 2005;105:921.
6. Davis GD, Thillet E, Lindemann J. Clinical characteristics of adolescent endometriosis. *J Adolesc Health* 1993;14:362–8.
7. Olive D, Henderson D. Endometrosis and Müllerian anomalies. *Obstet Gynecol* 1987;69:412–5.
8. Davis AR, Westhoff C, O'Connell K, Gallagher N. Oral contraceptives for dysmenorrhea in adolescent girls. *Obstet Gynecol* 2005;106:97–104.
9. Templeman C. Adolescent endometriosis. *Obstet Gynecol Clin North Am* 2009;36:177–86.
10. DiVasta AD, Laufer MR, Gordon C. Bone density in adolescent treated with a GnRH agonist and add-back therapy for endometriosis. *J Pediatr Adolesc Gynecol* 2007;20:293–7.
11. Vercellini P, Fedele L, Arcaini L, Bianchi S, Rognoni M, Candiani G. Laparoscopy in the diagnosis of chronic pelvic pain in adolescent women. *J Reprod Med* 1989;34:827–30.
12. Emmert C, Romann D, Riedel HH. Endometriosis diagnosed by laparoscopy in adolescent girls. *Arch Gynecol Obstet* 1998;261:89–93.

13. Marsh EE, Laufer MR. Endometriosis in premenarcheal girls who do not have an associated obstructed anomaly. *Fertil Steril* 2005;83:758–60.

14. Greco D. Management of adolescent chronic pelvic pain from endometriosis: A pain center perspective. *J Pediatr Adolesc Gynecol* 2003;16(3 Suppl):S17–9.

15. Wayne PM, Kerr CE, Schnyer RN et al. Japanese-style acupuncture for endometriosis-related pelvic pain in adolescents and young women: Results of a randomized sham-controlled trial. *J Pediatr Adolesc Gynecol* 2008;21:247–5.

7

Infertility attributed to endometriosis

SHALINI GAINDER AND NEETHI MALA MEKALA

INTRODUCTION

Endometriosis, a common debilitating, estrogen-dependent disorder in women of reproductive age, is characterized by the presence of endometrial-like (glands and stroma) tissue outside the uterine cavity, provoking a chronic inflammatory reaction and subsequent formation of adhesions, fibrosis, and scar tissue that can deform pelvic anatomy. It is estimated to affect around 1 in 10 women globally [1].

The specific pathogenesis of endometriosis is elusive. Though a number of theories including retrograde menstruation and implantation (the most accepted theory), altered immunity, coelomic metaplasia, direct transplantation, and vascular dissemination are well documented; stem cell, epigenetic, and genetic origins draw a special focus as evident from certain studies [2–10].

Although multiple mechanisms are involved in the initiation and spread of the disease, irrespective of the cause that incites the disease, there are still a few unanswered questions regarding why endometriosis develops in only a few, when retrograde menstruation is observed in around 90% of women [11]. Individual susceptibility influenced by anatomical, genetic, environmental, and hormonal factors, may explain it to a certain extent [12].

Infertility is one of the significant worrisome consequences of endometriosis, which imposes physical, psychological, and social issues for women.

EPIDEMIOLOGY

- In reference to certain population-based studies, the estimated prevalence of endometriosis ranges from 0.8% to 6% in women in the reproductive age group [13–15]; these figures rise drastically to as high as 20%–50% in subfertile women, with variations according to age of patients and over time periods [16,17].
- According to cited statistical information, the rate of prevalence of infertility, as a symptom, in women with endometriosis ranges from 30% to 50% [18–20].
- The estimated fecundity rates in normal couples in the reproductive age group are 15%–20%, while in those with untreated endometriosis, it ranges from 2% to 20% [19,22].

- Comparing natural conception rates between infertile women with mild endometriosis and those with unexplained infertility, the former group has experienced significantly lower conception rates over 3 years than the latter group (36% vs. 55%, respectively) [23].
- The results of a large prospective cohort study by Prescott et al. has shown that when compared with women (less than 35 years age) not having endometriosis, the likelihood of infertility was increased twofold in women with endometriosis [24].
- Although there is highly variable strength of association between the extent of the disease and reduced spontaneous conception rates in endometriosis, approximately 50% of them with minimal/mild disease and 25% of women with moderate disease conceive spontaneously. Only a few women with severe disease conceive without any treatment [25].

Taken together, all these observations give an inference that endometriosis reduces fertility that may roughly correlate with extent of the disease.

Nevertheless, certain cross-sectional studies have shown that age, superficial peritoneal endometriosis, and previous surgery for endometriosis have significantly higher association with infertility related to endometriosis compared with isolated endometriomas [26].

BIOLOGICAL MECHANISMS IN ENDOMETRIOSIS-ASSOCIATED INFERTILITY

Various mechanisms have been proposed to illustrate association of endometriosis and infertility. The relationship between two entities is obtained from comparisons of fertile and infertile women, animal models, donor sperm studies, and in vitro fertilization study results [27]. Although there is a well-documented association reported in the literature, the substantial cause–effect relationship is highly debatable and as remained controversial until now.

This chapter discusses current evidence and proposed pathophysiological mechanisms that explain how endometriosis may adversely affect fertility.

IMMUNOBIOLOGY AND MOLECULAR MECHANISMS

It is very important to understand the underlying basic immunological and molecular mechanisms as they form a backbone in initiating all consequences of endometriosis, particularly and significantly related to fertility.

Peritoneal fluid—a liquid that acts as a lubricant in the abdominal cavity—is rich in various inflammatory cells, cytokines, and growth factors. Multiple defective cellular and humoral immunological factors regulate the growth of ectopic endometrial implants and modulate their inflammatory behavior in endometriosis [28–32]. As a result, women with endometriosis not only have an increased amount of peritoneal fluid but also there are increased concentrations of various activated macrophages, inflammatory cytokines (TNF), interleukins (IL-1), prostaglandins, and reactive oxygen species, and there are decreased concentrations of antioxidants [33,34]. All these variations in endometriosis may affect fertility by several pathways through detrimental effects on the sperm, oocyte, embryo, or tubal functions (each will be described under the respective headings).

After resolution of acute inflammatory reaction induced by endometrial peritoneal implants, the activated macrophages continue a chronic inflammation reaction, which leads to the formation of peritoneal adhesions and angiogenesis and resistance to apoptosis [35–40]. All these observations are inferred from animal experiments and some human data. Therefore, endometriosis is characterized by typical chronic intraperitoneal inflammation [35,41,42]. An ovum capture inhibitor (OCI) identified in the peritoneal fluid of these patients may explain failure of fimbria to capture the ovum [33]. Apoptosis resistance exhibited by ectopic implants circumvents immune surveillance of the body, facilitating a self-perpetuating cycle.

DISTORTION OF PELVIC ANATOMY

Pelvic adhesions and peritubal adhesions disturb the relative anatomy of the ovaries and the fallopian tubes, which further hampers the ovum pickup. Chronic salpingitis may lead to the potential risk of tubal occlusion and can result in hydrosalpinx, and elevated levels of inflammatory cytokines impair tubal motility and hinder tubal patency; all of these affect the transport and interaction of gametes and embryo transport [44,45]. Fecundity is reduced due to all these mechanical disruptions.

ENDOCRINE AND OVULATORY ABNORMALITIES IN ENDOMETRIOSIS

The most common site of endometriosis are the ovaries. Altered levels of cytokines impair granulosa cellular function, follicular growth, and oocyte maturation and are also associated with decreased secretion of estradiol and reduction in follicular count. Apoptosis of these cells was also observed to increase in relation to extent of the disease and was found to reduce the pregnancy rates with the higher stage of disease. In patients with endometriosis, raised markers of oxidative stress were observed in the cytoplasm of granulosa cells [46,47].

Decreased receptors of luteinizing hormone (LH) in the follicles and altered LH surge affect ovulation. The follicular phase is lengthened due to disruption of the hypothalamo-pituitary-ovarian axis [48,49]. Luteal phase deficiency with decreased LH levels is observed in patients with endometriosis and the LH surge is delayed, which further intervenes with follicular growth, secretion of estrogen, the formation of corpus luteum, and secretion of progesterone [48,49]. Decreased expression of progesterone receptors in the endometrium may explain progesterone resistance in endometriosis [50–52].

Pituitary dysfunction in endometriosis could predict impaired folliculogenesis, decreased oocyte quality, or/and an altered endometrial receptivity [48,49,53,54]. Lower follicular count and decreased oocyte yield have been observed in women with bilateral chocolate cysts undergoing in vitro fertilization (IVF) [55].

Normally, the oocyte–cumulus complex is released from the ruptured dominant follicle within 38 hours after the LH surge. Sometimes, the luteinized follicle fails to rupture and release the ovum; this condition is known as luteinized unruptured follicle syndrome (LUF). This can only be demonstrated by visualization of unruptured follicles on serial pelvic ultrasonographic scans. Its prevalence is higher in women with endometriosis than those without the disease [56–58]. It

was also observed that use of nonsteroidal anti-inflammatory drugs in treating dysmenorrhea have increased the risk of LUF syndrome. These drugs inhibit cyclooxygenase enzyme, which will result in decreased ovarian prostaglandin production and inhibition of matrix metalloproteinases, thereby hindering follicle rupture [59].

FERTILIZATION AND IMPLANTATION DEFECTS

Effect on gametes

As mentioned above, inflammatory responses hinder oocyte production and ovulation from the affected ovary. It has been proposed that the alterations in peritoneal fluid not only impair sperm quality (as evident from increased DNA fragmentation due to oxidative stress) and function (binding of sperm to the inner lining of the affected tube, thus capacitation is impaired) but also enhance phagocytosis of sperm by activated macrophages [34,60].

Effect on embryos

Abnormal concentrations of inflammatory cells in peritoneal fluid have toxic effects, even on embryos [61]. It has been postulated that chocolate cysts secrete certain products specific to developing oocytes that may affect cleavage of the embryo, which results in developmental arrest at a cleavage or four-cell stage, attributing to the decreased quality of embryos in women with endometriosis [62–65].

Certain studies have shown that there is aberrant expression of catalase and glutathione peroxidase in the endometrium of women with endometriosis which may result in an increase of endometrial free radicles imposing a negative effect on the viability of an embryo [62,63].

Studies have shown that the embryos from women with endometriosis exhibit aberrant cytoplasmic and nuclear events such as abnormal distribution of microtubules, nuclear and cytoplasmic fragmentation, and increased cellular stress [64–66].

It is hypothesized that macrophages and inflammatory mediators present in the fluid of hydrosalpinx exert toxic effects on the embryo and intervene with its development and implantation (the proximal end of tube in hydrosalpinx is free which allows the fluid to drain, hampering implantation) [45,67–69].

Uterotubal dysperistalsis

In the uterus, coordinated muscular contractions augment the sperm transport to the tubes, where they undergo capacitation and hyperactivation in order to reach the ampullary part of the tube to fertilize the ovum. Postfertilization, passive transportation of the embryo to the uterine cavity occurs through the fallopian tubes.

Impaired tubal motility and abnormal uterine contractions mediated by the inflammatory cascade (increased production and concentration of prostaglandins and cytokines) signaled from ectopic endometrial tissue can interrupt at any step such as transport of gametes, fertilization, transport of embryo, adhesion, and penetration of the embryo on a pre-decidualized endometrium, affecting implantation and subsequent maintenance of ongoing pregnancies [70–73].

Effect on the endometrium

Apart from the above-mentioned inflammatory effects of endometriosis, there is substantiable data supporting that endometriosis affects the eutopic endometrium and may lead to implantation failure. But the mechanism by which the specific signal reaches and causes alterations in the eutopic endometrium is not clearly characterized. Certain experimental studies in mice infer that there was migration of experimental endometriotic tissue to the uterine endometrium, establishing bidirectional movement of cells between ectopic and eutopic endometrial tissue. The reprogrammed cells that have returned to the eutopic endometrium may generate signals leading to aberrant gene expression and cause implantation failure [74–76].

One of the examples of aberrant gene expression is the Hoxa 10/*HOXA10* gene. It is a gene which is associated with embryogenesis of the uterus and in regeneration of the endometrium in every menstrual cycle, and its expression is necessary for endometrial receptivity in women. Its expression peaks during the period of implantation under the influence of progesterone and estrogen.

Women with endometriosis do not show expected mid-luteal rise, which may partially describe their infertility [6,7].

It has been described that abnormal levels of aromatase were present in both eutopic endometrium (where it is normally absent) and endometriotic implants, resulting in raised estradiol production. Such increased production of estrogen in the endometrium may also impair endometrial development and receptivity [77].

Progesterone has a significant role in normal pregnancy, as it induces decidualization of the endometrium in the luteal phase. Its resistance and the dysregulation of its receptors in both ectopic and eutopic endometrium leads to an unopposed estrogen state, which is not suitable for proper implantation [51,52]. Delayed and out-of-phase histological maturation of the endometrium also impairs implantation [78,79].

Matrix metalloproteinases (MMPs), which break down extracellular matrices, are normally inhibited in the secretory phase under the influence of progesterone. But in endometriosis, their disinhibition due to progesterone resistance would theoretically lead to degradation of the extracellular matrix which makes the endometrium unfavorable for implantation [80].

Women with endometriosis have decreased expression of αvβ3-integrin (an adhesion molecule) that interferes with embryo attachment to pre-decidualized endometrium [41,78,79,81]. L-Selectin (a protein that covers the trophoblast on blastocyst) levels are poorly expressed in endometriosis [43].

Increased levels of anti-endometrial antibodies were detected in the serum and the endometrium of women with endometriosis, and further binding of those antibodies to endometrial antigens may affect endometrial receptivity and implantation [21,43].

As mentioned above, there is a complex system of immunological, molecular, and various hormonal factors, all interlinked together, hampering implantation in women with endometriosis.

EARLY PREGNANCY LOSS

The proximal end of the tube in the hydrosalpinx is free which allows the fluid to drain into the uterine cavity, intervening with implantation and increasing the abortion rate [45,67–69].

Table 7.1 Possible mechanisms explaining reduced fertility in women with endometriosis

1. IMMUNOBIOLOGY AND MOLECULAR MECHANISMS
   - Altered peritoneal function
     1. Increased production and concentration of prostaglandins and cytokines
     2. Increased number of activated macrophages
     3. Cytotoxic effects on gametes and embryos
   - Alterations in systemic immune response—increased prevalence of auto-antibodies and cell-mediated injury to gametes and embryos

2. DISTORTION OF PELVIC ANATOMY
   - Pelvic and peritubal adhesions
   - Chronic salpingitis
   - Hydrosalpinx
   - Impaired tubal motility
   - Disturbed tubo-ovarian liaison

3. ENDOCRINE AND OVULATORY ABNORMALITIES
   - Impaired folliculogenesis, poor ovarian reserve
   - Luteal phase defect
   - Luteinized unruptured follicle syndrome
   - Progesterone resistance
   - Hyperprolactinemia

4. FERTILIZATION AND IMPLANATATION DEFECTS
   - Effect on gametes and embryo
     1. Decreased oocyte production
     2. Poor oocyte quality
     3. Impaired sperm quality and function (capacitation)
     4. Enhanced phagocytosis of sperm
     5. Impaired embryogenesis and reduced quality of embryos
     6. Cytotoxic effects on embryo from toxic fluid of hydrosalpinx and aberrant expression of free radicles in endometrium
   - Uterotubal dysperistalsis—disrupted transport of gametes and embryo
   - Effect on endometrium
     1. Progesterone resistance
     2. Abnormal levels of aromatase—unopposed estrogen state
     3. Aberrant gene expression, e.g., Hoxa 10/*HOXA10* gene
     4. Disinhibition of matrix metalloproteinases
     5. Decreased expression of adhesion molecules (e.g., $\alpha v \beta 3$-integrin, L-selectin)
     6. Increased levels of anti-endometrial antibodies

5. EARLY PREGNANCY LOSS
   - Defective embryogenesis
   - Altered endometrial receptivity and abnormal uterine contractions
   - Toxic fluid from hydrosalpinx

6. Others: Decreased coital frequency due to dyspareunia

Defective embryogenesis or inadequate endometrial support to the developing embryo results in an increased incidence of spontaneous abortions that may occur at different gestational ages [51,52,64,65].

OTHER FACTORS

Others factors that contribute to reduced fertility rates in women with endometriosis are decreased coital frequency due to varying degrees of pelvic pain and dyspareunia.

CONCLUSION

However, as evidenced above, infertility associated with endometriosis can be explainable by two main mechanisms:

1. Distorted pelvic anatomy that prevents ovum pickup after ovulation and transportation of gametes
2. Increased production and concentration of prostaglandins, inflammatory mediators (cytokines, chemokines), and metalloproteinases leading to chronic inflammation that affects tubal, ovarian, and endometrial functions, resulting in impaired folliculogenesis, fertilization, or implantation

The first mechanism appears to be a logical explanation of decreased fertility in women with advanced stages of endometriosis, whereas the latter one may be applicable in women with minimal/mild disease. Diagnostic approaches based on endometrial changes associated with endometriosis are also providing insights into possible mechanisms of infertility, especially in women with milder forms of the disease [27].

Hence, the association of endometriosis with infertility appears to be multifactorial, including various mechanical, molecular, immunological, and genetic factors which are interlinked to a greater extent and operate simultaneously. (These mechanisms are summarized in Table 7.1.)

REFERENCES

1. Eskenazi B, Warner ML, Epidemiology of endometriosis. *Obstet Gyne Clin N Am* 1997;24;235–258.

2. Du H, Taylor HS. Contribution of bone marrow-derived stem cells to endometrium and endometriosis. *Stem Cells.* 2007;25(8):2082–2086.

3. Taylor HS. Endometrial cells derived from donor stem cells in bone marrow transplant recipients. *JAMA.* 2004;292(1):81–85.

4. Simpson JL, Elias S, Malinak LR, Buttram VC Jr. Heritable aspects of endometriosis. I. Genetic studies. *Am J Obstet Gynecol.* 1980;137(3):327–331.

5. Bedaiwy MA, Falcone T, Mascha EJ, Casper RF. Genetic polymorphism in the fibrinolytic system and endometriosis. *Obstet Gynecol.* 2006;108(1):162–168.

6. Taylor HS, Bagot C, Kardana A, Olive D, Arici A. HOX gene expression is altered in the endometrium of women with endometriosis. *Hum Reprod.* 1999;14(5):1328–1331.

7. Zanatta A, Rocha AM, Carvalho FM et al. The role of the Hoxa10/HOXA10 gene in the etiology of endometriosis and its related infertility: A review. *J Assist Reprod Genet.* 2010;27(12):701–710.

8. Lee B, Du H, Taylor HS. Experimental murine endometriosis induces DNA methylation and altered gene expression in eutopic endometrium. *Biol Reprod.* 2009;80(1):79–85.

9. Kim JJ, Taylor HS, Lu Z et al. Altered expression of HOXA10 in endometriosis: Potential role in decidualization. *Mol Hum Reprod.* 2007;13(5):323–332.

10. Grechukhina O, Petracco R, Popkhadze S et al. A polymorphism in a let-7 microRNA binding site of KRAS in women with endometriosis. *EMBO Mol Med.* 2012;4(3):206–217.

11. Halme J, Hammond MG, Hulka JF, Raj SG, Talbert LM. Retrograde menstruation in healthy women and in patients with endometriosis. *Obstet Gynecol.* United States. 1984;64(2):151–154.

12. Taylor RN, Lebovic DI. Endometriosis. In: Strauss JF Barbieri RL (eds). *Yen & Jaffe's Reproductive Endocrinology,* 7th edn. Philadelphia, PA: Elsevier Saunders, 2014. pp. 565–585.

13. Moen MH, Schei B. Epidemiology of endometriosis in a Norwegian county. *Acta Obstet Gynecol Scand.* 1997;76:559–5562.

14. Abbas S, Ihle P, Koster I, Schubert I. Prevalence and incidence of diagnosed endometriosis and risk of endometriosis in

patients with endometriosis-related symptoms: Findings from a statutory health insurancebased cohort in Germany. *Eur J Obstet Gynecol Reprod Biol.* 2012;160:79–83.

15. Fuldeore MJ, Soliman AM. Prevalence and symptomatic burden of diagnosed endometriosis in the United States: National estimates from a cross-sectional survey of 59,411 women. *Gynecol Obstet Invest.* 2016; DOI:10.1159/000452660. [Epub ahead of print]

16. Mahmood TA, Templeton A. Prevalence and genesis of endometriosis. *Hum Reprod.* 1991;6:544–549.

17. Meuleman C, Vandenabeele B, Fieuws S, Spiessens C, Timmerman D, D'Hooghe T. High prevalence of endometriosis in infertile women with normal ovulation and normospermic partners. *Fertil Steril.* 2009;92:68–74.

18. Verkauf BS. Incidence, symptoms, and signs of endometriosis in fertile and infertile women. *J Fla Med Assoc.* 1987;74(9):671–675.

19. American Society for Reproductive Medicine. Endometriosis and infertility: A committee opinion. *Fertil Steri* 2012;98:591–598.

20. Carvalho LF, Rossener R, Azeem A, Malvezzi H, Simoes Abrao M, Agarwal A. From conception to birth - how endometriosis affects the development of each stage of reproductive life. *Minerva Ginecol* 2013;65:181-198.

21. Sarapik A, Haller-Kikkatalo K, Utt M, Teesalu K, Salumets A, Uibo R. Serum anti-endometrial antibodies in infertile women—Potential risk factor for implantation failure. *Am J Reprod Immunol.* 2010;63:349–357.

22. Hughes EG, Fedorkow DM, Collins JA. A quantitative overview of controlled trials in endometriosis-associated infertility. *Fertil Steril.* 1993;59(5):963–970.

23. Akande VA, Hunt LP, Cahill DJ, Jenkins JM. Differences in time to natural conception between women with unexplained infertility and infertile women with minor endometriosis. *Hum Reprod.* 2004;19(1):96–103.

24. Prescott J, Farland LV, Tobias DK et al. A prospective cohort study of endometriosis and subsequent risk of infertility. *Hum Reprod* 2016;31:1475–82.

25. Olive DL, Stohs GF, Metzger DA, Franklin RR. Expectant management and hydrotubations in the treatment of endometriosis-associated infertility. *Fertil Steril.* 1985;44:35–41.

26. Santulli P, Lamau MC, Marcellin L et al. Endometriosis-related infertility: Ovarian endometrioma per se is not associated with presentation for infertility. *Hum Reprod.* 2016;31:1765–75.

27. Holoch KJ, Lessey BA. Endometriosis and infertility. *Clin Obstet Gynecol.* 2010;53(2):429–438.

28. Steele RW, Dmowski WP, Marmer DJ. Immunologic aspects of human endometriosis. *Am J Reprod Immunol.* 1984;6(1):33–36.

29. Oosterlynck DJ, Cornillie FJ, Waer M, Vandeputte M, Koninckx PR. Women with endometriosis show a defect in natural killer activity resulting in a decreased cytotoxicity to autologous endometrium. *Fertil Steril.* 1991;56(1):45–51.

30. Harada T, Iwabe T, Terakawa N. Role of cytokines in endometriosis. *Fertil Steril.* 2001;76(1):1–10.

31. Lebovic DI, Mueller MD, Taylor RN. Immunobiology of endometriosis. *Fertil Steril.* 2001;75(1):1–10.

32. Witz CA. Interleukin-6: Another piece of the endometriosis-cytokine puzzle. *Fertil Steril.* 2000;73(2):212–214.

33. Suginami H, Yano K. An ovum capture inhibitor (OCI) in endometriosis peritoneal fluid: An OCI-related membrane responsible for fimbrial failure of ovum capture. *Fertil Steril.* 1988;50(4):648–653.

34. Gupta S, Goldberg JM, Aziz N, Goldberg E, Krajcir N, Agarwal A. Pathogenic mechanisms in endometriosis-associated infertility. *Fertil Steril.* United States. 2008;90(2):247–257.

35. Ahn SH, Monsanto SP, Miller C, Singh SS, Thomas R, Tayade C. Pathophysiology and immune dysfunction in endometriosis. *Biomed Res Int.* 2015;2015:795976.

36. Braundmeier A, Jackson K, Hastings J, Koehler J, Nowak R, Fazleabas A. Induction of endometriosis alters the peripheral and endometrial regulatory T cell population in the non-human primate. *Hum Reprod.* 2012;27:1712–1722.

37. Borrelli GM, Carvalho KI, Kallas EG, Mechsner S, Baracat EC, Abrão MS. Chemokines in the pathogenesis of endometriosis and infertility. *J Reprod Immunol.* 2013;98:1–9.

38. Olkowska-Truchanowicz J, Bocian K, Maksym RB et al. CD4+ CD25+ FOXP3+ regulatory T cells in peripheral blood and peritoneal fluid of patients with endometriosis. *Hum Reprod.* 2013;28:119–124.

39. Li MQ, Wang Y, Chang KK et al. CD4+Foxp3+ regulatory T cell differentiation mediated by endometrial stromal cell-derived TECK promotes the growth and invasion of endometriotic lesions. *Cell Death Dis.* 2014;5:e1436.

40. Takebayashi A, Kimura F, Kishi Y et al. Subpopulations of macrophages within eutopic endometrium of endometriosis patients. *Am J Reprod Immunol.* 2015;73:221–231.

41. Giudice LC, Kao LC. Endometriosis. *Lancet.* 2004;364:1789–1799.

42. Lousse JC, Van Langendonckt A, Defrere S, Ramos RG, Colette S, Donnez J. Peritoneal endometriosis is an inflammatory disease. *Front Biosci (Elite Ed).* 2012;4:23–40.

43. Practice Committee of the American Society for Reproductive Medicine (ASRM). Endometriosis and Infertility. *Fertil Steril.* 2006;14:S156–60.

44. Macer ML, Taylor HS. Endometriosis and infertility: A review of the pathogenesis and treatment of endometriosis-associated infertility. *Obstet Gynecol Clin North Am.* United States. 2012;39(4):535–549.

45. David A, Garcia CR, Czernobilsky B. Human hydrosalpinx: Histologic study and chemical composition of fluid. *Am J Obstet Gynecol.* 1969;105(3):400–411.

46. Nakahara K, Saito H, Saito T et al. Incidence of apoptotic bodies in membrana granulosa of the patients participating in an *in vitro* fertilization program. *Fertil Steril.* United States. 1997;67(2):302–308.

47. Saito H, Seino T, Kaneko T, Nakahara K, Toya M, Kurachi H. Endometriosis and oocyte quality. *Gynecol Obstet Invest.* Switzerland. 2002;53(Suppl 1):46–51.

48. Cahill DJ, Wardle PG, Maile LA, Harlow CR, Hull MG. Pituitary-ovarian dysfunction as a cause for endometriosis-associated and unexplained infertility. *Hum Reprod.* England. 1995;10(12):3142–3146.

49. Cahill DJ, Hull MG. Pituitary-ovarian dysfunction and endometriosis. *Hum Reprod Update.* 2000;6:56–66.

50. Bulun SE, Cheng YH, Yin P et al. Progesterone resistance in endometriosis: Link to failure to metabolize estradiol. *Mol Cell Endocrinol.* 2006;248:94–103.

51. Lessey BA, Ilesanmi AO, Castelbaum AJ et al. Characterization of the functional progesterone receptor in an endometrial adenocarcinoma cell line (Ishikawa): Progesterone-induced expression of the alpha1 integrin. *J Steroid Biochem Mol Biol.* 1996;59(1):31–39.

52. Lessey BA, Yeh I, Castelbaum AJ et al. Endometrial progesterone receptors and markers of uterine receptivity in the window of implantation. *Fertil Steril.* 1996;65(3):477–483.

53. Pellicer A, Oliveira N, Ruiz A, Remohí J, Sim_on C. Exploring the mechanism(s) of endometriosis-related infertility: An analysis of embryo development and implantation in assisted reproduction. *Hum Reprod* 1995;10(Suppl 2):91–97.

54. Opøien HK, Fedorcsak P, Omland AK et al. In vitro fertilization is a successful treatment in endometriosis-associated infertility. *Fertil Steril.* 2012;97:912–918.

55. Benaglia L, Bermejo A, Somigliana E et al. In vitro fertilization outcome in women with unoperated bilateral endometriomas. *Fertil Steril.* United States. 2013;99(6):1714–1719.

56. Dmowski WP, Rao R, Scommegna A. The luteinized un-ruptured follicle syndrome and endometriosis. *Fertil Steril.* 1980;33:30–34.

57. Koninckx PR, Brosens IA. Clinical significance of the luteinized unruptured follicle syndrome as a cause of infertility. *Eur J Obstet Gynecol Reprod Biol.* Netherlands. 1982;13(6):355–368.

58. Qublan H, Amarin Z, Nawasreh M et al. Luteinized unruptured follicle syndrome: Incidence and recurrence rate in infertile women with unexplained infertility undergoing intrauterine insemination. *Hum Reprod.* England. 2006;21(8):2110–2113.

59. Smith G, Roberts R, Hall C, Nuki G. Reversible ovulatory failure associated with the development of luteinized unruptured follicles in women with inflammatory arthritis taking non-steroidal anti-inflammatory drugs. *Br J Rheumatol.* 1996;35:458–462.

60. Oral E, Arici A, Olive DL, Huszar G. Peritoneal fluid from women with moderate or severe endometriosis inhibits sperm motility: The role of seminal fluid components. *Fertil Steril.* 1996;66(5):787–792.

61. Morcos RN, Gibbons WE, Findley WE. Effect of peritoneal fluid on *in vitro* cleavage of 2-cell mouse embryos: Possible role in infertility associated with endometriosis. *Fertil Steril.* 1985;44(5):678–683.

62. Ota H, Igarashi S, Sato N, Tanaka H, Tanaka T. Involvement of catalase in the endometrium of patients with endometriosis and adenomyosis. *Fertil Steril.* 2002;78(4):804–809.

63. Ota H, Igarashi S, Kato N, Tanaka T. Aberrant expression of glutathione peroxidase in eutopic and ectopic endometrium in endometriosis and adenomyosis. *Fertil Steril.* 2000;74(2):313–318.

64. Stilley JA, Birt JA, Nagel SC, Sutovsky M, Sutovsky P, Sharpe-Timms KL. Neutralizing TIMP1 restores fecundity in a rat model of endometriosis and treating control rats with TIMP1 causes anomalies in ovarian function and embryo development. *Biol Reprod.* United States;2010;83(2):185–194.

65. Yanushpolsky EH, Best CL, Jackson KV, Clarke RN, Barbieri RL, Hornstein MD. Effects of endometriomas on oocyte quality, embryo quality, and pregnancy rates in *in vitro* fertilization cycles: A prospective, case controlled study. *J Assist Reprod Genet.* 1998;15(4):193–197.

66. Brizek CL, Schlaff S, Pellegrini VA, Frank JB, Worrilow KC. Increased incidence of aberrant morphological phenotypes in human embryogenesis—an association with endometriosis. *J Assist Reprod Genet.* United States. 1995;12(2):106–112.

67. Mukherjee T, Copperman AB, McCaffrey C, Cook CA, Bustillo M, Obasaju MF. Hydrosalpinx fluid has embryotoxic effects on murine embryogenesis: A case for prophylactic salpingectomy. *Fertil Steril.* 1996;66(5):851–853.

68. Mansour RT, Aboulghar MA, Serour GI, Riad R. Fluid accumulation of the uterine cavity before embryo transfer: A possible hindrance for implantation. *J In Vitro Fert Embryo Transf.* United States. 1991;8(3):157–159.

69. Oehninger S, Scott R, Muasher SJ, Acosta AA, Jones Jr. HW, Rosenwaks Z. Effects of the severity of tubo-ovarian disease and previous tubal surgery on the results of *in vitro* fertilization and embryo transfer. *Fertil Steril.* 1989;51(1):126–130.

70. Leyendecker G, Kunz G, Wildt L, Beil D, Deininger H. Uterine hyperperistalsis and dysperistalsis as dysfunctions of the mechanism of rapid sperm transport in patients with endometriosis and infertility. *Hum Reprod.* 1996;11:1542–1551.

71. Bulletti C, de Ziegler D, Polli V, Diotallevi L, Del Ferro E, Flamigni C. Uterine contractility during menstrual cycle. *Hum Reprod.* 2000;15:81–89.

72. Ijland MM, Evers JL, Dunselman GA, Hoogland HJ. Endometrial wavelike activity, endometrial thickness, and ultrasound texture in controlled ovarian hyperstimulation cycles. *Fertil Steril.* 1998;70(2):279–83.

73. IJland MM, Evers JL, Dunselman GA, Volovics L, Hoogland HJ. Relation between endometrial wavelike activity and fecundability in spontaneous cycles. *Fertil Steril.* 1997;67(3):492–496.

74. Santamaria X, Massasa EE, Taylor HS. Migration of cells from experimental endometriosis to the uterine endometrium. *Endocrinology.* 2012;153 Epub 2012/09/13.

75. Hou X, Tan Y, Li M, Dey SK, Das SK. Canonical Wnt signaling is critical to estrogen-mediated uterine growth. *Mol Endocrinol.* 2004;18(12):3035–3049.

76. Mohamed OA, Jonnaert M, Labelle-Dumais C, Kuroda K, Clarke HJ, Dufort D. Uterine Wnt/betacatenin signaling is required for implantation. *Proc Natl Acad Sci U S A.* 2005;102(24):8579–8584.

77. Zeitoun KM, Bulun SE. Aromatase: A key molecule in the pathophysiology of endometriosis and a therapeutic target. *Fertil Steril.* 1999;72(6):961–969.

78. Lessey BA. Implantation defects in infertile women with endometriosis. *Ann N Y Acad Sci.* United States. 2002;955:265:396-406.

79. ASRM. Practice Committee of the American Society for Reproductive Medicine (ASRM). Endometriosis and Infertility. *Fertil Steril.* 2006;14:156–160.

80. Osteen KG, Keller NR, Feltus FA, Melner MH. Paracrine regulation of matrix metalloproteinase expression in the normal human endometrium. *Gynecol Obstet Invest.* 1999;48(Suppl 1):2–13.

81. Lessey BA, Castelbaum AJ, Sawin SW et al. Aberrant integrin expression in the endometrium of women with endometriosis. *J Clin Endocrinol Metab.* 1994;79(2):643–649.

8

Medical management of endometriosis

BHARTI JOSHI AND NEELAM AGGARWAL

BACKGROUND

Endometriosis is a challenging chronic and recurrent medical condition. More so, it is a diagnostic dilemma as it mimics malignancy that can metastasize to local and distant sites and invade and damage other tissues. Despite its description since 1860, etiopathogenesis remains poorly understood. The classic triad of dysmenorrhea, dyschezia, and dyspareunia can make one suspicious of the disease entity. The incidence is reported to be 6%–10% in women of reproductive age with a much higher prevalence of 20%–50% in women with infertility and 30%–80% in women with chronic pelvic pain [1–3].

The diagnosis of endometriosis is suspected based on the history and the symptoms and signs, is corroborated by physical examination and imaging techniques, and is finally proved by histological examination of specimens collected during laparoscopy. The combination of laparoscopy and the histological verification of endometrial glands and stroma is considered to be the gold standard for the diagnosis of the disease.

MECHANISMS OF PAIN

The mechanisms involved in the pain associated with endometriosis are difficult to ascertain

for a number of reasons. Pain itself is a subjective parameter, difficult to measure, and influenced by hormonal milieu. It can be diffuse in the pelvis or more localized, often in the area of the rectum. Low backache, too, may be due to endometriosis. Pain associated with mild endometriosis more likely relates to the effects of focal bleeding from endometriotic implants and inflammatory actions of cytokines in the peritoneal cavity, whereas in deep endometriosis, irritation or direct infiltration of pelvic nerves are said to be the attributing mechanisms for pain. Impaired immune molecular functions in endometriotic implants result in increased production of proinflammatory cytokines, prostaglandins, and metalloproteinases leading to pain and a failure of the immune system to suppress and clear the inflammatory response. There is a role of cytokines, especially interleukin (IL-1b) and angiogenic factors such as vascular endothelial growth factor (VEGF) in inducing COX-2 expression and increased prostaglandin production in endometriotic implants [3,4].

The intensity of pain associated with deep infiltrating endometriosis is directly proportional to the level of penetration and invasion of nerves. There is no relationship among stage, site appearance of endometriosis, and pain. The explanation for the observation that many women with advanced disease remain asymptomatic whereas those with mild disease experience incapacitating pain remains unclear. In addition, it has been seen that women with midline disease are more symptomatic.

TREATMENT OF ENDOMETRIOSIS

Medical management most often is the first-line treatment for pain relief and prevention of recurrence after surgery [5]. Treatment strategies for endometriosis are based on its clinical manifestations, that is, pelvic pain and infertility. As both are difficult to assess objectively, one has to direct and interpret treatment response carefully in order to achieve the therapeutic targets with the available options. The endometriotic lesions are hormonally active, and a continuous estrogen is required for the growth and persistence of these implants; therefore, they can be suppressed by changing the hormonal milieu.

Nonsurgical treatment options for endometriosis can be expectant, analgesics, or can have one or more combination of medical treatments. Expectant management remains an option for the women approaching menopause and for those without significant symptoms.

MEDICAL TREATMENT

Women with suspected endometriosis with clinical manifestation of pelvic pain and no other indications for surgical treatment can be considered for medical therapy without establishing histological diagnosis. While going for empirical medical therapy, one has to keep in mind that positive response to treatment does not confirm the diagnosis of endometriosis. Despite significant improvement in symptoms, medical therapies have no measurable effect on endometriomas, infertility, and pelvic adhesions. The traditional medical therapy has been based on Sampson's theory of retrograde menstruation with the objective of eliminating or decreasing cyclical menstruation, thereby suppressing or preventing growth of new implants. Although these operational concepts of medical therapy have been there for decades, new upcoming perceptions of etiopathogenesis of endometriosis at the molecular level are now bringing new treatment modalities aimed at the mechanisms of disease.

TREATMENT IN CURRENT PRACTICE

There are various pharmacological agents used for the treatment of endometriosis. These act by anti-inflammatory action, inhibiting ovulation, reducing estradiol levels, causing decidualization, and modulating immunological function and progesterone receptor activity [6]. Nonsteroidal anti-inflammatory drugs are invariably used for the relief of primary dysmenorrhea. Various agents used are as follows.

Ovarian suppression

ESTROGEN PROGESTIN CONTRACEPTIVES

The oral combined estrogen and progestin contraceptives, taken cyclically or in a continuous manner, have been the mainstay of treatment for endometriosis-associated pelvic pain for a long time. Continuous therapy induces anovulation and endometrial decidualization through negative hypophyseal feedback, thereby dubbing a state of pseudopregnancy. They are said to be the first choice for women with mild endometriosis to suppress or improve endometriosis who are not desirous of conception. They are expected to provide pain relief in the majority of patients if take taken in a continuous manner [6,7]. There is no consensus on the role of estrogen–progesterone formulations in prevention of endometriosis. No preparation is superior to another and they can be taken for a long time due to better tolerance and lower metabolic impact. A large multicenter trial from Japan has shown low-dose oral contraceptive pills to be effective for dysmenorrhea, nonmenstrual pain, and deep dyspareunia, including patient satisfaction. In subfertile women with painful endometriosis, nonsteroidal anti-inflammatory drugs (NSAIDs) appear to be the only option as no improvement in natural conception after ovarian suppression is seen in many randomized trials [8,9].

Progesterone resistance

There is robust literature supporting the role of progesterone resistance in the etiopathogenesis of endometriosis. This progesterone resistance mechanism has been the explanation for the preference of progestogens rather than oral contraceptives by some authors [10]. An overall reduction in progesterone receptor activity, along with the absence of the progesterone type B receptor (PR-B), is seen in endometriotic implants. The available drugs targeting the progesterone receptors are progestins and progesterone receptor modulators.

PROGESTINS (ORAL/INTRAVAGINAL/SUBCUTANEOUS/INTRAUTERINE)

Oral administration of different progestins addresses various pathologies of endometriosis: it causes decidualization, inhibits angiogenesis, and alters estrogen receptors, inducing atrophy of ectopic endometrium. Improvement in pain varies from 60% to 94%, as reported in various retrospective studies.

Medroxyprogesterone acetate (MPA) given orally (20–100 mg/day) has been found to relieve endometriosis-associated dysmenorrhea, dyspareunia, and intermenstrual pain in the majority of patients. Nausea, breast tenderness, irregular bleeding, and depression are commonly observed side effects. Studies have shown the same efficacy of oral MPA as that of gonadotropin-releasing hormone (GnRH) analogues in reducing endometriosis-associated pain, thereby improving quality of life [10]. High doses of medroxyprogesterone can adversely affect the lipoprotein profile. Megestrol acetate (40 mg/day) and norethindrone acetate are other oral progestins used with similar side effects.

Norethisterone acetate (NETA), a 19-nortestosterone derivative (5–15 mg/day) suppresses ovulation, thereby eventually causing decidualization and atrophy of the endometrium. This progestin has been proved effective for reducing chronic pelvic pain, dysmenorrhea, dyspareunia, and dyschezia similar to combined pills and, in patients with colorectal endometriosis, improves gastrointestinal symptoms. NETA seems to be an inexpensive, effective, tolerable, good alternative for the long-term treatment of endometriosis. It has a positive effect on control of uterine bleeding and calcium metabolism [11–13].

Depot medroxyprogesterone acetate (DMPA), given 150 mg every 3 months, has been found to be an effective alternative for reducing pain symptoms in endometriosis. This progestin has shown better results in terms of patient satisfaction and pain relief compared with low-dose danazol, but with more side effects [14]. Subcutaneous preparation of DMPA (104 mg) has also been studied and has shown equivalent results to that of leuprolide acetate [15].

Dienogest (DNG) is structural derivative of the norethindrone family, having a cyanomethyl group at the C-17 position. There is enough evidence supporting a 2 mg daily dose of dienogest in endometriosis-associated dysmenorrhea and pelvic and premenstrual pain in various randomized and other clinical studies [16–19]. An equivalent efficacy to GnRH analogues with better safety and low incidence of hypoestrogenic symptoms was confirmed in another studies. It has positive effect on quality of life and on pelvic pain when given as pre- or postoperative therapy [20–22]. Long-term use has shown a favorable efficacy with progressive decrease in bleeding irregularities and pelvic pain. The positive effect on pain was seen even after 6 months of discontinuation of treatment. Dienogest used in patients with deep infiltrating endometriosis has shown a decrease in the size of implants after a period of 10–12 months of use and immediate relief in symptoms [23,24]. This can be considered as an alternative to surgery in bladder endometriosis in reducing pain and other urinary symptoms [25]. Similar to other progestins, irregular bleeding is common but decreases over a period of time and resolves after stoppage of treatment [26]. The only drawback for use of dienogest is its cost.

The dienogest-estradiol (DNG-EE) combination pill is an emerging contraceptive. This has also shown an equal effect to that of GnRH analogues in relieving chronic pelvic pain in patients with endometriosis. Continuous administration of the DNG-EE pill led to significant improvement in pain. Overall progestogens can be used when oral contraceptives are not tolerated or are contraindicated and should be preferred in deep lesions.

Levonorgestrel-releasing intrauterine device (LNG-IUD) is a potent contraceptive steroid which releases LNG in the uterine cavity. Apart from endometrial atrophy, long-term use decreases expression of estrogenic receptors and cellular proliferation. A number of studies has proved the role of LNG-IUD in pain relief and reduction in the size of peritoneal and rectosigmoid endometriotic implants [31,32]. It was observed that LNG-IUD decreases the severity of the disease over a period of time and has the potential to provide long-term therapy in a number of patients [33,34]. Randomized trials found better pain relief with immediate treatment with LNG-IUD to that of expectant management of endometriosis. When the LNG group was compared with a GnRH analogue, equivalent efficacy was seen but better compliance and lesser hypoestrogenic symptoms in the former group [34,35]. There is a need for future studies to confirm the role of LNG-IUD in the postoperative period to reduce the recurrence of painful periods. To conclude, LNG-IUD seems to be a very good option for long-term treatment of endometriosis-associated pelvic pain in women not desiring conception; however, more literature is desired.

SELECTIVE PROGESTERONE RECEPTOR MODULATORS

Selective progesterone receptor modulators (SPRMs) are novel ligands with the potential of greater flexibility and efficacy to interact with progesterone receptors to block or modify downstream effects. They exhibit agonistic or mixed or antagonistic effects based on target tissue and presence of progesterone receptors. They induce atrophy of the endometrium by reversible suppression of blood vessels and prostaglandin production, with possible benefits on pain. Their potential benefit over other modalities in terms of maintaining hormonal milieu make them patient friendly. A number of SRPMs including, asoprisnil, mifepristone, ulipristal acetate, telapristone acetate, tanaproget, and lonaprisan have been studied on human cell lines. No drug-related serious events have been reported with their treatment.

Mifepristone (RU486): Its use, apart from medical abortions, is also studied in the management of pain associated with endometriosis. Small trials have shown that both mifepristone in a dose of 50 mg and onapristone demonstrated significant reduction in visible disease and clinical symptoms [36,37]. On the other hand, mifepristone 5 mg/day resulted in pain improvement but no regression of endometriotic implants [38]. They modulate the action of progesterone on eutopic and ectopic epithelium. Mifepristone subdermal implants are the alternative effective option for endometriosis [39]. More randomized trials are needed to confirm the utility of mifepristone in women with endometriosis.

A randomized controlled trial of asoprisnil demonstrated that all doses (i.e., 5, 10, and 25 mg/day) reduce pelvic pain in endometriosis, but the bleeding pattern is different [40]. The minimum effective dose for pain relief is 5 mg in women with proven endometriosis [41].

Ulipristal acetate is approved for treatment of fibroids in a few countries. It decrease cellular proliferation and has an anti-inflammatory effect [41–43]. Its role in endometriosis has yet to be determined. Also, safety concerns are still there as atypical proliferation at ectopic endometrial sites may increase the risk of ovarian endometroid cancers. Therefore, more data are needed for long-term outcome and overall safety.

GnRH analogues

Leuprolide, goserelin, nafarelin, triptorelin, and buserelin are various GnRH analogues found to be effective in endometriosis-associated pain [44]. They are still considered the gold standard treatment in women with endometriosis [45,46]. GnRH therapy may reduce pain and delay recurrence of symptoms in women with residual endometriosis [47]. Their prolonged use is limited by various side effects associated with a hypoestrogenic state: depression, loss of libido, hot flashes, genitourinary atrophy, and altered lipid profile. The long-term consequences of the hypoestrogenic state on calcium metabolism and bone are of concern. It is recommended to monitor bone density during the GnRH therapy. The addition of add-back therapy minimizes side effects; therefore, they can be given for up to 2 years [48]. The GnRH antagonists may appear superior to agonists because of immediate suppression of LH and follicle-stimulating hormone (FSH). A subcutaneous administration of cetrorelix has shown significant improvement in clinical symptoms and staging of disease [49]. A weekly dose of 3 mg given for 8 weeks has been found to induce regression of endometriotic implants. An oral GnRH antagonist, elagolix, demonstrated acceptable response in endometriosis-associated pain in a phase 2 randomized trial [50].

Aromatase inhibitors

Aromatase is a key enzyme regulating the conversion of c-19 steroids to estrogen. Its activity is expressed in testicular Leydig cells, granulosa cells, and the placental syncytiotrophoblasts. Targeting the aromatase activity seems to be a rational approach for treating endometriosis. It has been seen that endometriotic implants exhibit high aromatase activity due to inflammatory mediators as compared to that of uterine endometrium. Aromatase inhibitors by irreversible binding result in decreased estradiol production, thereby suppressing the growth of endometriotic implants [51]. Among various available aromatase inhibitors, anastrozole and letrozole have substantial advantages over other agents in terms of efficacy and tolerability.

Selective estrogen receptor modulators (SERMs)

SERMs are nonsteroidal anti-estrogens and can act as either agonists or antagonists depending on the target tissue [52]. SERMs are best known for their use in menopause and breast cancer. Raloxifene is a second-generation SERM that has been shown to have an antiestrogenic effect on endometrial tissue. There are emerging data indicating the use of this medication to treat endometriosis. Studies have demonstrated the efficacy of SERMs in the treatment of endometriosis in mice but, in humans, clinical studies are not yet known [53]. The reduction in size of the experimental endometriotic implants was similar to that of anastrazole [54,55].

Other drugs

Danazol is an orally administered isoxazole derivative of 17α-ethinyltestosterone. It eliminates mid-cycle luteinizing hormone (LH) surge, induces anovulation, modulates immunological function, and inhibits steroidogenesis. The recommended doses (400–800 mg/day) create substantial androgenic and hypoestrogenic environments that suppress the growth of endometriosis and are useful to relieve the pain of endometriosis. Many side effects such as weight gain, fluid retention, breast atrophy, hirsutism, hot flushes, and muscle cramps limit its clinical utility. Danazol has been associated with virilization of the female fetus if taken during pregnancy, adverse changes in lipid profile, and irreversible hoarseness of the voice. Liver functions should be monitored during treatment as it is metabolized largely in the liver, and in some patients may cause hepatocellular damage. The majority of the patients treated with danazol show recurrence within the first year after discontinuation of the drug. The success of danazol treatment is greatest in cases of peritoneal endometriosis or those with small lesions of the ovary.

Endometriomas larger than 1.0 cm are less likely to respond to danazol, although quite surprisingly, regression of endometriomas larger than 1.0 cm is sometimes seen. Danazol-loaded intra-uterine systems and vaginal rings are other routes of administration with fewer side effects [27,28]. Due to local administration, negligible serum levels are seen and the majority of the side effects are seldom observed. Danazol administered vaginally 200 mg/day for 12 months has found to relieve painful symptoms with similar efficacy to the oral route and with fewer side effects [29,30].

CRITICAL APPRAISAL OF CURRENT TREATMENT MODALITIES

Endometriosis, being a chronic disease, needs long-term therapy and the treatment choice is based on patient preference, age, conception desire, pain severity, and extent of disease. Medical therapy often employed as first line has shown promising results but is associated with the temporary relief of symptoms, and on discontinuation, recurrence is the rule. For instance, endometriosis-associated pain can continue after medical treatment or conservative surgery. After medical treatment or surgical treatment, the recurrence of endometriosis is estimated to be 21.5% at 2 years and 40%–50% at 5 years. After surgical treatment, the recurrence rate of clinically detectable endometriosis tends to be higher in older women with advanced stages of the disease and lower in women with infertility. In a 7-year follow-up study, the reoperation rate increased with increasing time since the initial surgery.

Nonsteroidal anti-inflammatory drugs, because of their anti-inflammatory and analgesic effects, have been widely used for pain relief in primary dysmenorrhea. Patient receiving naproxen and tolfenamic acid, compared with placebo, had significant pain relief in dysmenorrhea associated with mild to moderate endometriosis, but high-quality evidence favoring NSAIDs is lacking, and prolonged use of these drugs causes adverse events [56,57].

Combined oral contraceptives (COCs) and progestins administered through different routes (orally, depot injections, transdermal, implants, and LNG-IUS) are effective first-line modalities with better tolerability and efficacy. While COCs have been favored for decades in patients of endometriosis, there is emerging consensus for progesterone monotherapy [58]. In fact, the supra-physiological level of estrogen in COCs may lead to growth of endometriotic implants, thereby causing progression of disease [10]. The adherence to progestin treatment is likely to be more because the potential adverse events of abnormal bleeding usually decrease with continuous use and modification of dosage and schedule. They are better tolerated and have lower thrombotic risk compared with combined oral contraceptives. A pooled analysis on the use of DNG 2 mg/day found a much lower discontinuation rate due to abnormal bleeding [60]. Why 25%–35% women do not respond to first-line therapy is not very clear, but failed response has been linked to several molecular mechanisms and different estrogen and progesterone receptor subtypes [61].

The next line of therapy in the form of GnRH analogues has been found tobe effective when first-line treatment is contraindicated or unresponsive. Few studies evaluating dosage and schedule of GnRH analogues concluded the safety until 6 months, and beyond this period, GnRH should be complemented with add-back therapy with COCs or norethisterone acetate [62]. Recently, GnRH antagonists have come into play due to their property to maintain sufficient estrogen levels; therefore, there are fewer adverse effects. The effectiveness of elagolix has been proved in multicenter trials, but the most effective dosage remains unclear [59]. To date, no SERM has been found to be effective and safe for endometriosis-associated pain.

FUTURE DIRECTIONS

Current treatment for symptomatic endometriosis is based on patient preferences, efficacy treatment goals, the side effect profile, associated comorbidities, and the costs. A few related recent reports are noteworthy, and discoveries in tumorigenesis, neurogenesis neuroendocrinology, and genomics will greatly transform the current management approaches for endometriosis. Multidisciplinary approaches to the sensitized patient should also be considered, such as physiotherapy and cognitive treatment, although more clinical trials specifically in endometriosis are required. In addition, endometriosis has been associated with local neurogenesis, which in combination with central sensitization would further amplify pain signaling.

CONCLUSION

In conclusion, although current medical treatments are helpful for many women with endometriosis, these treatments have limitations that include side effects in some women and contraceptive action for women desiring to conceive. Emerging medical treatments range from GnRH antagonists, SPRM/SERM, aromatase inhibitors, immunomodulators, and antiangiogenic drugs. More research into local neurogenesis, central sensitization, and the genetics of endometriosis may provide future targets. Endometriosis has a highly variable phenotype, and thus a wide variety of medical treatments targeting different pathways is likely to be important to move toward precision health (personalized medicine) in endometriosis but also for optimizing novel hormonal agents to treat different disease phenotypes.

REFERENCES

1. Giudice LC, Kao L. Endometriosis. *Lancet* 2004;364:1789–99.
2. Ilangavan K, Kalu E. High prevalence of endometriosis in infertile women with normal ovulation and normospermic partners [letter]. *Fertil Steril* 2010;93:e10.
3. Guo SW, Wang Y. The prevalence of endometriosis in women with chronic pelvic pain. *Gynecol Obstet Invest* 2006;62:121–30.
4. Ferrero S, Barra F, Maggiore ULR. Current and emerging therapeutics for the management of endometriosis. *Drugs* 2018 Jul;78(10):995–1012.
5. Vercellini P, Buggio L, Frattaruolo MP, Borghi A, Dridi D, Somigliana E. Medical treatment of endometriosis-related pain. *Best Pract Res Clin Obstet Gynaecol* 2018;51:68–91.
6. Han SJ, O'Malley BW. The dynamics of nuclear receptors and nuclear receptor coregulators in the pathogenesis of endometriosis. *Hum Reprod Update* 2014;20(4):467–84.
7. Seracchioli R, Mabrouk M, Manuzzi L et al. Post-operative use of oral contraceptive pills for prevention of anatomical relapse or symptom-recurrence after conservative surgery for endometriosis. *Hum Reprod* 2009;24:2729–35.
8. Harada T, Kosaka S, Elliesen J, Yasuda M, Ito M, Momoeda M. Ethinylestrdiol 20 μg/drospirenone 3 mg in a flexible extended regiment for the management of endometriosis-associated

pelvic pan: A randomized, controlled trial. *Fertil Steril* 2017;108:798–805.

9. Henzl MR, Corson SL, Moghissi K, Buttram VC, Berqvist C, Jacobson J. Administration of nasal nafarelin as compared with oral danazol for endometriosis. *N Engl J Med* 1988;318:485–9.

10. Casper RF. Progestin-only pills may be a better first-line treatment for endometriosis than combined estrogen-progestin contraceptive pills. *Fertil Steril* 2017 Mar;107(3):533–6.

11. Muneyyirci-Delaleand O, Karacan M. Effect of norethindrone acetate in the treatment of symptomatic endometriosis. *Int J FertilWomens Med* 1998;43(1):24–7.

12. Vercellini P, Pietropaolo G, DeGiorgi O, Pasin R, Chiodini A, Crosignani PG. Treatment of symptomatic rectovaginal endometriosis with an estrogen–progestogen combination versus low-dose norethindrone acetate. *FertilSteril* 2005;84(5):1375–87.

13. Chwalisz K, Surrey E, Stanczyk FZ. The hormonal profile of norethindrone acetate: Rationale for add-back therapy with gonadotropin-releasing hormone agonists in women with endometriosis. *Reprod Sci.* 2012 Jun;19(6):563–71.

14. Ferrero S, Camerini G, Ragni N, Venturini PL, Biscaldi E, Remorgida V. Norethisterone acetate in the treatment of colorectal endometriosis: A pilot study. *Hum Reprod* 2010;25(1):94–100

15. Vercellini P, De Giorgi O, Oldani S, Cortesi I, Panazza S, Crosignani PG. Depot medroxyprogesterone acetate versus an oral contraceptive combined with very-low-dose danazol for long-term treatment of pelvic pain associated with endometriosis. *Am J ObstetGynecol* 1996;175:396–401.

16. Crosignani PG, Luciano A, Ray A, Bergqvist A. Subcutaneous depot medroxyprogesterone acetate versus leuprolide acetate in the treatment of endometriosis-associated pain. *Hum Reprod* 2006;21:248–56. Tosti C et al. *Eur J Obstet Gynecol Reprod Biol* 2017;209:61–66 65.

17. Schlaff WD, Carson SA, Luciano A, Ross D, Bergqvist A. Subcutaneous injection of depot medroxyprogesterone acetate compared with leuprolide acetate in the treatment of endometriosis-associated pain. *FertilSteril* 2006;85:314–25

18. Kohler G, Faustmann TA, Gerlinger C, Seitz C, Mueck AO. A dose-ranging study to determine the efficacy and safety of 1, 2, and 4 mg of dienogest daily for endometriosis. *Int J Gynaecol Obstet* 2010;108:21–5.

19. Momoeda M, Taketani Y, Terakawa N. A randomized double-blind, multicenter, parallel, dose-response study of dienogest in patients with endometriosis. *Jpn Pharmacol Ther* 2007;35:796–883. 17. Harada T, Taniguchi F. Dienogest: A new therapeutic agent for the treatment of endometriosis. *Womens Health (LondEngl)* 2010;6:27–35.

20. Strowitzki T, Faustmann T, Gerlinger C, Seitz C. Dienogest in the treatment of endometriosis-associated pelvic pain: A 12-week, randomized, double-blind, placebo-controlled study. *Eur J ObstetGynecolReprodBiol* 2010;151:193–8.

21. Harada T, Momoeda M, Taketani Y et al. Dienogest is as effective as intranasal buserelin acetate for the relief of pain symptoms associated with endometriosis-a randomized, double-blind, multicenter, controlled trial. *FertilSteril* 2009;91:675–81.

22. Strowitzki T, Marr J, Gerlinger C, Faustmann T, Seitz C. Dienogest is as effective as leuprolide acetate in treating the painful symptoms of endometriosis: A 24-week, randomized, multicentre, open-label trial. *Hum Reprod* 2010; 25:633–41

23. Luisi S, Parazzini F, Angioni S et al. Dienogest treatment improves quality of life in women with endometriosis. *J Endometr Pelvic Pain Dis* 2015.

24. Harada M, Osuga Y, Izumi G et al. Dienogest, a new conservative strategy for extragenital endometriosis: A pilot study. *Gynecol Endocrinol* 2011 Sep;27(9):717–20.

25. Angioni S, Nappi L, Pontis A et al. Dienogest. A possible conservative approach in bladder endometriosis. Results of a pilot study. *Gynecol Endocrinol* 2015;31(May (5)):406–8.

26. Cosson M, Querleu D, Donnez J et al. Dienogest is as effective as triptorelin in the treatment of endometriosis after laparoscopic surgery: Results of a prospective, multicenter, randomized study. *FertilSteril* 2002;77:684–92.

27. Igarashi M, Abe Y, Fukuda M et al. Novel conservative medical therapy for uterine adenomyosis with a danazol-loaded intrauterine device. *FertilSteril* 2000;74(October (4)):851.

28. Igarashi M, Iizuka M, Abe Y, Ibuki Y. Novel vaginal danazol ring therapy for pelvic endometriosis, in particular deeply infiltrating endometriosis. *Hum Reprod* 1998;13(July (7)):1952–6.

29. Cobellis L, Razzi S, Fava A, Severi FM, Igarashi M, Petraglia F. A danazol-loaded intrauterine device decreases dysmenorrhea, pelvic pain, and dyspareunia associated with endometriosis. *FertilSteril* 2004;82(July (1)):239–40.

30. Razzi S, Luisi S, Calonaci F, Altomare A, Bocchi C, Petraglia F. Efficacy of vaginal danazol treatment in women with recurrent deeply infiltrating endometriosis. *FertilSteril* 2007;88(October (4)):789–94.

31. Fedele L, Bianchi S, Zanconato G, Portuese A, Raffaelli R. Use of a levonorgestrel-releasing intrauterine device in the treatment of rectovaginal endometriosis. *FertilSteril* 2001;75:485–8.

32. Vercellini P, Aimi G, Panazza S, De Giorgi O, Pesole A, Crosignani PG. A levonorgestrel-releasing intrauterine system for the treatment of dysmenorrhea associated with endometriosis: A pilot study. *FertilSteril* 1999;72:505–8.

33. Lockhat FB, Emembolu JO, Konje JC. The evaluation of the effectiveness of an intra-uterine-administered progestogen (levonorgestrel) in the symptomatic treatment of endometriosis and in the staging of the disease. *Hum Reprod* 2004;19:179–84.

34. Petta CA, Ferriani RA, Abrao MS, Hassan D, Rosa E, Silva JC, Podgaec S, Bahamondes L. Randomized clinical trial of a levonorgestrel-releasing intrauterine system and a depot GnRH analogue for the treatment of chronic pelvic pain in women with endometriosis. *Hum Reprod* 2005;20:1993–8.

35. Abou-Setta AM, Al-Inany HG, Farquhar C. Levonorgestrel-releasing intrauterine device (LNG-IUD) for symptomatic endometriosis following surgery. *Cochrane Database of Systematic Reviews* 2006;(4):Art. No.: CD005072. doi: 10.1002/ 14651858.CD005072.pub2.

36. Kettel LM, Murphy AA, Morales AJ, Ulmann A, Baulieu EE, Yen SS. Treatment of endometriosis with the antiprogesterone mifepristone (RU486). *FertilSteril* 1996;65:23–8.

37. Kettel LM, Murphy AA, Morales AJ, Yen SS. Preliminary report on the treatment of endometriosis with low-dose mifepristone (RU 486). *Am J ObstetGynecol* 1998;178:1151–6.

38. Kettel LM, Murphy AA, Mortola JF et al. Preliminary report on the treatment of endometriosis with low-dose mifepristone (RU 486). *Am J ObstetGynecol* 1998;178:1151–6.

39. Mei L, Bao J, Tang L et al. A novel mifepristone-loaded implant for long-term treatment of endometriosis: In vitro and in vivo studies. *Eur J Pharm Sci* 2010;39:421–7.

40. Chwalisz K, Larsen L, McCrary K, Edmonds A. Effects of the novel selective progesterone receptor modulator (SPRM) asoprisnil on selected hormonal parameters in subjects with leiomyomata. *FertilSteril* 2004;82(Suppl. 2):S306.

41. Chwalisz K, Perez MC, Demanno D, Winkel C, Schubert G, Elger W. Selective progesterone receptor modulator development and use in the treatment of leiomyomata and endometriosis. *Endocr Rev* 2005;26:423–38.

42. Huniadi CA, Pop OL, Antal TA, Stamatian F. The effects of ulipristal on Bax/Bcl-2, cytochrome c, Ki-67 and cyclooxygenase-2 expression in a rat model with surgically induced endometriosis. *Eur J ObstetGynecolReprodBiol* 2013;169:360–5.

43. Bruner-Tran KL, Zhang Z, Eisenberg E, Winneker RC, Osteen KG. Downregulation of endometrial matrix metalloproteinase-3 and -7 expression in vitro and therapeutic regression of experimental endometriosis in vivo by a novel nonsteroidal progesterone receptor agonist, tanaproget. *J Clin Endocrinol Metab* 2006;91:1554–60,

44. Surrey ES. Gonadotropin-releasing hormone agonist and add-back therapy: What do the data show? *Curr Opin Obstet Gynecol* 2010;22:283–8.

45. Somigliana E, Vigano P, Barbara G, Vercellini P. Treatment of endometriosis-related pain: Options and outcomes. *Front Biosci* 2009;1:455–65.

46. Ferrero S, Alessandri F, Racca A, Leone Roberti Maggiore U. Treatment of pain associated with deep endometriosis: Alternatives and evidence. *FertilSteril* 2015;104(October (4)):771–92.

47. Angioni S, Pontis A, Dessole M, Surico D, De Cicco Nardone C, Melis I. Pain control and quality of life after laparoscopic en-block resection of deep infiltrating endometriosis (DIE) vs. incomplete surgical

treatment with or without GnRHa administration after surgery. *Arch Gynecol Obstet* 2015;291(February (2)):363–70.

48. Magon N. Gonadotropin releasing hormone agonists: Expanding vistas. *Indian J Endocrinol Metab* 2011;15:261–7.

49. Kupker W, Felberbaum RE, Krapp M, Schill T, Malik E, Diedrich K. Use of GnRH antagonists in the treatment of endometriosis. *Reprod Biomed Online* 2002;5:12–6.

50. Diamond MP, Carr B, Dmowski WP et al. Elagolix treatment for endometriosis-associated pain: Results from a phase 2, randomized, double-blind, placebo-controlled study. *Reprod Sci* 2014;21:363–71.

51. Zeitoun KM, Bulun SE. Aromatase: A key molecule in the pathophysiology of endometriosis and a therapeutic target. *Fertil Steril* 1999;72:961–9.

52. Vogelvang TE, van der Mooren MJ, Mijatovic V, Kenemans P. Emerging selective estrogen receptor modulators: Special focus on effects on coronary heart disease in postmenopausal women. *Drugs* 2006;66:191–221.

53. Harris HA, Bruner-Tran KL, Zhang X et al. A selective estrogen receptor-b agonists causes lesion regression in an experimentally induced model of endometriosis. *Hum Reprod* 2005;20:936–41.

54. Altintas D, Kokcu A, Kandemir B, Tosun M, Cetinkaya MB. Comparison of the effects of raloxifene and anastrozole on experimental endometriosis. *Eur J Obstet Gynecol Reprod Biol* 2010;150:84–7.

55. Yavuz E, Oktem M, Esinler I, Toru SA, Zeyneloglu HB. Genistein causes regression of endometriotic implants in the rat model. *Fertil Steril* 2007; 88:1129–34.

56. Brown J, Crawford TJ, Allen C et al. Nonsteroidal anti-inflammatory drugs for pain in women with endometriosis. *Cochrane Database Syst Rev* 2017 Jan 23;1.

57. Cobellis L, Razzi S, De Simone S et al. The treatment with a COX-2 specific inhibitor is effective in the management of pain related to endometriosis. *Eur J Obstet Gynecol Reprod Biol* 2004 Sep 10;116 (1):100–2.

58. Barra F, Scala C, Ferrero S. Current understanding on pharmacokinetics, clinical efficacy and safety of progestins for treating pain associated to endometriosis. *Expert Opin Drug Metab Toxicol* 2018 Apr;4. PubMed PMID: 29617576. DOI:10.1080/17425255.2018.1461840.

59. Hornstein MD. An oral GnRH antagonist for endometriosis – a new drug for an old disease. *N Engl J Med* 2017 Jul 6;377(1): 81–3.

60. Strowitzki T, Faustmann T, Gerlinger C et al. Safety and tolerability of dienogest in endometriosis: Pooled analysis from the European clinical study program. *Int J Women's Health* 2015;7:391–401

61. Patel BG, Rudnicki M, Yu J et al. Progesterone resistance in endometriosis: Origins, consequences and interventions. *Acta Obstet Gynecol Scand* 2017 Jun;96(6):623–32.

62. DiVasta AD, Laufer MR. The use of gonadotropin releasing hormone analogues in adolescent and young patients with endometriosis. *Curr Opin Obstet Gynecol* 2013 Aug;25 (4):287–92.

9

Surgical exploration as the primary modality of treatment

SUJATA SIWATCH AND INDU SAROHA

Endometriosis is characterized by the presence of tissue resembling endometrium in sites other than the uterine cavity. It affects 6%–10% of women in the reproductive age group [1]. Endometriosis presents in three different entities, which are usually found together—peritoneal lesions, deep endometriosis, and endometrioma [2]. It usually presents in reproductive aged women with pain or subfertility, though, rarely, it may be an incidental finding or may have extrapelvic disease presentation such as catamenial pneumothorax.

Management options include medical, expectant, and surgical options, which depend on symptoms; age; previous treatment; desire for fertility; availability, risks, and side effects of treatment options; and desires of the patient.

Though surgery has long been considered as the mainstay of management, the availability of new medical options for pain relief and artificial reproductive techniques has opened up newer alternatives that can be individualized. Though surgery aims at removing the endometrial tissue for histopathological confirmation and helps alleviate pain, the chances of recurrence, reduction of the ovarian reserve, especially in women with infertility, and the risks of surgery need careful consideration requiring good counseling and discussion with the patient.

SURGERY AS THE PRIMARY MODALITY

Surgery may be required as a primary modality when medical management fails or cannot be administered, or as an adjunct to medical management:

- For diagnosis of disease
- Laparoscopy with histologic examination is the gold standard for diagnosis of disease. It involves examination of the pelvis clockwise and counterclockwise so that no lesion is missed. Number, size, location of lesion, endometriotic cyst, and type of adhesions are noted
- In adolescents with severe, incapacitating pain symptoms and significant functional impairments [3]
- Severe and advanced disease with significant anatomic impairment [3]
- Contraindications to medical management
- Acute abdomen such as torsion or rupture of endometrioma
- Endometriosis leading to obstructive uropathy or bowel obstruction
- Ultrasonographic diagnosis of large ovarian mass with radiological suspicion of malignancy
- Bilateral or unilateral hydrosalpinx or large endometrioma >3 cm prior to assisted reproductive technology (ART) (after due discussion on chances of compromise of ovarian reserve and ovarian removal)
- Symptomatic women who have completed their families and not ready for follow-up [4]
- Denial for medical treatment

WHEN TO SHIFT FROM MEDICAL TO SURGICAL MANAGEMENT

- Symptoms do not improve with medical treatment (incomplete response with medical management)
- Intolerable side effects of medical therapy such as headaches, mood changes, and abnormal bleeding
- Noncompliance, patient not desirous of medical treatment
- Develops radiological signs suspicious of malignancy during the expectant/medical treatment
- Develops acute abdomen on medical management such as intestinal obstruction or obstructive uropathy
- Infection of endometriotic cyst fluid during oocyte retrieval
- Surgery planned before ART

- Pain associated with deeper endometriotic lesions
- Abnormal uterine bleeding associated with adenomyosis

COUNSELING AND CONSENT FOR SURGERY

The role of patient counseling cannot be over-emphasized. A careful discussion of the patient's symptomatology, prior treatment, medical and surgical comorbidities, desires of pregnancy, pathology of disease, progression, recurrence of the disease, and management options available, with their benefits and risks, should be clearly discussed and documented.

In women desiring fertility, risks associated with surgery, risk of laparoscopic procedure, reduction in ovarian reserve, risk of loss of ovary, reduction in future fertility, requirement of ART, and possibility of preoperative freezing of oocytes should be explained [4]. Women undergoing repeat surgery and with bilateral ovarian cysts should be especially involved in decision making for surgery. Sociocultural and religious considerations affect the desires and decisions of the patient and should be considered prior to definitive surgery. A frank discussion between care provider and patient should occur regarding the patients thoughts on ART options, especially in an infertile woman, and should be discussed prior to surgery.

In women who have completed their families, while preparing the patient for hysterectomy, consent explaining unimprovement of painful symptoms, recurrence, possibility of experiencing menopausal symptoms, and the need and effects of hormone replacement therapy (HRT) should be explained and due decision taken.

The risk of missing of all the disease sites, incomplete resection or relief, especially in women with deep endometriosis, risk of recurrence, and need for postoperative medical therapy should be explained to women undergoing surgery for pain. A total intraoperative and postoperative complication rate of 2.1% and 13.9%, respectively (4.6% major and 9.5% minor complications) have been reported, especially where bowel surgery is needed [5].

The risk of a missed occult malignancy is very low without any radiological features suggestive of malignancy. However, the risk of ovarian cancer in later life with lifetime increased probability of

1%–2%, in the presence of endometrioma, should also be explained for follow-up of cases on conservative management.

SURGERY FOR ACUTE PAIN

Endometriosis may be present in an emergency as a ruptured cyst in an unstable patient or as an interstinal obstruction or obstructive uropathy in cases of extragenital involvement or acute pelvic inflammatory disease (PID) with tubo-ovarian masses after infection of endometrioma after hysterosalpingography or oocyte retrieval. In that situation, the intraoperative findings should be carefully documented, the acute issue tackled as per the situation, and long-term planning for further medical or surgical treatment for the patient should be done.

SURGERY FOR CHRONIC PAIN

Pain in endometriosis may present as congestive dysmenorrhea, dyspareunia, and chronic pelvic pain. Other causes of pain like PID, cystitis, and irritable bowel syndrome need to be considered.

In a study published by Wullschleger et al., the authors compared the pre- and postoperative effects of health on quality of work life in women with endometriosis undergoing minimally invasive surgery. They concluded that negative effects of endometriosis are clearly reduced in women undergoing indicated surgery. Related absence from work, negative impact on work, loss in working performance is reduced. It also improves quality of life. Thus, timely diagnosis and subsequent treatment of the patient by the indicated suitable surgery may help to minimize suffering and to reduce economic costs at once [6].

Laparoscopy is usually preferable to laparotomy for endometriosis-associated pain. A "see and treat" approach is advocated, and operative laparoscopy, rather than diagnostic laparoscopy, should be done to help alleviate the patient's symptoms. Excision of the endometriotic tissue should be done to obtain tissue for confirming the histopathology. Excision and fulguration of endometriotic spots in mild to moderate endometriosis helps in reducing the pain symptom of the woman. Cystectomy and fulguration of the endometriotic tissue should be done for endometriomas of the ovary (Figure 9.1). If unilateral involvement, unilateral oophorectomy can be done in women who have completed their families.

In woman with severe pain and dyspareunia, a careful vaginal examination should be done to palpate for nodularity in the uterosacrals. Preoperatively, there is a growing focus on advanced imaging for diagnosing deep endometriosis prior to surgery. In the case of deep endometriosis, the surgery should be done in expert hands with the right equipment, time, and other assistance that may be required for the disease expected.

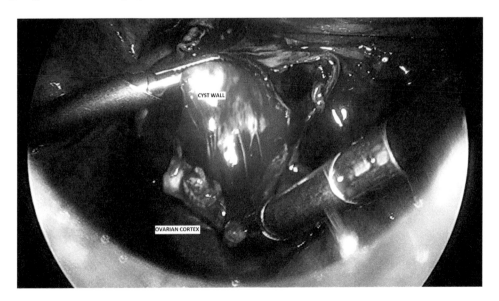

Figure 9.1 Laparoscopic endometrioma cystectomy.

In the case that endometriosis is discovered incidentally during surgery, concomitant with other pathologies, appropriate surgical excision should be done for biopsy or treatment, considering the risks and benefits of the procedure, known symptoms, and wishes of the patient, and consent taken for surgery.

Incidence of appendicular involvement in bowel endometriosis is up to 17%. Indication of appendectomy involves chronic right-sided pain in endometriosis. It may lead to complete relief in pain in up to 97% of patients [7].

ADENOMYOMECTOMY

Hysterectomy is definitive surgical treatment for adenomyosis with endometriosis. Focal adenomyosis can be managed by laparoscopic, hysteroscopic, or open adenomyomectomy. High-level surgical expertise is needed in doing conservative adenomyotic surgery to preserve fertility. Magnetic resonance guided focussed ultrasound (MRgFUS) and uterine artery embolization are other treatment modalities for adenomyosis [8].

HYSTERECTOMY WITH BILATERAL SALPINGO-OOPHORECTOMY

Definitive surgery should be considered in women who have completed their families and had failed to respond to conservative treatment. It should be explained to woman that it will not necessarily cure the symptoms or disease. If hysterectomy is indicated, excise all visible endometriotic lesions at the time of surgery.

LUNA AND PRESACRAL NEURECTOMY

Laparoscopic uterosacral nerve ablation (LUNA) is no longer recommended as an additional procedure to conservative surgery for reducing endometriosis-associated pain. However, presacral neurectomy is an effective additional procedure to conservative surgery to reduce endometriosis-associated midline pain [9]. It requires a high degree of skill and is a potentially hazardous procedure.

SCAR ENDOMETRIOSIS

Scar endometriosis is very rare disease. It has nonspecific symptoms such as pain and swelling at the scar site during menstruation. Incidence of scar endometriosis is 0.03%–0.1% [10]. It usually develops after cesarean section. Trucut biopsy aids in confirmation of diagnosis. Wide excision of the mass is the first-line management. If recurrence occurs, the clinician should maintain high suspicion of malignancy. For prevention of scar site endometriosis, decidua should be excluded while closing the uterus and using separate mops or needles while closing different layers.

SURGERY FOR SUSPECTED MALIGNANCY IN OVARIAN ENDOMETRIOMA

In a large epidemiological study, the frequency of ovarian cancer in a patient with endometriosis was 0.3%–0.8%, a risk that was two to three times higher than controls [11]. This information supports that clear cell ovarian and endometrioid ovarian carcinomas may arise from endometriosis. Other neoplasms such as seromucinous borderline, low-grade serous ovarian carcinomas [12], adenosarcomas, and endometrial stromal sarcomas may also arise from endometriosis [13].

Women undergoing expectant or medical treatment of endometriosis need to be followed, both clinically and radiologically. Raised levels of tumor markers and radiological findings of malignancy should be considered seriously. Elevated levels of CA-125 may not be the specific biomarker since it can be raised in the presence of various gynecologic pathologies, such as endometriosis, ovarian cancers, or inflammation [14]. In some cases, levels of HE4 as a serum biomarker can be used to distinguish endometriosis from ovarian and endometrial cancers [15].

In careful consideration with the patient, staging laparotomy and surgery need to be done.

SURGERY FOR WOMEN WITH INFERTILITY

Various factors in endometriosis have been proposed to contribute to infertility. Among others, the most accepted are an abnormal chronic inflammation and reduced ovarian reserve that affect ovulation and distorted anatomy due to adhesions that affect the tubo-ovarian relationship. Nevertheless, women with infertility and endometriosis should be evaluated for other causes of infertility, including a male factor, before planning any surgery for endometriosis.

In a Cochrane review published in 2014, Duffy et al. [40] propose that laparoscopic treatment of mild to moderate endometriosis improves ongoing pregnancy rates and live births. Nezhat et al. [41] and Vercellini et al. [42], in their large prospective cohort studies, showed that surgery in moderate to severe endometriosis increased the crude spontaneous pregnancy rates from 0% to 57%–69% and 33% to 52%–68% in moderate to severe endometriosis, respectively. However, others authors report that reproductive outcomes have not been shown to be improved by the excision of deeply infiltrating endometriosis.

BEFORE ART

Surgery before artificial reproductive techniques is controversial. Hamdan et al. [43], in their meta-analysis found that outcome of IVF/intracytoplasmic sperm injection (ICSI) did not differ in women who had surgical removal of endometrioma versus no surgery. Opoien et al. [44] reported a higher implantation rate, pregnancy rate, and live birth rate in women undergoing operative laparoscopy for minimal to mild endometriosis. Though some authors propose cystectomy for endometriomas more than 3 cm before ART, quoting easier access to oocyte removal, to reduce endometriosis-associated pain and to resolve any concern of malignancy, others caution as cystectomy leads to reduced ovarian reserve, as evidenced by reduction in anti-müllerian hormone (AMH) levels and subsequent responsiveness to gonadotropin stimulation, especially in cases of bilateral endometriomas and repeat surgeries. In recurrent endometriosis with infertility, cyst aspiration is recommended when the ovarian reserve is poor. The minimal risk of infection in the endometrioma (0%–1.9%) and contamination of follicular fluid with endometrioma contents (2.8%–6.1%) do not rationalize surgery for endometriomas before IVF treatment [16].

HYDROSALPINX REMOVAL

Endometriosis leads to disruption of anatomy and may lead to hydrosalpinx, which harbors inflammatory milieu, leading to decreased IVF success rate. Thus, multiple studies suggest removal of hydrosalpinges prior to IVF for improving outcomes. It may also help by improving accessibility for oocyte retrieval in ART [17].

MODE OF SURGERY

Various factors need to be taken into consideration while planning for surgery and choosing the mode of surgery, including age, symptoms (pain, infertility, abnormal uterine bleeding [AUB]), aim of treatment (elimination of pain, improving fertility, ruling out malignancy), previous surgeries, and existing comorbidities of the patient.

Laparoscopy

Laparoscopy is preferred, unless contraindicated. Laparoscopic surgery with histological examination is the gold standard for diagnosis and treatment simultaneously. Both laparoscopy and laparotomy are equally effective for management of endometriosis-associated pain, but laparoscopy has the advantage of less pain, shorter hospital stay, rapid recovery, and better cosmetic outcome. Laparoscopy has the advantage of magnification, especially of difficult to access spaces during surgery. However, it is a compromise on the tactile differentiation of various structures during surgery.

"See and treat policy" should be followed at laparoscopy [18]. Operative rather than diagnostic laparoscopy is more effective in increasing ongoing pregnancy rates, even in mild to moderate endometriosis [19]. Excision of the lesion is preferential as it may yield a sample for histology. Both ablation and excision of peritoneal endometriotic implants to reduce endometriosis-associated pain should be considered [20]. Laparoscopic surgery has a limitation in treatment of moderate to severe endometriosis because of obliteration of surgical planes, deeper implants, and dense adhesions which require expert surgical skills.

Menakaya et al. gave the ultrasonography-based endometriotic staging system (UBESS) [21] to assess the severity of pelvic endometriosis, based on the histological phenotypes of endometriosis, the anatomical locations of deep infiltrating endometriosis, and their sonographic markers of local invasiveness. This system has three stages correlating to three levels of incremental complexity of surgery required. This scale would help triage women to appropriate levels of surgical expertise for laparoscopic surgery.

Laparotomy

With the growing popularity of laparoscopy, laparotomy is rarely needed for the management of benign endometrioma, regardless of adhesions. However, the need for conversion to laparotomy, if required, should always be included in the consent for surgery in cases of dense and extensive adhesions that make delineation of anatomy difficult or in cases of suspected or actual inadvert injury in the case of surgery. Some authors, on the other hand, believe that if the procedure of endometrioma removal is too difficult, it is advised to stop the procedure after drainage of the endometrioma, take a biopsy, and to prescribe GnRH for 3 months and then to re-operate 3–6 months later and complete the surgery [22].

A two- or three-step procedure can be considered for managing large endometrioma: opening and closing after examining cyst cavity, taking a biopsy which is followed by GnRH administration for 3 months, and lastly completing surgery using laparoscopic cystectomy or ablation methods [23].

Robotic surgery

Traditional laparoscopy has gained popularity for the management of this disease but has limitations in the surgical treatment of the most difficult cases of endometriosis.

As both experience and technology expand, it has been suggested that the robotic surgery platform enables more complex dissections and may be the ideal modality of the surgical management of deeply infiltrating endometriosis [24].

SURGICAL TECHNIQUES

Both adhesiolysis with excision and ablation of lesions have a role in the surgical management of endometriosis. Excision also provides tissue for histopathology. Cystectomy scores better than drainage and coagulation for endometriosis-associated pain [25]. Cystectomy is preferred over CO_2 laser vaporization in women with endometriomas as it has a lower recurrence rate. Both ablation and excision of peritoneal endometriosis is beneficial in reducing endometriosis-associated pain [26].

In stage I/II endometriosis, CO_2 laser vaporization is associated with a higher cumulative spontaneous pregnancy rate than electrocoagulation with monopolar cautery [27].

During ablation, the entire inner surface of the cyst wall is ablated using a laser beam at power settings of 30–35 W for the CO_2 laser beam and 6–10 W for the CO_2 fiber. The aim is to vaporize the endometriotic cyst lining until hemosiderin pigment stained tissue is no longer visible and there is change of color of implants from red to yellowish white [28]. It should be set on ablation mode to widen the beam. Endometriotic tissue is present only superficially, so the entire depth of the tissue doesn't need to be coagulated.

Plasma energy ablation can also be done with the coagulation mode set at 10–40 W, at a distance about 5 mm from the tip of the hand piece. Apply plasma at an angle perpendicular to the cyst wall. Electrocoagulation using monopolar or bipolar energy sources can be used to ablate endometriotic lesions. However, when using electrocoagulation, the ovary should be cooled frequently with irrigation fluid as tissue damage is deeper [29].

Electrocoagulation using different techniques and electrodes leads to different voltage levels. Tissue damage with electrocoagulation techniques is usually deeper than with laser or plasma energy. The impact of energy on superficial tissue may be visible due to change of color; however, damage to deeper tissue is difficult to assess. Uncontrolled use can lead to damage to primordial follicles and destruction of structure and function of healthy ovarian tissue.

- *Bipolar forceps*—Used commonly at a setting of 25–40 W. Its penetration into the tissue can be up to the depth of 10–12 mm. It should be used for short coagulation time to minimize damage to ovarian tissue.
- *Monopolar energy*—Generally used at a power setting of 15–20 W in areas of fibrotic endometriotic tissue at the hilum.
- *Argon beam coagulation*—Effect on tissue is similar to monopolar coagulation, but it has benefit of using it over the wider superficial areas.

CYSTECTOMY

Cystectomy should be preferred over drainage and coagulation in reducing pain associated with endometriosis as it has lower recurrence rates as compared to CO_2 vaporization [28] and in improving the postoperative spontaneous pregnancy rates. Several European Society of Human Reproduction and Embryology (EHSRE) studies have evaluated the usefulness of cystectomy prior to ART in women with endometriosis. Based on no difference in pregnancy rate, some advise cystectomy while others advise caution with cystectomy because of harmful effects on ovarian reserve as a result of stripping of the cyst wall carrying healthy ovarian tissue.

Anatomical consideration—Ovaries and endometriotic cysts are usually adherent to pelvic side walls and ovarian fossa where the ureter might be involved. Blood supply of the ovary is from the ovarian artery and ascending branch of the uterine artery in the ovarian ligament. Thus, large intra-ovarian vessels are found on anterolateral aspect of the ovary at the hilum near the insertion of the meso-ovarium.

Extent of disease and baseline ovarian reserve should be evaluated for prognostication in infertile women using bimanual examination, radiological imaging modalities, antral follicle count (AFC), and anti-Müllerian hormone levels.

Method of cystectomy [30]

- Three-port laparoscopic surgery is preferred.
- Inspect pelvic organs, upper abdomen, and appendix.
- In case of suspicion of malignancy, peritoneal washings and biopsy from the suspected area should be taken before mobilizing ovary.
- Separate ovary and endometriotic cyst from pelvic side wall.
- Visualize course of ureter.
- If the cyst ruptures during separation, extend the opening in the cyst wall to expose cyst cavity. Any suspicious area should be biopsied. Turn cyst inside out to facilitate further removal of cyst wall and achieve hemostasis.
- Multiple incisions should be avoided over cyst.
- When ovary is nonadherent, incision should be made on thinnest part of endometrioma on antimesenteric border.
- Vasopressin and saline injections in cyst capsule can be done to reduce blood loss during cystectomy.
- If cleavage plane is not identified, send cyst wall for histology, and use ablation method, rather than stripping of ovarian stroma.
- Careful dissection plane and precise spot bipolar coagulation is the key to achieve hemostasis.
- After removal of large cyst, reconstruction of ovary may be needed using monofilament suture.

- Cyst wall is retrieved through laparoscopy ports and rarely through posterior colpotomy.
- Ovarian suspension and anti-adhesive measures should be used to prevent postoperative adhesion formation.
- Irrigation, aspiration, and removal of blood clots are done to check hemostasis.

ADHESION PREVENTION

Using regenerated cellulose during operative laparoscopy for endometriosis helps in adhesion prevention [31]. Icodexrin (4%) derivative of maltodextrin, which is a colloid osmotic agent, can be used for peritoneal lavage during laparoscopy/laparotomy. It remains in the peritoneal cavity for 4 days and helps in prevention of adhesion formation by hydrofloatation of peritoneal organs, thus keeping them apart during the probable time of adhesion formation in the postoperative period [32]. Other agents like polytetrafluoroethylene (PTFE) surgical membrane and hyaluronic acid supresses the engraftment of inoculated endometrial fragments by preventing the interaction of CD44 positive endometrial cells with peritoneum thus preventing the further endometriotic implant formation [33].

HOW MUCH RESECTION IS NOT TOO MUCH?

If fertility is desired [34]

- Offer excision/ablation and adhesiolysis to women with endometriosis not involving bowel, bladder, and ureter to increase the pregnancy rates.
- Offer laparoscopic cystectomy to women with endometrioma.
- Do not offer hormonal treatment to women with endometriosis who want to conceive.
- Cystectomy is associated with reduced ovarian reserve, and the same should be discussed with the patient before surgery, especially in cases of bilateral endometriomas and recurrent surgeries.

If fertility is not desired [34]

- Consider excision rather than ablation of endometriosis lesions.

- For deeper endometriosis involving bladder, bowel, and ureter, consider doing MRI and a 3-month course of GnRH before operative laparoscopy [34].
- Consider outpatient department (OPD) follow-up if deep infiltrating endometriosis or one or more endometrioma >3 cm.
- If hysterectomy is indicated, excise all visible endometriotic lesions with hysterectomy.

ROLE OF PREOPERATIVE/ POSTOPERATIVE MEDICAL MANAGEMENT

Preoperative hormonal therapy does not improve the surgical outcome in women undergoing surgery for pain nor to improve spontaneous pregnancy rates [35]. Likewise, postoperative hormonal therapy in the first 6 months does not improve the surgical outcome of pain relief. Postoperative additional hormonal therapy does not improve spontaneous pregnancy rates and should not be given.

Nonetheless, hormonal therapy prescribed after surgery is helpful for contraception or secondary prevention. Secondary prevention is described as interventions aimed to prevent the recurrence of endometriosis and associated symptoms such as pain, more than 6 months after surgery [36]. LNG-IUS or combined hormonal contraceptives can be used for secondary prevention of endometriosis-associated dysmenorrhea, though not for dyspareunia and nonmenstrual pelvic pain. Contraceptives are also recommended for secondary prevention of endometriomas [37].

In women undergoing surgical menopause for endometriosis, combined estrogen/progesterone therapy or tibolone may be given until the age of natural menopause [38]. However, the risk of reactivation of disease or malignant transformation of the same and the side effects of hormone replacement therapy should be considered and discussed with the patient [39].

REFERENCES

1. Giudice LC. Clinical practice. Endometriosis. *N Engl J Med* 2010;362:2389–2398.
2. Nisolle M, Donnez J. Peritoneal endometriosis, ovarian endometriosis, and adenomyotic nodules of the rectovaginal septum are three different entities. *Fertil Steril* 1997;68:585–596.
3. Bedaiwy MA, Barker NM. Evidence based surgical management of endometriosis. *Middle East Fertil Soc J.* 2012;17:57–60.
4. Somigliana E, Vigano P, Filippi F, Papaleo E, Benaglia L, Candiani M, Vercellini P. Fertility preservation in women with endometriosis: For all, for some, for none? *Hum Reprod* 2015;30:1280–1286.
5. Kondo, W, Bourdel N, Tamburro S, Cavoli D, Jardon K, Rabischong B, Botchorishvili R, Pouly J, Mage G, Canis M. Complications after surgery for deeply infiltrating pelvic endometriosis. *BJOG* 2011;118:292–298.
6. Wullschleger MF, Imboden S, Wanner J, Mueller, MD. Minimally invasive surgery when treating endometriosis has a positive effect on health and on quality of work life of affected women. *Hum Reprod* 2015;30(3):553–557.
7. AlSalilli M, Vilos GA. Prospective evaluation of laparoscopic appendectomy in women with chronic right lower quadrant pain. *J Am Assoc Gynecol Laparosc* 1995;2:139–142.
8. Taran FA, Stewart EA, Brucker S. Adenomyosis: Epidemiology, risk factors, clinical phenotype and surgical and interventional alternatives to hysterectomy. *Geburtshilfe Frauenheilkd* 2013 Sep;73(9):924–931.
9. Proctor ML, Latthe PM, Farquhar CM, Khan KS, Johnson NP. Surgical interruption of pelvic nerve pathways for primary and secondary dysmenorrhoea. *Cochrane Database Syst Rev.* 2005 Oct 19;(4):CD001896.
10. Wolf GC, Singh KB. Cesarean scar endometriosis: A review. *Obstet Gynecol Surv* 1989 Feb;44(2):89–95.
11. Wei JJ, William J, Bulun S. Endometriosis and ovarian cancer: A review of clinical, pathologic, and molecular aspects. *Int J Gynecol Pathol* 2011;30(6):553–568. doi: 10.1097/ PGP.0b013e31821f4b85. [PMC free article] [PubMed] [CrossRef] [Google Scholar]
12. Pearce CL, Templeman C, Rossing MA et al. Association between endometriosis and risk of histological subtypes of ovarian cancer: A pooled analysis of case-control studies. *Lancet Oncol* 2012;13(4):385–394. doi: 10.1016/S1470-2045(11)70404-1. [PMC free article] [PubMed] [CrossRef] [Google Scholar]
13. Masand RP, Euscher ED, Deavers MT et al. Endometrioid stromal sarcoma: A clinicopathologic study of 63 cases. *Am J Surg*

Pathol 2013;37(11):1635–1647. doi: 10.1097/PAS.0000000000000083. [PubMed] [CrossRef] [Google Scholar]

14. Moss EL, Hollingworth J, Reynolds TM. The role of CA125 in clinical practice. *J Clin Pathol* 2005;58(3):308–312. doi: 10.1136/jcp.2004.018077. [PMC free article] [PubMed] [CrossRef] [Google Scholar]

15. Huhtinen K, Suvitie P, Hiissa J et al. Serum HE4 concentration differentiates malignant ovarian tumours from ovarian endometriotic cysts. *Br J Cancer* 2009;100(8):1315–1319. doi: 10.1038/sj.bjc.6605011. [PMC free article] [PubMed] [CrossRef] [Google Scholar]

16. Jayaprakasan K, Becker C, Mittal M on behalf of the Royal College of Obstetricians and Gynaecologists. The effect of surgery for endometriomas on fertility. Scientific Impact Paper No. 55. *BJOG* 2017;125:e19–e28.

17. Johnson N, van Voorst S, Sowter MC, Strandell A, Mol BW. Surgical treatment for tubal disease in women due to undergo *in vitro* fertilisation. *Co-Chrane Database Syst Rev* 2010 Jan 20;(1):CD002125.

18. Jacobson TZ, Duffy JM, Barlow D, Koninckx PR, Garry R. Laparoscopic surgery for pelvic pain associated with endometriosis. *Cochrane Database Syst Rev* 2009 Oct 7;(4):CD001300.

19. Jacobson TZ, Duffy JM, Barlow D, Farquhar C, Koninckx PR, Olive D. Laparoscopic surgery for subfertility associated with endometriosis. *Cochrane Database Syst Rev* 2010 Jan 20;(1):CD001398.

20. Healey M, Ang WC, Cheng C. Surgical treatment of endometriosis: A prospective randomized double-blinded trial comparing excision and ablation. *FertilSteril* 2010;94:2536–2540.

21. Menakaya U, Reid S, Lu C, Gerges B, Infante F, Condous G. Performance of ultrasound-based endometriosis staging system (UBESS) for predicting level of complexity of laparoscopic surgery for endometriosis. *Ultrasound Obstet Gynecol* 2016 Dec;48(6):786–795. doi: 10.1002/uog.15858

22. Johnson NP, Hummelshoj L, World Endometriosis Society Montpellier C. Consensus on current management of endometriosis. *Hum Reprod* 2013;28:1552–1568.

23. Donnez J, Nisolle M, Gillet N, Smets M, Bassil S, Casanas-Roux F. Large ovarian endometriomas. *Hum Reprod* 1996;11:641–646.

24. Zanotti KM, Abdelbadee AY. Robotic management of Endometriosis: Where do we stand? *Minerva Gynecol* 2015;67(3):257–272.

25. Hart RJ, Hickey M, Maouris P, Buckett W. Excisional surgery versus ablative surgery for ovarian endometriomata. *Cochrane Database Syst Rev* 2008 Apr 16;(2):CD004992.

26. Wright J, Lotfallah H, Jones K, Lovell D. A randomized trial of excision versus ablation for mild endometriosis. *FertilSteril* 2005;83:1830–1836.

27. Chang FH, Chou HH, Soong YK, Chang MY, Lee CL, Lai YM. Efficacy of isotopic 13CO$_2$ laser laparoscopic evaporation in the treatment of infertile patients with minimal and mild endometriosis: A life table cumulative pregnancy rates study. *J Am Assoc Gynecol Laparosc* 1997;4:219–223.

28. Carmona F, Martinez-Zamora MA, Rabanal A, Martinez-Roman S, Balasch J. Ovarian cystectomy versus laser vaporization in the treatment of ovarian endometriomas: A randomized clinical trial with a five-year follow-up. *Fertil Steril* 2011;96:251–254.

29. Roman H, Auber M, Bourdel N, Martin C, Marpeau L, Puscasiu L. Postoperative recurrence and fertility after endometrioma ablation using plasma energy: Retrospective assessment of a 3-year experience. *J Minim Invasive Gynecol* 2013;20:573–582.

30. Working group of ESGE, ESHRE and WES. Recommendations for the surgical treatment of endometriosis. Part 1: Ovarian endometrioma. *Hum Reprod Open* 2017;2017(4):hox016. doi:10.1093/hropen/hox016

31. Ahmad G, Duffy JM, Farquhar C, Vail A, Vandekerckhove P, Watson A, Wiseman D. Barrier agents for adhesion prevention after gynaecological surgery. *Cochrane Database Syst Rev* 2008 Apr 16;(2):CD000475.

32. Trew G, Pistofidis G, Pados G et al. Gynaecological endoscopic evaluation of 4% icodextrin solution: A European, multicentre, double-blind, randomized study of the efficacy and safety in the reduction of *de novo* adhesions after laparoscopic gynaecological surgery. *Hum Reprod* 2011;26:2015–2027.

33. Hoo WL, Stavroulis A, Pateman K, Saridogan E, Cutner A, Pandis G, Tong EN, Jurkovic D. Does ovarian suspension following laparoscopic surgery for endometriosis reduce postoperative adhesions? An RCT. *Hum Reprod* 2014;29:670–676.

34. NICE National institute for health and care excellence. Endometriosis: Diagnosis and management. nice.org.uk/guidance/ng73. 2017

35. Dunselman GA, Vermeulen N, Becker C et al. ESHRE guideline: Management of women with endometriosis. *Hum Reprod* 2014;29:400–441.

36. Yap C, Furness S, Farquhar C. Pre and postoperative medical therapy for endometriosis surgery. *Cochrane Database Syst Rev* 2004;(3):CD003678.

37. Vercellini P, Somigliana E, Vigano P, De Matteis S, Barbara G, Fedele L. Postoperative endometriosis recurrence: A plea for prevention based on pathogenetic, epidemiological and clinical evidence. *Reprod Biomed Online* 2010b;21:259–265.

38. Seracchioli R, Mabrouk M, Manuzzi L, Vicenzi C, Frasca C, Elmakky A, Venturoli S. Post-operative use of oral contraceptive pills for prevention of anatomical relapse or symptom-recurrence after conservative surgery for endometriosis. *Hum Reprod* 2009;24:2729–2735.

39. Al Kadri H, Hassan S, Al-Fozan HM, Hajeer A. Hormone therapy for endometriosis and surgical menopause. *Cochrane Database Syst Rev* 2009 Jan 21;(1):CD005997.

40. Duffy JM, Arambage K, Correa FJ, Olive D, Farquhar C, Garry R, Barlow DH, Jacobson TZ. Laparoscopic surgery for endometriosis. *Cochrane Database Syst Rev.* 2014 Apr 3;(4):CD011031.

41. Nezhat C, Crowgey S, Nezhat F. Videolaseroscopy for the treatment of endometriosis associated with infertility. *Fertil Steril.* 1989 Feb;51(2):237–240.

42. Vercellin P, Somigliana E, Daguati R, Barbara G, Abbiati A, Fedele L. The second time around: Reproductive performance after repetitive versus primary surgery for endometriosis. *Fertil Steril.* 2009 Oct;92(4):1253–1255.

43. Hamdan M, Dunselman G, Li TC, Cheong Y. The impact of endometrioma on IVF/ICSI outcomes: A systematic review and meta-analysis. *Hum Reprod Update.* 2015 Nov–Dec;21(6):809–825.

44. Opøien HK, Fedorcsak P, Byholm T, Tanbo T. Complete surgical removal of minimal and mild endometriosis improves outcome of subsequent IVF/ICSI treatment. *Reprod Biomed Online.* 2011 Sep;23(3):389–395.

10

Management of deep infiltrative endometriosis (DIE) causing gynecological morbidity: A urologist's perspective

ADITYA PRAKASH SHARMA AND GIRDHAR SINGH BORA

INTRODUCTION AND EPIDEMIOLOGY

Endometriosis has been classically classified as follows: ovarian endometriosis, superficial peritoneal endometriosis, and deep infiltrating endometriosis (DIE). DIE is one of the most severe forms of endometriosis and the prevalence of DIE is about 1% among females in the reproductive age group [1]. DIE is defined as endometriosis infiltration of more than 5 mm beneath the peritoneum. The common locations of DIE include the following: uterine body, posterior fornix, vagina, rectum, and urinary tract. The presence of endometrium (glandular and stromal components) in or around the urethra, bladder, ureters, or kidney entails the urinary tract involvement by DIE. Urinary tract endometriosis (UTE) per se is rare, with an incidence of 1%–5.5% in patients with endometriosis [1–4]. However, the prevalence of UTE in DIE ranges from 19% to 53% [3–6]. Involvement of the bladder is the most common form of UTE, occurring in 70%–85% of cases, followed by ureteral involvement in 9%–23% of UTE cases with DIE [6]. The age group commonly affected is the fourth decade [6,7]. Abeshouse and Abeshouse, in their review of 147 patients with UTE, noted involvement of the bladder, ureter, kidney, and urethra to be 85%, 10%, 4%, and 2%, respectively [8].

ETIOPATHOGENESIS

The pathophysiology of endometriosis pertaining to urinary tract involvement remains unclear. Various theories have been proposed to explain the endometrial "tissue transport" outside the uterus and involvement of the urinary tract [4,9–11]. These include direct extension (transplantation theory) outside the uterine wall, hematogenous or lymphatic spread, retrograde menstruation through the fallopian tube (migratory or metastatic theory), metaplasia of the Wolffian and

Müllerian remnants (embryonal theory), and iatrogenic mechanisms (after cesarean section).

The anterior cul-de-sac is the most common site of implantation and hence responsible for bladder involvement in the majority of cases. After implantation, the inflammatory process causes adhesions to develop between the adjacent contiguous organs and forms a fibrotic nodule underneath the peritoneum. The metaplasia theory, although questioned, is supported by reports of 11 cases of male endometriosis [6]. Four of them were reported to develop endometriosis of the bladder concomitant with high estrogen exposure for the treatment of prostate cancer [12–15].

Some evidence also suggests that the prevalence of endometriosis is higher than usual in patients' undergoing pelvic surgeries, providing support to the theory of direct extension [4,16]. Immunological reaction has also been postulated in the etiology of endometriosis [10]. With a number of theories available, it may still be possible that more than one process leads to development of UTE in a single patient.

HISTORY AND EXAMINATION

Bladder endometriosis

The most prevalent symptoms of DIE include dysmenorrhea, dyspareunia, and pelvic pain [17–19]. Lower urinary tract symptoms (LUTS) have been variably reported, ranging from 2% to 77% [20–22]. Panel et al. found no difference in the rate of LUTS (urgency, frequency, and pain in bladder) between patients with posterior endometriosis with or without bladder endometriosis (BE) [22]. Symptoms specific to BE include dysuria, frequency, bladder pain, hematuria, urgency, and urinary incontinence [3,4,23,24]. Dysuria is found in 21%–69% of patients with BE [3,4,24]. The severity of dysuria depends upon the size of the lesion [38]. Bladder lesions rarely infiltrate the mucosa, and thus, cyclical hematuria, although classical, is found less commonly, ranging from 0% to 35% in various series [3,4].

Due to common symptomatology, BE mimics other common urological conditions such as bacterial cystitis, tubercular cystitis, overactive bladder, carcinoma bladder, and interstitial cystitis/bladder pain syndrome. Studies have shown a coexistence (16%–78%) of bladder endometriosis and interstitial

cystitis, given the term "evil twin syndrome" by Chung et al. [25,26]. Physical examination including a vaginal examination is the first step in making the diagnosis of DIE and BE [6,7]. Physical findings include a palpable nodule, a thickening along the anterior vaginal wall with tender points [6–8]. In women in the reproductive age group complaining of LUTS, particularly in combination with pain and positive findings on vaginal examination, endometriosis should be strongly suspected and further investigations should be done.

Ureteric endometriosis

Ureteral endometriosis (UE) differs from BE in being oligosymptomatic [27]. Ureteral endometriosis can present with the symptoms associated with classical gynecological endometriosis or urological symptoms related directly to the presence of endometrial tissue in and around the ureter. There are two major pathological types of ureteral endometriosis—extrinsic and intrinsic. Extrinsic endometriosis is the commoner form (80%) and has endometrial tissue within the submucosa and adventitia of the ureter [27–29]. In contrast, intrinsic endometriosis (20%) involves the urothelium and submucosa [30]. Both types of ureteral endometriosis may be present simultaneously or may be independent of each other.

Ureteral involvement should be suspected in patients with gynecological endometriosis. The incidence of hematuria in patients with ureteral endometriosis is 15% [27]. The ectopic endometrial tissue is hormone responsive and its sloughing may occur in the ureter, giving rise to microscopic or gross hematuria. As a consequence, a cyclical hematuria may arise in the intrinsic form of ureteral endometriosis [31]. UE may present with uremic symptoms in bilateral ureteric obstruction, with hypertension in unilateral ureteral obstruction, anuria in a solitary kidney with obstruction, and cyclical ureteral obstruction [27,32–33]. Isolated reports of endometriosis mimicking sigmoid carcinoma associated with ureteral obstruction and hypertension and isolated totally painless gross hematuria without accompanying pelvic symptoms have been described [34].

A proposed classification of ureteral endometriosis was provided by Knabben et al. [4] and is provided as follows:

Grade	Description
0	Peritoneal endometriosis overlying the ureter
1	Retroperitoneal endometriosis with entanglement of the ureter but no dilatation
2	Dilatation of the ureter and/or hydronephrosis without functional impairment (urodynamic no relevant obstruction)
3	Urodynamically relevant obstruction with symmetrical renal split clearance in renal furosemide scintigraphy and normal total clearance
4	Urodynamically relevant obstruction with impaired split clearance in renal furosemide scintigraphy or impaired total clearance
5	Silent kidney

Renal endometriosis

Renal endometriosis is extremely rare and has been described in case reports [35,36]. It may present with abdominal pain due to periodic bleeding giving rise to hemorrhagic cysts or invasion of the renal capsule [35]. Gross hematuria with clot colic may arise when the lesions break into the renal pelvicalyceal system and cause ureteral obstructions [27]. Rarely, renal endometriosis can result in asymptomatic kidney dysfunction if a large endometriotic lesion involves directly the renal pelvis, resulting in hydronephrosis [35]. Anecdotal reports of incidentally detected asymptomatic renal endometriosis have been published while investigating patients for some other disease. The lesions in this case involved only the renal cortex with no involvement of the pelvicalyceal system.

Urethral endometriosis

Cabral Ribeiro et al. described a case of a 32-year-old nulliparous woman who presented with a painful suburethral mass causing symptoms of obstruction during voiding [37]. A couple of cases have been described with endometriosis in the urethral diverticulum as well [38,39].

EVALUATION

Questionnaires

Questionnaires used for evaluation of lower urinary tract symptoms (LUTS) in males for benign enlargement of prostate, such as the American Urological Association Symptom Index (AUASI) and the International Prostate Symptom Score (IPPS), have been evaluated for describing LUTS in women [40]. Fedele et al. [41] modified the AUASI/IPSS by replacing three questions concerning obstructive symptoms with three other questions for irritative symptoms and found this modified questionnaire useful in evaluating symptoms specifically related to BE in patients with high suspicion for this disease. The questionnaire was effective in identifying BE with an area under the curve of 0.95 [41].

Ballester et al. found IPSS and the Bristol Female LUTS (BFLUTS) useful in patients with DIE to identify the degree of urinary dysfunction before and after surgery [21,42]. The BFLUTS questionnaire has three domains: symptom questions, sexual function questions, and quality-of-life questions. The use of these validated questionnaires may be found to be useful in managing BE patients. Maggiore et al., in their systematic review, stated that the modified AUASI questionnaire by Fedele et al. can be utilized during the diagnostic workup to improve the detection of BE [6,41]. These questionnaires are useful in primary evaluation as well as in monitoring changes in symptom complex after treatment. However, the administration and answering of these questionnaires are time consuming and cumbersome in routine clinical practice, thus limiting their use as a research tool only.

Hematological investigations

All patients should be assessed for anemia, which may arise because of hematuria. Renal function tests should be performed as mentioned above, as there may be a silent loss of renal function [7].

Urinalysis

The urine routine microscopy should be ordered to look for microscopic hematuria and cultured to rule out an infectious etiology for LUTS [7]. Urine cytology may be performed if high-grade urothelial carcinoma is a differential [7].

IMAGING

Ultrasonography

Ultrasonography (USG) is the first modality used in evaluation of BE. USG characterizes the location of endometriotic nodules, determines the size of nodules, can estimate the distance between the lesion and ureteric orifice, and can also be used to differentiate these nodules from a malignant lesion (Figure 10.1a) [44]. BE is seen as a filling defect located most commonly on the posterior

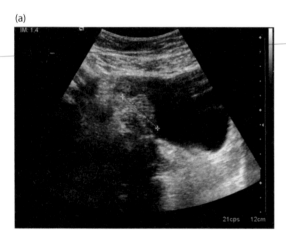

(a)

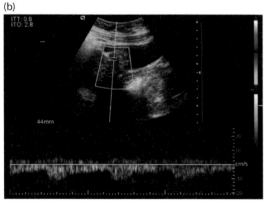

(b)

Figure 10.1 (a) Sagittal transabdominal ultrasound image of the endometriotic mass located at the right posterolateral bladder wall. (b) Power Doppler imaging reveals the presence of a large amount of blood vessels inside the lesion. (From Barrabino R et al. *J Surg Open Access* 2016;2(2): http://dx.doi.org/10.16966/2470-0991.114.)

wall and protruding into the lumen in a full bladder. The nodules vary in shape. They may appear regular with a spherical or comma-shaped outline or they may be irregular, raising a suspicion of malignancy. The lesions are iso/hypoechoic and lack a vascular core much more consistent with a vascular tumor. However, a major distinguishing feature remains the location of BE nodules, which are usually submucosal in contrast to the mucosal lesions in malignancy of the urinary bladder. The malignant lesions on the other hand will show papillary projections causing an interruption in the layers of the bladder wall. Color or power Doppler shows internal blood flow which is minimal compared with a malignant lesion in patients with BE (Figure 10.1b) [44].

Studies have shown transvaginal sonography (TVS) to be the most accurate modality for defining the size of the lesions, infiltration of the detrusor muscle, and continuity with extravesical lesions (Figure 10.2) [45]. Both transabdominal USG and TVS may be used to detect BE. As gynecologists are much more familiar with TVS, it remains the preferred technique in clinical practice.

A recent systematic review and meta-analysis revealed overall pooled sensitivity of 62% (95% CI, 40%–80%) and specificity of 100% (95% CI, 97%–100%) for TVS detection of BE. The study establishes TVS as a useful first-line method for diagnosing BE in clinical practice. Studies evaluating the operator dependency of USG have demonstrated [46] high reproducibility, good accuracy and specificity, and fair sensitivity for detection of DIE and BE [46]. A three-dimensional (3D) TVS with color Doppler is an improvement in the TVS modality. The 3D TVS was found to be as effective as MRI and superior to scopy in diagnosing and surgical planning for BE.

Intravenous pyelography

Intravenous pyelography (IVP) is one of the most commonly used tests for assessing the intrinsic UE [27,28]. It is usually a first-line investigation for evaluation of a patient with hematuria and flank. Renal colic arising from obstruction due to clots can trigger the clinician to order an IVP or computed tomography (CT) urography.

IVP can help in localizing the degree, level, and site of ureteral obstruction. Intrinsic endometriosis takes a shape of filling defect inside the

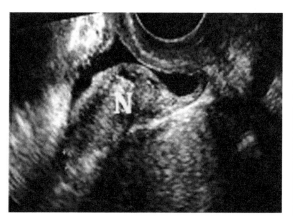
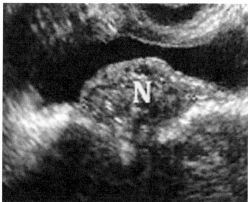

Figure 10.2 Transvaginal ultrasound with endometriotic endovesical lesion. N-Nodule. (From Stopiglia RM et al. *Int Braz J Urol* 2017;43:87–94.)

ureteric lumen mimicking other common urological conditions such as radiolucent calculus or urothelial carcinoma. In addition, IVP can reflect the function of the involved moiety. Coupled with retrograde pyelogram (Figure 10.3), IVP helps in identifying most ureteral strictures secondary to intrinsic or extrinsic endometriosis [27,28].

Computed tomography

Computed tomography (CT) is as useful as IVP in diagnosing BE and ureteral endometriosis [27,47]. Similar to IVP, a CT urography identifies the extent of disease in extrinsic ureteral endometriosis, together with the degree, site, and level of obstruction (Figure 10.3). Ureteral endometriosis

appearance on CT has been described by Plous et al. [47]. CT scan usually show soft tissue density with poor enhancement at the site of transition from dilated to the narrowed ureter [47].

Magnetic resonance imaging

Magnetic resonance imaging (MRI) is the second-line imaging modality used for assessment of BE after USG. It provides a high-contrast resolution for delineation of layers of bladder wall and tissue characterization to distinguish malignancy from BE lesions [48]. BE appears to be of low signal intensity on T2-weighted with intermediate or high-signal intensity on T1-weighted image (Figure 10.4) [49]. A systemic review and metanalysis conducted

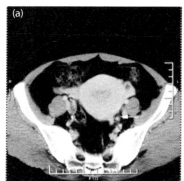
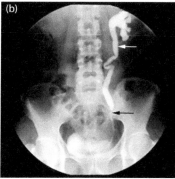
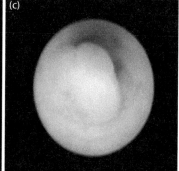

Figure 10.3 Enhanced CT scan of patients. (a) White arrow shows the space-occupying lesion in lower part of left ureter. (b) Retrograde pyelography of patients. White arrow shows hydronephrosis in left kidney and dilatation in upper part of ureter. Black arrow shows the filling defect in lower part of left ureter. (c) Ureteroscopy shows the papillary neoplasm in lower part of left ureter. (From Mu D et al. *Urol J* 2014;11(4):1806–12.)

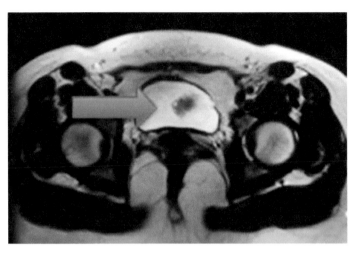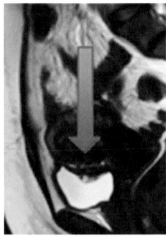

Figure 10.4 T2W MRI of the pelvis depicting hypointense lesion of endometriosis. Arrow depicts the nodule. (From Stopiglia RM et al. *Int Braz J Urol* 2017;43:87–94.)

by Medeiros et al. [50] estimated the accuracy of pelvic MRI in the diagnosis of DIE. Pelvic MRI was found to have pooled sensitivity of 0.64 (95% CI, 0.48–0.77) and pooled specificity of 0.98 (95% CI, 0.96–0.99) for detection of BE. The area under the curve was 0.93 [50]. MRI pelvis using a 3-Tesla system provides high spatial and contrast resolution. It provides us with information about the endometrial implants, helping to provide a road map for surgery by accurately delineating the lesions involving bowel, bladder, and uterine ligaments.

CYSTOSCOPY AND URETEROSCOPY

Cystoscopy is a diagnostic, office-based procedure and gives accurate diagnosis of hematuria of bladder origin. The bladder endometrial lesion, when it involves the mucosa, appears as an adenomatous and nodular red or bluish mass; ulcerations are rare [51]. The cystoscopy should be scheduled before menstruation as the endometriosis lesions will be congested, allowing for optimal characterization. Cystoscopy also provides accurate estimation of the distance of the lesion from the ureteral orifice and helps in planning the most appropriate surgical approach [6,51].

Furthermore, cystoscopy is helpful in ruling out the common differential diagnosis of hematuria such as varices, bladder carcinoma, and other benign tumors of the bladder. It can be an adjunct in case of intrinsic endometriosis of the ureter and guide further imaging or endoscopy by lateralizing

the hematuria by observing efflux from the ureteric orifices. Ureteroscopy using semi-rigid or flexible ureteroscopy can be used in the case of lateralizing hematuria and diagnosing the intrinsic ureteral endometriosis. Transurethral resection of the nodule should be done for diagnosis as a cold cup biopsy is seldom diagnostic for endometriosis [52].

URODYNAMICS

Urodynamics is the one of the less studied investigations in characterization of voiding dysfunction in DIE [21,22]. A systematic review by Bonneau et al. [20] assessed the incidence of urinary dysfunction in patients with DIE, both pre- and postoperatively. They found that patients with DIE have at least one abnormal urodynamic finding in 48.0%–83.3% [21]. Panel et al. [22] studied the characteristics of LUTS and urodynamic findings in 30 patients with DIE. They correlated the findings to the anatomic location of nodules found intraoperatively. All patients were found to have posterior endometriosis and 10 (33.3%) patients had BE. Urodynamics study revealed changes in 29 (96.7%) women. Patients with BE had a higher rate of bladder sensation (90.0% vs. 45.0%) and painful bladder filling (70.0% vs. 30.0%). Voiding symptoms (70.0% vs. 55.0%), urgency (80.0% vs. 40.0%), frequency (60.0% vs. 45.0%), and bladder pain (60.0% vs. 25.0%) were significantly similar in the two study groups [22]. Urodynamics again remains a research tool in patients with DIE.

TREATMENT

There is no consensus on the management of UTE since there are no randomized trials because of rarity of this disease. Several factor such as age, extent of urinary tract involvement, urinary symptoms. and pregnancy preference may dictate the choice of treatment. The management of UTE consists of medical therapy, surgical therapy, or both.

Medical therapy

The aim of the medical (hormonal) therapy is to cause regression of the growth of the endometrial tissue. However, until recently, hormonal treatment was considered ineffective for DIE, and radical excision was the mainstay of treatment. Hormonal therapy was usually considered for the residual disease. In recent years, estrogen–progestin and progestin therapy have emerged as successful treatment options, even in patients with DIE lesions including BE, except the subocclusive ureteral endometriotic lesions [6,53]. Combined hormonal contraceptives and progestogens have shown good results in relieving the pain and improving the quality of life in two-thirds of the patients [53]. The expression of estrogen and progesterone receptors in the DIE nodules was analyzed and all 10 patients of BE showed expression, suggesting a role of these compounds in BE [54]. However, there is paucity of data regarding the choice and the superiority of one formulation over the other, and no guideline can be made on the long-term use of these compounds [55]. Various studies done with deferent hormonal agents on BE showed both symptomatic as well as anatomical improvement; however, follow-up and recurrence data are not available [56,57]. Not only recurrence, but also a rebound phenomenon, has been described, leading to development of highly vascularized polyps following sudden withdrawal of hormonal agents [58]. Therefore, long term use of hormonal therapy until menopause or as a combination with surgical intervention is indicated.

Moreover, Carmen Maccagnano et al. suggested that hormonal therapy may be less effective in scarred endometriotic tissue in detrusor muscle of BE [7]. The authors suggested hormonal therapy alone only for BE lesions <5 mm in postmenopausal women due to the high recurrence

rate following the cessation of the treatment. In ureteral endometriosis, hormonal therapy should also be tried in very selected patients as the risk of upper tract damage is high [59,60]. A very few studies have shown some benefit, but with a high relapse rate and the requirement of adjuvant surgical interventions [59,60].

Medical management, though, decreases the symptom severity as well the lesions, but temporarily. Therefore, before deciding on hormonal therapy alone, the high recurrence rate and the need for long-term use (maybe until menopause) and stringent follow-up need to be discussed with the patient.

Surgical treatment

BLADDER ENDOMETRIOSIS

Cystoscopy is to be performed in all patients with BE, which can demonstrate bluish intraluminal mass at the dome or the posterior wall. Cystoscopy is crucial before planning any surgical intervention. The location and size of the tumor, as well as distance from the ureteric orifices, should be assessed [7]. Preoperative stenting can be done if the ureteric orifice is close, and a biopsy can be planned when urothelial malignancy or other bladder tumors are suspected.

Transurethral resection (TUR) is usually attempted in younger patients in whom partial cystectomy is deemed more radical. However, literature doesn't support this modality of treatment [7,61–63]. To prevent BE recurrence, the surgical procedure should be able to completely excise the disease. Since BE, unlike transitional cell carcinoma (TCC), grows from peritoneum to inside the bladder wall [52], complete excision of the disease with TUR is not possible, leading to high recurrence of symptoms and disease. Moreover, in an attempt to complete the resection, one may lead to more radical resection with risk of bladder perforation [62–64]. Even when TUR is combined with hormonal therapy, the recurrence rates are up to 25%–30% [7]. Therefore, the current evidence does not suggest this modality of treatment.

Segmental resection/partial cystectomy: Partial cystectomy involves full-thickness removal of the endometrial nodule with a normal bladder margin. It is generally a safe procedure when the lesion is at the dome and away from the ureteric orifices, though the technique may vary from laparotomy

[61,64,67–70] to laparoscopy [62,64,71–75] or, more recently, robotic assistance [76–81]. However, the steps of the technique are essentially similar, that is, dissection of the vesicouterine pouch, cystotomy with complete full-thickness removal of the nodule, and watertight closure of the bladder with absorbable sutures. Laparoscopy has all the advantages of minimally invasive surgery including less magnified vision, postoperative pain, fewer wound-related problems, and early recovery. Robotic assistance has the added advantage of 3D vision and ease of intracorporeal suturing in the deep pelvis. The need for ureteric stenting can be assessed during the cystoscopy and is required when the nodule is close to the ureteric orifice (<2 cm) or recurrent nodules with scarring [82]. Patients may require ureteric re-implantation when complete excision of the nodule required excision of the vesicoureteral junction. All techniques have demonstrated excellent outcomes and recurrence rates following partial cystectomy, irrespective of the surgical approach used.

There are few reports of cystoscopy-assisted partial cystectomy in which margins of the nodule can be better delineated and there is less loss of normal bladder wall [83]. A combined approach of TUR with partial cystectomy has been described, especially in larger tumors to avoid excision of a larger area of normal bladder tissue [84]. However, there is paucity of the data on the combined technique of management.

URETERAL ENDOMETRIOSIS

The treatment of ureteral endometriosis is aimed at relief of symptoms and resection of the tissue around the ureter to remove the obstruction and preservation of renal function (Figure 10.5). The choice of treatment depends on the severity and extent of ureteral involvement as well as the function of the affected renal moiety. Hormonal therapy is less effective in scarred endometriotic tissue, and most of the cases will require surgical intervention to remove the scarred tissue [27]. The hormonal therapy that is most popular in ureteral endometriosis is danazol or GnRH agonists. It can be given in a very select group of patients with minimal scarring around the ureter who desire pregnancy, or postmenopausal women. However, it requires strict follow-up and imaging for upper-tracts function [85]. Hormonal therapy should not be attempted in the presence of hydronephrosis and is not a good modality for ureteric endometriosis because of high recurrence and risk of renal damage [27,60].

With the advancement in end urological techniques, ureteroscopic ablation of the intrinsic endometriosis with laser, balloon dilatation, or stent placement has been attempted [86–88]. Although these techniques can relieve the ureteral obstruction, they do not treat the actual pathology, that is, entrapment/compression of the ureter. Patients may require prolonged stenting/re-stenting, need for hormonal therapy (duration and timing not

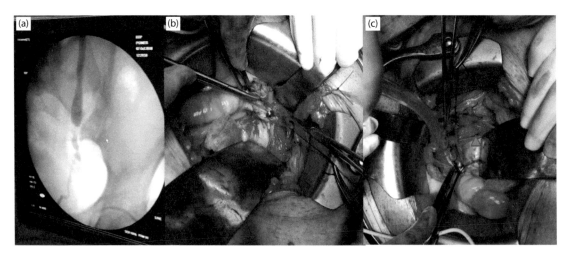

Figure 10.5 (a) Retrograde pyelogram showing dilated upper ureter and narrowed lower ureter due to encasement by DIE. (b) Chocolate cyst seen during ureterolysis (arrow). (c) Dilated ureter seen after utererolysis (arrowhead).

defined), and stringent follow-up with imaging and ureteroscopy to detect early recurrence and preservation of renal function [89].

Conventionally, laparotomy was the approach for extensive ureteral endometriosis and consisted of surgical castration with or without hysterectomy and ureterolysis/ureteric resection or nephrectomy [27,90]. With the advent of minimally invasive surgery, there are reports of decreased morbidity with equivalent outcomes by laparoscopic and robotic surgery [91–93]. The studies on the robotic platform suggest that robotic assistance is better than laparoscopy, mainly in severe endometriosis (stage IV) with low conversion rate to laparotomy [93,94]. Operative procedures include ureterolysis, ureteral resection with ureteral reconstruction, and nephrectomy depending on the type, extent, and location of the disease, as well as the renal functional status.

Ureterolysis is done in cases with extrinsic UE, with disease extending <3 cm of the ureteric length and no associated upper tract dilatation [95]. However, in a systematic review by J. Cavaco-Gomesa et al., even in patients with preoperative hydronephrosis, the recurrence rate after ureterolysis was very low (3.6%). The authors suggested ureterolysis was sufficient in 86.7% of patients in relieving the obstruction and symptoms with a low rate of postoperative complication [92]. The technique of laparoscopic ureterolysis includes (1) preoperative ureteral stenting for identification of the ureter during surgery as well as identification of ureteric injury, (2) dissection of the peritoneum over the normal part of the ureter, (3) dissection caudally toward the uterosacral ligaments up to the ureteric canal, and (4) ureterolysis with removal of fibrotic tissue till the lower part of the normal ureter.

Ureteric resection is required in intrinsic endometriosis, lesions larger than 3 cm with significant hydronephrosis, failure of ureterolysis, and ureteric injury during ureterolysis. The techniques of reconstruction after resection include uretero-ureterostomy and ureteroneocystostomy. Since disease involves the ureter in the ureteric canal, a good length of the healthy distal ureter can be found, and when a tension free anastomosis is possible, ureteroureterostomy can be done [96–98].

Ureteroneocystostomy is the operation of choice in cases of extensive disease where tension-free uretero-ureterostomy is not possible or disease extending close to vesicoureteral junction [99]. The modified Lich–Gregoire or Leadbetter–Politano technique with or without psoas hitch/Boari flap may be used [100–102]. Anna Stepniewska et al., in a series of 20 patients of ureteroneocystostomy, showed good functional outcome (100%) at 6 months of follow-up [102]. Nonetheless, the psoas hitch/Boari flap technique can place the anastomosis and the ureter away from the pelvis, which is the usual site of recurrence [103].

Up to 50% of patients with ureteral stenosis can be asymptomatic [97], and a delay in diagnosis of ureteral endometriosis can lead to eventual loss of renal function requiring nephrectomy [104]. The transperitoneal route is preferred as it allows simultaneous removal of pelvic endometriosis and the specimen can be delivered by opening the vagina [66].

CONCLUSION

A high index of suspicion is required to detect the urinary tract endometriosis, as the symptoms mimic other common urological conditions. Ultrasound (abdominal and TVS) remains the first line of investigation for diagnosing DIE, including BE. MRI is regarded as a second-line imaging technique for assessment of BE with better tissue delineation and guide for therapy. Hormonal therapy alone is less effective in UTE and should be applied in very select group of patients. Partial cystectomy is better than TUR in BE in terms of long-term disease control. Early diagnosis and treatment is required to preserve the renal function in ureteral endometriosis. The surgical approach and technique should be individualized based on the extent and severity of the disease and renal function status. A multimodality team including gynecologists, a urologist, and a gastrointestinal surgeon can improve the outcome in DIE.

REFERENCES

1. Koninckx PR, Ussia A, Adamyan L, Wattiez A, Donnez J. Deep endometriosis: Definition, diagnosis, and treatment. *Fertil Steril* 2012;98:564–71.
2. Berlanda N, Vercellini P, Carmignani L, Aimi G, Amicarelli F, Fedele L. Ureteral and vesical endometriosis. Two different clinical entities sharing the same pathogenesis. *Obstet Gynecol Surv* 2009;64:830–42.

3. Gabriel B, Nassif J, Trompoukis P, Barata S, Wattiez A. Prevalence and management of urinary tract endometriosis: A clinical case series. *Urology* 2011;78:1269–74.

4. Knabben L, Imboden S, Fellmann B, Nirgianakis K, Kuhn A, Mueller MD. Urinary tract endometriosis in patients with deep infiltrating endometriosis: Prevalence, symptoms, management, and proposal for a new clinical classification. *Fertil Steril* 2015; 103:147–52.

5. Chapron C, Fauconnier A, Vieira M et al. Anatomical distribution of deeply infiltrating endometriosis: Surgical implications and proposition for a classification. *Hum Reprod* 2003;18:157–61.

6. Maggiore UL, Ferrero S, Candiani M, Somigliana E, Viganò P, Vercellini P. Bladder endometriosis: A systematic review of pathogenesis, diagnosis, treatment, impact on fertility, and risk of malignant transformation. *Eur Urol* 2017 May 1;71(5):790–807.

7. Maccagnano C, Pellucchi F, Rocchini L, Ghezzi M, Scattoni V, Montorsi F, Rigatti P, Colombo R. Diagnosis and treatment of bladder endometriosis: State of the art. *Urol Int* 2012;89(3):249–58.

8. Abeshouse BS, Abeshouse G. Endometriosis of the urinary tract: A review of the literature and a report of four cases of vesical endometriosis. *J Int Coll Surg* 1960;34:43–63.

9. Young RH, Scully RE. Testicular and paratesticular tumors and tumor-like lesions of ovarian common epithelial and Müllerian types. A report of four cases and review of the literature. *Am J Clin Pathol* 1986;86:146–52.

10. Beckman EN, Pintado SO, Leonard GL, Sternberg WH. Endometriosis of the prostate. *Am J Surg Pathol* 1985;9:374–9.

11. Taguchi S, Enomoto Y, Homma Y. Bladder endometriosis developed after long-term estrogen therapy for prostate cancer. *Int J Urol* 2012;19:964–5.

12. Jabr FI, Mani V. An unusual cause of abdominal pain in a male patient: Endometriosis. *Avicenna J Med* 2014;4:99–101.

13. Pinkert TC, Catlow CE, Straus R. Endometriosis of the urinary bladder in a man with prostatic carcinoma. *Cancer* 1979;43:1562–7.

14. Schrodt GR, Alcorn MO, Ibanez J. Endometriosis of the male urinary system: A case report. *J Urol* 1980;124:722–3.

15. Oliker AJ, Harris AE. Endometriosis of the bladder in a male patient. *J Urol* 1971; 106:858–9.

16. Fukunaga M. Paratesticular endometriosis in a man with a prolonged hormonal therapy for prostatic carcinoma. *Pathol Res Pract* 2012;208:59–61.

17. Fauconnier A, Chapron C, Dubuisson JB, Vieira M, Dousset B, Breart G. Relation between pain symptoms and the anatomic location of deep infiltrating endometriosis. *Fertil Steril* 2002;78:719–26.

18. Fauconnier A, Chapron C. Endometriosis and pelvic pain: Epidemiological evidence of the relationship and implications. *Hum Reprod Update* 2005;11:595–606.

19. Sinaii N, Plumb K, Cotton L et al. Differences in characteristics among 1,000 women with endometriosis based on extent of disease. *Fertil Steril* 2008;89:538–45.

20. Bonneau C, Zilberman S, Ballester M et al. Incidence of pre- and postoperative urinary dysfunction associated with deep infiltrating endometriosis: Relevance of urodynamic tests and therapeutic implications. *Minerva Ginecol* 2013;65:385–405.

21. Ballester M, Dubernard G, Wafo E et al. Evaluation of urinary dysfunction by urodynamic tests, electromyography and quality of life questionnaire before and after surgery for deep infiltrating endometriosis. *Eur J Obstet Gynecol Reprod Biol* 2014; 179:135–40.

22. Panel P, Huchon C, Estrade-Huchon S, Le Tohic A, Fritel X, Fauconnier A. Bladder symptoms and urodynamic observations of patients with endometriosis confirmed by laparoscopy. *Int Urogynecol J* 2016;27:445–51.

23. Villa G, Mabrouk M, Guerrini M et al. Relationship between site and size of bladder endometriotic nodules and severity of dysuria. *J Minim Invasive Gynecol* 2007;14:628–32.

24. Leone Roberti Maggiore U, Ferrero S, Salvatore S. Urinary incontinence and bladder endometriosis: Conservative management. *Int Urogynecol J* 2015;26:159–62.

25. Tirlapur SA, Kuhrt K, Chaliha C, Ball E, Meads C, Khan KS. The "evil twin syndrome" in chronic pelvic pain: A systematic review of prevalence studies of bladder pain syndrome and endometriosis. *Int J Surg* 2013; 11:233–7.

26. Chung MK, Chung RP, Gordon D. Interstitial cystitis and endometriosis in patients with chronic pelvic pain: The "evil twins" syndrome. *J Soc Laparoendosc Surg* 2005;9:25–9.

27. Yohannes P. Ureteral endometriosis. *J Urol* 2003 Jul 1;170(1):20–5.

28. Pollack HM, Willis JS. Radiographic features of ureteral endometriosis. *AJR Am J Roentgenol* 1978;131:627.

29. Olive DL. Endometriosis: Advances in understanding and management. *Curr Opin Obstet Gynecol* 1992;4:380.

30. Takeuchi S, Minoura H, Toyoda N, Ichio T, Hirano H, Sugiyama Y. Intrinsic ureteric involvement by endometriosis: A case report. *J Obstet Gynaecol Res* 1997;23:273.

31. Sakellariou PG, Protopapas AG, Kyritsis NI, Voulgaris ZG, Akrivos TN, Maraki SN. Retroperitoneal endometriosis causing cyclical obstruction. *Eur J Obstet Gynecol Reprod Biol* 1996;67:59.

32. Lam AM, French M, Charnock FM. Bilateral ureteric obstruction due to recurrent endometriosis associated with hormone replacement therapy. *Aust N Z J Obstet Gynaecol* 1992;32:83.

33. Esen T, Akinci M, Ander H, Tunc M, Tellaloglu S, Narter I. Bilateral ureteric obstruction due to endometriosis. *Br J Urol* 1990;66:98.

34. Zanetta G, Webb M, Segura JW. Ureteral endometriosis diagnosed at ureteroscopy. *Obstet Gynecol* 1998;91:857.

35. Shook TE, Nyberg LM. Endometriosis of the urinary tract. *Urology* 1988;31:1–6.

36. Giambelluca D, Albano D, Giambelluca E et al. Renal endometriosis mimicking complicated cysts of kidney: Report of two cases. *Il Giorn Chir* 2017 Sep;38(5):250.

37. Cabral Ribeiro J, Pérez García D, Martins Silva C, Ribeiro Santos A. Endometrioma suburetral. *Actas Urol Esp* 2007 Feb;31(2):153–6.

38. Palagiri A. Urethral diverticulum with endometriosis. *Urology* 1978 Mar 1;11(3):271–2.

39. Chowdhry AA, Miller FH, Hammer RA. Endometriosis presenting as a urethral diverticulum: A case report. *J Reprod Med* 2004 Apr;49(4):321–3.

40. Scarpero HM, Fiske J, Xue X, Nitti VW. American Urological Association Symptom Index for lower urinary tract symptoms in women: Correlation with degree of bother and impact on quality of life. *Urology* 2003;61:1118–22.

41. Fedele L, Bianchi S, Carmignani L, Berlanda N, Fontana E, Frontino G. Evaluation of a new questionnaire for the presurgical diagnosis of bladder endometriosis. *Hum Reprod* 2007;22:2698–701.

42. Ballester M, Santulli P, Bazot M, Coutant C, Rouzier R, Darai E. Preoperative evaluation of posterior deep-infiltrating endometriosis demonstrates a relationship with urinary dysfunction and parametrial involvement. *J Minim Invasive Gynecol* 2011;18:36–42.

43. Mu D, Li X, Zhou G, Guo H. Diagnosis and treatment of ureteral endometriosis: Study of 23 cases. *Urol J* 2014;11(4):1806–12.

44. Guerriero S, Condous G, Van den Bosch T et al. Systematic approach to sonographic evaluation of the pelvis in women with suspected endometriosis, including terms, definitions and measurements: A consensus opinion from the International Deep Endometriosis Analysis (IDEA) group. *Ultrasound Obstet Gynecol* 2016;48:318–32.

45. Fedele L, Bianchi S, Raffaelli R, Portuese A. Pre-operative assessment of bladder endometriosis. *Hum Reprod* 1997;12:2519–22.

46. Tammaa A, Fritzer N, Lozano P et al. Interobserver agreement and accuracy of non-invasive diagnosis of endometriosis by transvaginal sonography. *Ultrasound Obstet Gynecol* 2015;46:737–40.

47. Plous RH, Sunshine R, Goldman H, Schwartz IS. Ureteral endometriosis in post-menopausal women. *Urology* 1985;26:408.

48. Mallampati GK, Siegelman ES. MR imaging of the bladder. *Magn Reson Imaging Clin N Am* 2004;12:545–55.

49. Kruger K, Gilly L, Niedobitek-Kreuter G, Mpinou L, Ebert AD. Bladder endometriosis: Characterization by magnetic resonance imaging and the value of documenting

ureteral involvement. *Eur J Obstet Gynecol Reprod Biol* 2014;176:39–43.

50. Medeiros LR, Rosa MI, Silva BR et al. Accuracy of magnetic resonance in deeply infiltrating endometriosis: A systematic review and meta-analysis. *Arch Gynecol Obstet* 2015;291:611–21.

51. Vercellini P, Frontino G, Pisacreta A, De Giorgi O, Cattaneo M, Crosignani PG. The pathogenesis of bladder detrusor endometriosis. *Am J Obstet Gynecol* 2002;187:538–42.

52. Vercellini P, Carmignani L, Rubino T, Barbara G, Abbiati A, Fedele L. Surgery for deep endometriosis: A pathogenesis-oriented approach. *Gynecol Obstet Investig* 2009;68:88–103.

53. Vercellini P, Buggio L, Berlanda N, Barbara G, Somigliana E, Bosari S. Estrogen-progestins and progestins for the management of endometriosis. *Fertil Steril* 2016;106:1552–71.

54. Noël JC, Chapron C, Bucella D et al. Estrogen and progesterone receptors in smooth muscle component of deep infiltrating endometriosis. *Fertil Steril* 2010;93:1774–7.

55. Hirsch M, Duffy JM, Kusznir JO, Davis CJ, Plana MN, Khan KS, International Collaboration to Harmonize Outcomes and Measures for Endometriosis. Variation in outcome reporting in endometriosis trials: A systematic review. *Am J Obstet Gynecol* 2016;214:452–64.

56. Westney OL, Amundsen CL, McGuire EJ. Bladder endometriosis: Conservative management. *J Urol* 2000;163:1814–7.

57. Fedele L, Bianchi S, Montefusco S, Frontino G, Carmignani L. A gonadotropin-releasing hormone agonist versus a continuous oral contraceptive pill in the treatment of bladder endometriosis. *Fertil Steril* 2008;90:183–4.

58. Othman NH, Othman MS, Ismail AN, Mohammad NZ, Ismail Z. Multiple polypoid endometriosis—a rare complication following withdrawal of gonadotrophin releasing hormone (GnRH) agonist for severe endometriosis: A case report. *Aust N Z J Obstet Gynaecol* 1996;36:216.

59. Matsuura K, Kawasaki N, Oka M, Ii H, Maeyama M. Treatment with danazol of ureteral obstruction caused by endometriosis. *Acta Obstet Gynecol Scand* 1985;64:339.

60. Rivlin ME, Miller JD, Krueger RP, Patel RB, Bower JD. Leuprolide acetate in the management of ureteral obstruction caused by endometriosis. *Obstet Gynecol* 1990;75:532.

61. Antonelli A, Simeone C, Zani D et al. Clinical aspects and surgical treatment of urinary tract endometriosis: Our experience with 31 cases. *Eur Urol* 2006;49:1093–7.

62. Perez-Utrilla Perez M, Aguilera Bazan A, Alonso Dorrego JM et al. Urinary tract endometriosis: Clinical, diagnostic, and therapeutic aspects. *Urology* 2009;73:47–51.

63. Fuentes Pastor J, Ballestero Diego R, Correas Gomez MA et al. Bladder endometriosis and endocervicosis: Presentation of 2 cases with endoscopic management and review of literature. *Case Rep Urol* 2014;2014:296908.

64. Fedele L, Bianchi S, Zanconato G, Bergamini V, Berlanda N, Carmignani L. Long-term follow-up after conservative surgery for bladder endometriosis. *Fertil Steril* 2005;83:1729–33.

65. Barrabino R, Fernández-Sánchez A, Gil Julio H. Bladder endometriosis: An under diagnosed cause of bladder pain syndrome: Report of two new cases managed with endoscopic resection. *J Surg Open Access* 2016;2(2): http://dx.doi.org/10.16966/2470-0991.114

66. Jadoul P, Feyaerts A, Squifflet J, Donnez J. Combined laparoscopic and vaginal approach for nephrectomy, ureterectomy, and removal of a large rectovaginal endometriotic nodule causing loss of renal function. *J Minim Invasive Gynecol* 2007 Mar-Apr;14(2):256–9.

67. Chopin N, Vieira M, Borghese B et al. Operative management of deeply infiltrating endometriosis: Results on pelvic pain symptoms according to a surgical classification. *J Minim Invasive Gynecol* 2005;12:106–12.

68. Fleisch MC, Xafis D, De Bruyne F, Hucke J, Bender HG, Dall P. Radical resection of invasive endometriosis with bowel or bladder involvement—long-term results. *Eur J Obstet Gynecol Rep Biol* 2005;123:224–9.

69. Rozsnyai F, Roman H, Resch B et al. Outcomes of surgical management of deep infiltrating endometriosis of the ureter and urinary bladder. *J Soc Laparoendosc Surg* 2011;15:439–47.

70. Kjer JJ, Kristensen J, Hartwell D, Jensen MA. Full-thickness endometriosis of the bladder:

Report of 31 cases. *Eur J Obstet Gynecol Reprod Biol* 2014;176:31–3.

71. Nezhat CR, Nezhat F, Admon D, Seidman D, Nezhat CH. Laparoscopic management of genitourinary endometriosis. *J Am Assoc Gynecol Laparosc* 1994;1:S25.

72. Chapron C, Dubuisson JB. Laparoscopic management of bladder endometriosis. *Acta Obstet Gynecol Scand* 1999;78:887–90.

73. Seracchioli R, Mabrouk M, Montanari G, Manuzzi L, Concetti S, Venturoli S. Conservative laparoscopic management of urinary tract endometriosis (UTE): Surgical outcome and long-term follow- up. *Fertil Steril* 2010;94:856–61.

74. Chapron C, Bourret A, Chopin N et al. Surgery for bladder endometriosis: Long-term results and concomitant management of associated posterior deep lesions. *Hum Reprod* 2010;25:884–9.

75. Soriano D, Bouaziz J, Elizur S et al. Reproductive outcome is favorable after laparoscopic resection of bladder endometriosis. *J Minim Invasive Gynecol* 2016;23:781–6.

76. Nezhat C, Hajhosseini B, King LP. Robotic assisted laparoscopic treatment of bowel, bladder, and ureteral endometriosis. *JSLS* 2011;15:387–92.

77. Liu C, Perisic D, Samadi D, Nezhat F. Robotic-assisted laparoscopic partial bladder resection for the treatment of infiltrating endometriosis. *J Minim Invasive Gynecol* 2008;15:745–8.

78. Chammas MF Jr, Kim FJ, Barbarino A, Hubert N, Feuillu B, Coissard A, Hubert J. Asymptomatic rectal and bladder endometriosis: A case for robotic-assisted surgery. *Can J Urol* 2008;15:4097–100.

79. Collinet P, Leguevaque P, Neme RM et al. Robot-assisted laparoscopy for deep infiltrating endometriosis: International multicentric retrospective study. *Surg Endosc* 2014;28:2474–9.

80. Siesto G, Ieda N, Rosati R, Vitobello D. Robotic surgery for deep endometriosis: A paradigm shift. *Int J Med Robot* 2014;10:140–6.

81. Abo C, Roman H, Bridoux V et al. Management of deep infiltrating endometriosis by laparoscopic route with robotic assistance: 3-year experience. *J Gynecol Obstet Biol Reprod.* 2017 Jan 1;46(1):9–18.

82. Vercellini P, Pisacreta A, De Giorgi O, Yaylayan L, Zaina B, Crosignani PG. Management of advanced endometriosis. In: Kempers RD, Cohen J, Haney AF, Younger JB, editors. *Fertility and Reproductive Medicine.* Amsterdam: Elsevier Science; 1998, pp. 369–86.

83. Stopiglia RM, Ferreira U, Faundes DG, Petta CA. Cystoscopy-assisted laparoscopy for bladder endometriosis: Modified light-to-light technique for bladder preservation. *Int Braz J Urol* 2017;43:87–94.

84. Litta P, Saccardi C, D'Agostino G, Florio P, De Zorzi L, Bianco MD. Combined transurethral approach with Versapoint and laparoscopic treatment in the management of bladder endometriosis: Technique and 12 months follow-up. *Surg Endosc* 2012;26:2446–50.

85. Palla VV, Karaolanis G, Katafigiotis I, Anastasiou I. Ureteral endometriosis: A systematic literature review. *Indian J Urol* 2017 Oct-Dec;33(4):276–82.

86. Kulkarni RP, Bellamy EA. A new thermo-expandable shape-memory nickel-titanium alloy stent for the management of ureteric strictures. *BJU Int* 1999;83:755–9.

87. Pittaway DE, Daniell JF, Maxson WS, Winfield AC, Wentz AC. Recurrence of ureteral obstruction caused by endometriosis after danazol therapy. *Am J Obstet Gynecol* 1982;143:720–2.

88. Yamada, S., Ono, Y., Ohshima, S, Miyake, K. Transurethral ureteroscopic ureterotomy assisted by a prior balloon dilation for relieving ureteral strictures. *J Urol* 1995;153:1418.

89. Castaneda CV, Shapiro EY, Ahn JJ, Van Batavia JP, Silva MV, Tan Y, Gupta M. Endoscopic management of intraluminal ureteral endometriosis. *Urology* 2013;82:307e–312.

90. Antonelli A, Simeone C, Canossi E et al. Surgical approach to urinary endometriosis: Experience on 28 cases. *Arch Ital Urol Androl* 2006;78:35–8.

91. Ghezzi F, Cromi A, Bergamini V et al. Outcome of laparoscopic ureterolysis for ureteral endometriosis. *Fertil Steril* 2006; 86:418–22.

92. Cavaco-Gomesa J, Martinhoa M, Gilabert-Aguilarb J, Gilabert-Estéllesb J. Laparoscopic management of ureteral endometriosis: A systematic review. *J Obstet Gynecol Reprod Biol* 2017;210:94–101.

93. Nezhat C, Lewis M, Kotikela S, Veeraswamy A, Saadat L, Hajhosseini B, Nezhat C. Robotic versus standard laparoscopy for the treatment of endometriosis. *Fertil Steril* 2010;94:2758–60.

94. Marchal F, Rauch P, Vandromme J et al. Telerobotic-assisted laparoscopic hysterectomy for benign and oncologic pathologies: Initial clinical experience with 30 patients. *Surg Endosc* 2005;19:826–31.

95. Comiter CV. Endometriosis of the urinary tract. *Urol Clin North Am* 2002;29:625–35.

96. Mereu L, Gagliardi ML, Clarizia R, Mainardi P, Landi S, Minelli L. Laparoscopic management of ureteral endometriosis in case of moderate-severe hydroureteronephrosis. *Fertil and Steril* 2010;93:46–51.

97. Seracchioli R, Mabrouk M, Manuzzi L et al. Importance of retroperitoneal ureteric evaluation in cases of deep infiltrating endometriosis. *J Minim Invasive Gynecol* 2008;15:435–9.

98. Nezhat C, Nezhat F, Green B. Laparoscopic treatment of obstructed ureter due to endometriosis by resection and ureteroureterostomy: A case report. *J Urol* 1992;148:865–8.

99. Bosev D, Nicoll LM, Bhagan L et al. Laparoscopic management of ureteral endometriosis: The Stanford University hospital experience with 96 consecutive cases. *J Urol* 2009;182:2748–52.

100. Nezhat CH, Malik S, Nezhat F, Nezhat C. Laparoscopic ureteroneocystostomy and vesicopsoas hitch for infiltrative endometriosis. *JSLS* 2004;8(1):3–7.

101. Azioni G, Bracale U, Scala A et al. Laparoscopic ureteroneocystostomy and vesicopsoas hitch for infiltrative ureteral endometriosis. *Minim Invasive Ther Allied Technol* 2010;19(5):292–7.

102. Stepniewska A, Grosso G, Molon A et al. Ureteral endometriosis: Clinical and radiological follow-up after laparoscopic ureterocystoneostomy. *Hum Reprod* 2011; 26(1):112–6.

103. Bondavalli C, Dall'Oglio B, Schiavon L et al. Pathology of the gynecologic ureter: Our experience. *Arch Ital Urol Androl* 2002;74:25–6.

104. Arrieta Bretón S, López Carrasco A, Hernández Gutiérrez A, Rodríguez González R, de Santiago García J. Complete loss of unilateral renal function secondary to endometriosis: A report of three cases. *Eur J Obstet Gynecol Reprod Biol* 2013 Nov; 171(1):132–7.

11

Management of deep infiltrative endometriosis (DIE) causing gynecological morbidity: A colorectal surgeon's perspective

ADITYA KULKARNI AND RAJESH GUPTA

INTRODUCTION, DEFINITION, AND SCOPE OF THE PROBLEM

Endometriosis is defined as "the presence of endometrium-like tissue outside the confines of the uterine cavity that can incite a chronic inflammatory-fibroblastic reaction." It is a common cause of pelvic pain, dyspareunia, and infertility worldwide. It affects up to 10%–15% of all women in the reproductive age group and accounts for almost one-third of infertility cases [1].

Bowel endometriosis is defined as "endometrial-like glands and stroma infiltrating the bowel wall reaching at least the subserous fat tissue or adjacent to the neurovascular branches (subserous plexus)" [2]. Bowel involvement is seen in approximately 3.8%–37% of all patients with endometriosis [2]. Deep infiltrative endometriosis (DIE) is defined arbitrarily as "endometriotic lesion extending more than 5 mm below the surface of the peritoneum" [3].

Bowel endometriosis constitutes a major source of morbidity and mortality. Effective treatment is a formidable challenge for both the gynecologist and the colorectal surgeon. In this chapter, we aim to provide a brief review of the pathology, clinical features, investigations, and treatment of this incapacitating disease.

MORPHOLOGY AND PATTERNS OF INVOLVEMENT

Bowel involvement in endometriosis is associated with the presence of other endometriotic lesions in the pelvis in over 99% of patients [4]. In a study by Chapron et al., the rectum and rectosigmoid junction were involved in 65.7% of the cases, followed by the sigmoid colon (17.4%), cecum and ileocecal junction (4.1%), appendix (6.4%), small bowel (4.7%), and omentum (1.7%) [5]. Rare cases have been reported with involvement of the transverse

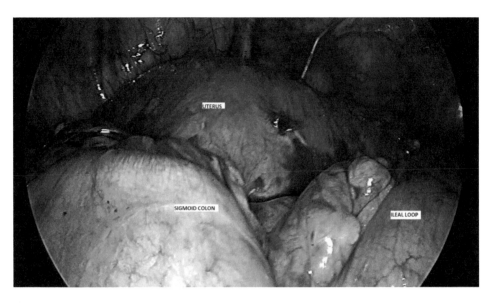

Figure 11.1 Deep infiltrating endometriosis with bowel involvement.

colon and stomach; however, endometriosis generally remains isolated to the lower abdomen and pelvis (Figure 11.1).

An important point to consider in the distribution of bowel involvement is the presence of multifocal and multicentric lesions [6]. Multifocality is defined as the presence of endometriotic lesions within a 2 cm area from the main lesion) and its multicentric involvement (defined as the presence of endometriotic lesions beyond 2 cm from the main lesion). Multifocality and multicentricity are observed in 62% and 38% of surgical en bloc specimens, respectively [6]. This point assumes significance in the surgical treatment, as will be discussed later.

CLINICAL FEATURES

Bowel endometriosis is probably the most commonly misdiagnosed form of endometriosis. The clinical spectrum and symptoms overlap with a number of varied conditions (Table 11.1), which may lead to a delay in diagnosis and treatment [7].

The majority of patients have symptoms of deep pelvic pain, dysmenorrheal, and dyspareunia [2]. Up to 25% of patients also suffer from infertility. The range of symptoms is wide and depends upon the distribution and extent of involvement of the bowel. A high index of suspicion is necessary to suspect bowel endometriosis and correlate lesions with symptoms. Generally, smaller serosal nodules

do not cause symptoms. However, the size of the lesions does not correlate with the clinical symptoms in most cases.

Rectal or rectosigmoid involvement is seen in nearly two-thirds of all patients. Rectal endometriosis may lead to dyschezia, tenesmus, hypogastric pain, bloating sensation, and alteration of bowel habit (which may include both diarrhea and constipation) [9]. Bulky rectal lesions with extensive surrounding fibrosis may lead to rectal stenosis and large bowel obstruction. Rectal bleeding is uncommon as the disease generally starts from the serosal aspect, and transmural infiltration is rare. However, around 5% of patients may manifest cyclical rectal bleeding [10].

As is characteristic of endometriosis at other locations, the severity of the bowel symptoms may vary according to the menstrual cycle. There may be a change in bowel habit one to two days prior to menstruation. Occasionally, patients may not have

Table 11.1 Differential diagnoses of bowel endometriosis [2,7,8]

Irritable bowel syndrome
Solitary rectal ulcer syndrome
Inflammatory bowel disease (ulcerative colitis, Crohn's disease)
Colon adenocarcinoma
Diverticular disease
Adhesions

bowel symptoms at all, and bowel involvement is diagnosed only when laparoscopy is performed.

On clinical examination, tender nodules may be felt occasionally in the pouch of Douglas. Per-rectal examination is usually unrevealing, as the disease generally does not affect the mucosa. Dragisic et al. reported that clinical examination had a sensitivity of 34%, a specificity of 96.7%, and a positive predictive value of 55.6% in detecting rectal involvement [11]. In a study by Koninckx et al., it was found that clinical examination may be more revealing if performed during menstruation [12].

Endometriotic nodules over the small bowel can be asymptomatic, can lead to adhesions, and, rarely, have been reported to cause intestinal obstruction [13]. Involvement of the appendix is very rare, with estimated prevalence of only around 0.8% [14]. Acute appendicitis [15,16], appendicular perforation [17], cecal intussusception [18], right lower quadrant cyclic pain, and melena have all been reported.

INVESTIGATIONS

Radiological investigations form a key element of the preoperative assessment, particularly because the symptoms and findings are often unrevealing [2,19]. The aim of investigations is to define the extent of involvement and size and location of the nodules, especially with regard to the distance of the nodules from the anal verge. With adequate staging, it is possible to involve key members of the team (urologist, colorectal surgeon, etc.) in patient management at an early stage and also to have a detailed discussion with the patient regarding possible options and complications. Planning of surgical intervention depends on good-quality, comprehensive imaging.

Transvaginal ultrasound

There have been several studies demonstrating the utility of transvaginal ultrasound (TVS) in demonstrating the presence and distribution of endometriotic nodules [19–21]. Indeed, TVS has been recommended as first-line modality for investigation of DIE [21]. TVS with bowel preparation can assess the size, number, location, and depth of infiltration of the nodules into the intestinal wall. Endometriotic nodules appear as irregular hypoechoic masses penetrating into the wall of the

intestine, sometimes with hyperechoic foci within [22]. On histologic analysis, the hypoechoic area corresponds to the thickened muscularis propria and the echogenic rim to serosa, submucosa, and mucosa of the bowel [23]. Distending the rectum with water prior to TVS may further improve the diagnostic yield [24].

Hudelist et al. [20], in their meta-analysis, reported overall sensitivity of 91% and specificity of 98% of TVS. TVS has a comparable efficacy as transrectal ultrasound in detecting posterior pelvic involvement [25]. Disadvantages of TVS include operator dependency, inability to assess lesions that are beyond the reach of the TVS probe, and inability to accurately judge distance from the anal verge, which is very important when surgical resection or excision is planned.

Transrectal ultrasound

The utility of transrectal ultrasound (TRUS) has been well described [26]. It scores over MRI in the diagnosis of rectal involvement [27]. In a large series, reported sensitivity and specificity of TRUS was 97% and 96%, respectively. TRUS offers the same advantages as TVS, that is, estimation of precise depth of involvement of the bowel wall layers and number of lesions and their location. It has an added advantage that the distance of the lesion from the anal verge can be estimated [26]. However, TRUS can be painful and uncomfortable, especially when assessing lesions near the rectosigmoid. This may necessitate general anesthesia in a few patients. In addition, TRUS is infrequently available and difficult to access for most gynecologists. Therefore, TRUS is supplanted by TVS in most instances.

Colonoscopy

Colonoscopy usually does not offer much in the way of diagnosis as lesions are usually submucosal and not well-visualized on endoscopy [1,2]. However, it may be performed in order to rule out alternative diagnoses or in the occasional patient who presents with per-rectal bleeding.

Double-contrast barium enema

Although rarely performed, double-contrast barium enema (DBCE) can be used to diagnose colonic involvement in endometriosis. Nodules can be seen as extrinsic impressions with a crenellated appearance [28]. However, the extrinsic mass effect is seen only in around 54% cases [29]. The other limitation of DBCE is that smaller nodules may not be visualized, and it is not possible to investigate the depth of penetration.

Magnetic resonance imaging

MRI is one of the commonly used techniques in the demonstration of DIE. The reported sensitivity, specificity, and accuracy for detection of rectosigmoid disease are 88%, 97.8%, and 94.9%, respectively [30]. Endometriotic nodules contain hemorrhagic fluid and appear as hyperintense on T1-weighted and hypointense on T2-weighted MR images [1]. MRI is very sensitive for detection of disease in the cul-de-sac and uterosacral ligaments. However, when it comes to detection of rectal involvement, MRI has a slightly lower sensitivity and specificity compared with endoluminal ultrasound [27]. Filling the rectum or vagina with jelly prior to examination has been reported to improve the accuracy of detection [31]. One of the limitations of MRI is the difficulty in picking up lesions with significant fibrosis and lacking blood-filled cysts, as the intermediate signal produced by fibrotic lesions is similar to the normal muscle layer [2,32].

Multidetector CT enteroclysis

Recently, multidetector CT enteroclysis (MDCTE) has been evaluated in the diagnosis of bowel endometriosis [33]. MDCTE involves bowel preparation and retrograde colonic distension by filling water. Peristaltic activity is suppressed by antispasmodic administration. The scan is then acquired after administration of intravenous contrast. Endometriotic deposits appear as solid nodules with positive contrast enhancement. Information regarding the size of nodules, their location, and even the depth of infiltration can be accurately obtained. A major advantage of MDCTE is that endometriotic lesions over the cecum, appendix, and ileum can be detected at the same time. MDCTE is reported to have a sensitivity of 98.7%, a specificity of 100%, a positive predictive value of 100%, and a negative predictive value of 95.7% in identifying women with bowel endometriosis [34].

SCORING SYSTEMS FOR BOWEL ENDOMETRIOSIS

The revised American Fertility Society (r-AFS) Score [35] is used to grade severity of endometriosis. However, bowel involvement is only indirectly included in this system. The system lacks correlation between pain symptoms and severity of disease. The Enzian classification system seeks to classify infiltration of bowel, rectum, and rectovaginal septum in a more detailed manner [35,36].

Bowel-specific classifications in this system are

- E1c: Isolated nodule in the rectovaginal space
- E2c: Infiltration of the rectum <1 cm
- E3c: Infiltration of the rectum 1–3 cm without stenosis
- E4c: Infiltration of the rectum >3 cm and/or rectal stenosis
- FI: Intestinal infiltration (other side than rectum or sigmoid)

TREATMENT

Principles of treatment of BE

The goal of treatment is to achieve improvement in the quality-of-life parameters, pain, and possibly the fertility rates. Multidisciplinary management at a high-volume center may achieve better outcomes [37]. Hence, a colorectal surgeon or urologist should be involved right from the stage of preoperative planning, particularly when the patient has disease involving the deep cul-de-sac or rectovaginal septum. The decision to intervene has to be taken on a case-by-case basis, keeping in mind the following factors before deciding the future plan of treatment (Table 11.2).

Conservative management

A conservative approach may be applied for patients approaching menopause, having mild or nondebilitating symptoms, in whom the family is already complete. These patients are likely to have spontaneous decrease in disease activity with the onset of menopause.

Table 11.2 Factors to consider while making a plan of treatment

Patient factors	Age
	Fertility status
	Hormonal status
Clinical factors	Pain intensity
	Features of bowel obstruction
Disease-related factors	Number and location of lesions
	Distance from the anal verge
	Size of deposits
	Relation and depth of penetration into the bowel wall
	Percentage of bowel circumference involved
	Multifocality

Medical management

The natural history and progression of bowel endometriosis is not well known. However, it is likely that size of the nodules and the surrounding fibrosis may increase with time, thus predisposing to stricture formation and obstruction [38]. Therefore, patients who desire medical management should be counseled regarding the risk of progression of lesions in the future, even while on medical management [1]. Careful monitoring by transvaginal ultrasound may be warranted to document any enlargement of the nodule while on treatment.

Not all patients are candidates for medical therapy. Patients who are severely symptomatic are probably better served by surgery. Women who wish to conceive cannot take oral medications, as these have the effect of ovulation inhibition. Commonly used drugs include GnRH analogues, progestins, and aromatase inhibitors. Triptorelin and tibolone have been shown to improve intestinal symptoms and pain in a small series [39].

Oral progestins (norethisterone) have also shown efficacy in menstrual-related symptoms such dysmenorrhea, cyclical rectal bleeding, and diarrhea. However, there was no or minimal improvement in obstructive features. Recently, aromatase inhibitors (letrozole), in combination with progestins, have also been utilized for treating bowel endometriosis [40]. However, many patients experience recurrent symptoms after discontinuation of therapy.

Surgical management

Surgery is indicated when patients have symptoms (pain, dyspareunia, dyschezia, or bowel obstruction) that hamper daily activities and impair quality of life [41,42]. The main aim of surgical treatment is the complete removal of all endometriotic deposits on the bowel. Recurrence rates after treatment depend upon the completeness of excision [43,44]. To this end, surgery by an experienced surgeon in resection of endometriosis has been shown to significantly decrease the recurrence rates [45].

PREOPERATIVE PREPARATION

There is a small yet significant chance of complications following surgery for BE. Thus all patients should be counseled prior to undergoing surgery, and proper written informed consent should be obtained, which should include consent for stoma. As bowel resection may need to be performed, mechanical bowel preparation should be administered before surgery. Stoma site marking is routinely performed, ideally in conjunction with an enterostomal therapist. Mechanical (stockings, pneumatic compression devices) and pharmacologic (LMW heparin) anti-thrombosis prophylaxis is instituted before surgery at our institution. Perioperative antibiotic prophylaxis appropriate for colorectal surgery is administered.

SURGERY

After administration of anesthesia, the surgery begins with the patient in the lithotomy position so as to allow access for per-vaginal and per-rectal examination by an assistant. A diagnostic laparoscopy and examination under anesthesia is performed to stage the disease process and identify the nodules to be excised.

Different options for excision of nodules include

- Partial-thickness excision or "shave"
- Full-thickness disc excision
- Segmental bowel resection

The type of resection to be performed for a particular patient depends upon the surgeon's preference and experience. In a large series of 169 patients treated surgically, the majority of patients (78%) underwent shave excision, followed by bowel resection (15%) and disc excision (7%) [46].

Partial-thickness resection or "shaving"

Resection of superficial lesions on the serosa can be carried out by sharp dissection after lifting the lesion with grasping forceps and using scissors. Use of thermal cautery is risky, as this can result in delayed ischemia and perforation. Alternatively, CO_2 laser can be used if available. Excision will leave a defect on the bowel wall that can be closed with interrupted sutures. The pelvis is filled with saline and an air leak test with per-rectal insufflation of air is done to rule out leakage. Donnez and Squifflet reported on 500 cases treated by shaving technique with high pregnancy rates (84%), low rate of recurrence (8%), and low rate of major complications (3.20%) [47].

Full-thickness disc excision

Lesions infiltrating into or beyond the muscularis propria can be resected by excising a full-thickness disc of bowel wall containing the lesion followed by primary suture closure of the defect in one or two layers [48,49]. Selection of lesions for this approach has to be done meticulously, as closure of too large a defect may result in rectal stenosis. Generally, single lesions, less than 3 cm and involving less than 40% of the rectal wall circumference, are considered to be amenable for this approach [50].

Even though full-thickness resection is a popular technique, there is a theoretical risk of higher pain recurrence with this approach. This is because the endometriotic lesions preferentially invade the bowel wall along the nerves up to 4–5 cm away from the actual nodule [51]. Full-thickness excision has been shown to result in incomplete clearance in up to 40% of patients [52]. Hence, these cells may be left behind, resulting in recurrence and pain.

Segmental bowel resection

The indications for segmental bowel resection include deep-penetrating nodules, nodules larger than 3 cm, nodules involving more than half of the circumference, nodules located in higher bowel segments, multifocal disease, and any lesion that cannot be adequately treated with the modalities mentioned above.

The surgery performed most commonly is anterior resection of the rectum. This may be done either laparoscopically or by laparotomy, depending upon the surgeon's experience. The laparoscopic approach carries a steep learning curve, and conversion rates of up to 20% have been reported. Darai et al. conducted a randomized controlled trial comparing laparoscopic and open approach for colorectal resection in endometriosis [53]. This trial showed that laparoscopy and open surgery were equivalent with regard to reduction in pain, digestive symptoms, and gynecological symptoms. However, the open approach was associated with more complications. Also, patients in the laparoscopy group had a higher pregnancy rate, probably related to less postoperative adhesion formation.

The surgery begins with insertion of a cannula into the uterus so as to lift and antevert it. The ureters are identified at the beginning of the dissection. Very often, fibrosis may cause medial displacement of the ureter, thus bringing them into harm's way. Therefore, in patients in whom significant adhesions are expected, it is better to place bilateral lighted ureteral stents preoperatively.

Since the surgery is performed for benign as opposed to malignant disease, it is acceptable to keep the dissection and vessel ligation close to the bowel wall. This avoids injury to surrounding vital structures. The dissection is started from an area of normal peritoneum away from the endometriotic nodule. Significant adhesions may be present between the sigmoid and left adnexal structures. The rectum is mobilized from its lateral and posterior attachments. The anterior dissection may be the most difficult part, as nodules in the cul-de-sac and rectovaginal septum incite dense fibrosis. Dissection is carried caudally, beyond the nodule into normal rectovaginal septum. A manipulator placed into the vagina and another into the rectum can help with this part. In case of severe adhesions, a cuff of posterior vaginal wall can be included with the bowel. The aim is to get below the lesion to a healthy, well-vascularized segment of the bowel wall. The branches of inferior mesenteric vessels are sequentially controlled with hem-o-lock clips or harmonic shears. Once the disease-free rectal wall is circumferentially mobilized, the rectum is transected with an Endo-GIA stapler (in laparoscopy) or a TA stapler (in open procedure). The proximal sigmoid colon is mobilized enough to come down to the pelvis for anastomosis. The proximal bowel is divided and the anvil of a circular stapler is inserted into the bowel and a purse-string suture applied. The colon is returned to the abdomen, the body of the stapler is inserted transanally, and a circular stapled anastomosis is constructed. Specimen extraction can be done by transvaginal route if the vagina has been opened in the course of the operation.

Endometriotic deposits involving the lower third of the rectum (less than 5–8 cm from the anal verge) presents a difficult scenario. Segmental bowel resection in this setting would mean performing a low or ultralow anterior resection. This has been shown to be associated with a higher rate of complications, including anastomotic leakage, rectovaginal fistulae, and bladder dysfunction [54–56]. These patients are better treated with an organ-preserving approach rather than rectal resection [57]. The use of parasympathetic nerve-sparing techniques has been shown to reduce functional problems such as bladder atony, constipation, and sexual dysfunction, which may be related to pelvic denervation after surgery [58].

A technique of full-thickness resection using a transanal circular stapler has been described in small lesions involving the lower rectum [59,60]. Recently, Roman and Tuech described a technique for combined transanal and laparoscopic nodule resection using a Contour Transtar stapler, which can resect a lesion as large as 8 cm and involving 50%–60% of the circumference [61].

POSTOPERATIVE MANAGEMENT

Postoperative recovery is hastened with an enhanced-recovery protocol. Postoperative pain is controlled with epidural analgesia and transdermal patches. Intravenous opioid use is minimized as much as possible. We do not use nasogastric tubes, and oral liquids *ad libitum* are allowed from the first day onward. Soft diet is resumed form the third or fourth postoperative day, once the bowel activity resumes. The urinary catheter is removed after 4 or 5 days.

Postoperative hormonal therapy has been shown to reduce the recurrence rate and pain [62,63]. However, it is prudent to wait for 2–4 months after surgery to observe for symptom relief, as immediate application of GnRH analogues has not been shown to offer any added advantage [64]. Persistence of symptoms should also prompt investigation for residual disease that may remain after excision.

TREATMENT OF ENDOMETRIOSIS AT OTHER SITES

It is rare for appendiceal, cecal, or small bowel endometriosis to be symptomatic. Small bowel obstruction has been reported due to fibrosis from nodules, which can cause bowel adhesions, strictures, and kinking [65,66]. The treatment is laparotomy and adhesiolysis. Nodulectomy with wedge excision and primary closure is appropriate for smaller lesions, while larger nodules involving more than half of the bowel circumference need bowel resection and end-to-end anastomosis. Appendiceal involvement may cause acute appendicitis, mucocele formation, or ileocecal intussusception [1]. Treatment is appendectomy.

OUTCOMES OF TREATMENT

Outcomes of treatment of bowel endometriosis have to be evaluated on three main parameters, namely, symptom relief, pregnancy rates, and recurrence rates. Several studies have shown significant improvement in overall quality of life among patients treated surgically [41,67,68]. Bassi et al. [41] reported on quality-of-life parameters in patients undergoing laparoscopic segmental resection of the rectosigmoid. After surgery, pain-related symptoms improved significantly. There was also a significant increase in scores in all the SF-36 domains.

Pregnancy rates are reported to be fairly high among patients who have undergone surgical resection. A large study of 288 women treated with nodulectomy reported an 84% spontaneous or assisted pregnancy rate at a median follow-up of 3.1 years [47]. Laparoscopic approach has been shown to have higher fertility rates than open surgery [69]. Meuleman et al. [70] showed nearly equivalent pregnancy rates in those who underwent bowel resection and those who did not. Cumulative pregnancy rates at 1, 2, and 3 years were 44%, 58%, and 73%, respectively. In a review of studies evaluating reproductive performance after surgery for rectovaginal and rectosigmoid endometriosis, Vercellini et al. [71] reported 39% mean pregnancy rate after surgery in all patients who wanted to become pregnant, out of which, in patients who conceived spontaneously, the pregnancy rate was 24%.

Pain relief has been reported to be excellent at the end of 1 year [72]. Bailey et al. [73] reported 5-year outcomes in 130 women after surgery for colorectal endometriosis: 86% of the patients reported almost complete symptom relief with no recurrence. Similar results were reported by Kavallaris et al. [6], with 72% symptom relief with a mean follow-up of 32 months. The risk of recurrence is quite low if the initial extirpation has been adequate. Koninckx et al. [67] reported that more than 85% of women showed improvement of symptoms and recurrence rates lower than 5%. In studies with more than a 2-year follow-up period, recurrence varies between 4% and 25% [74]. When comparing bowel resection anastomosis groups and mixed study groups (full-thickness disc excision, bowel resection anastomosis, shave/superficial excision), the recurrence rates were 5.8% and 17.6%, respectively [74].

Major complications include rectovaginal fistulae, anastomotic leak, pelvic abscess, and functional problems. In a review by Meuleman et al. [74], in patients undergoing bowel resection anastomosis, there was a 2.7% incidence of rectovaginal fistulae, a 1.5% incidence of anastomotic leakage, and a 0.34% incidence of pelvic abscess; whereas in the mixed surgical group (shave excision + full-thickness disc excision + bowel resection), the reported incidence of rectovaginal fistulae was 0.7%, anastomotic leakage was 0.7%, and abscess was 0.3%.

CONCLUSION

Bowel endometriosis is a complex problem for gynecologists and colorectal surgeons alike. The clinical presentation is varied and often deceptive. Transvaginal ultrasound and MR imaging remain the mainstays of diagnosis. Surgical resection is indicated when symptoms impair quality of life and activities of daily living. A multidisciplinary approach is indicated to improve patient outcomes. The laparoscopic approach has made postoperative recovery quicker and safer. Complete surgical excision results in significant improvement in quality of life, fertility, and pain.

REFERENCES

1. Ferrero S, Camerini G, Maggiore ULR, Venturini PL, Biscaldi E, Remorgida V. Bowel endometriosis: Recent insights and unsolved problems. *World J Gastroint Surg* 2011;3(3):31–8.

2. Remorgida V, Ferrero S, Fulcheri E, Ragni N, Martin DC. Bowel endometriosis: Presentation, diagnosis, and treatment. *Obstet Gynecol Surv* 2007;62(7):461–70.

3. Koninckx PR, Martin DC. Deep endometriosis: A consequence of infiltration or retraction or possibly adenomyosis externa? *Fertil Steril* 1992;58(5):924–8.

4. Redwine DB. Ovarian endometriosis: A marker for more extensive pelvic and intestinal disease. *Fertil Steril* 1999;72(2):310–5.

5. Chapron C, Chopin N, Borghese B et al. Deeply infiltrating endometriosis: Pathogenetic implications of the anatomical distribution. *Hum Reprod* 2006;21(7):1839–45.

6. Kavallaris A, Kohler C, Kuhne-Heid R, Schneider A. Histopathological extent of rectal invasion by rectovaginal endometriosis. *Hum Reprod* 2003;18(6):1323–7.

7. Kaufman LC, Smyrk TC, Levy MJ, Enders FT, Oxentenko AS. Symptomatic intestinal endometriosis requiring surgical resection: Clinical presentation and preoperative diagnosis. *Am J Gastroenterol* 2011;106(7):1325–32.

8. Haggag H, Solomayer E, Juhasz-Boss I. The treatment of rectal endometriosis and the role of laparoscopic surgery. *Curr Opin Obstet Gynecol* 2011;23(4):278–82.

9. Roman H, Ness J, Suciu N et al. Are digestive symptoms in women presenting with pelvic endometriosis specific to lesion localizations? A preliminary prospective study. *Hum Reprod* 2012;27(12):3440–9.

10. Ribeiro C, Nogueira F, Guerreiro SC, Leao P. Deep infiltrating endometriosis of the colon causing cyclic bleeding. *BMJ Case Rep* 2015;2015.

11. Dragisic KG, Padilla LA, Milad MP. The accuracy of the rectovaginal examination in detecting cul-de-sac disease in patients under general anaesthesia. *Hum Reprod* 2003;18(8):1712–5.

12. Koninckx PR, Meuleman C, Oosterlynck D, Cornillie FJ. Diagnosis of deep endometriosis by clinical examination during menstruation and plasma CA-125 concentration. *Fertil Steril* 1996;65(2):280–7.

13. Khwaja SA, Zakaria R, Carneiro HA, Khwaja HA. Endometriosis: A rare cause of small bowel obstruction. *BMJ Case Rep* 2012;2012.

14. Berker B, Lashay N, Davarpanah R, Marziali M, Nezhat CH, Nezhat C. Laparoscopic appendectomy in patients with endometriosis. *J Minim Invasive Gynecol* 2005;12(3): 206–9.

15. Laskou S, Papavramidis TS, Cheva A et al. Acute appendicitis caused by endometriosis: A case report. *J Med Case Rep* 2011;5:144.

16. Uncu H, Taner D. Appendiceal endometriosis: Two case reports. *Arch Gynecol Obstet* 2008;278(3):273–5.

17. Hasegawa T, Yoshida K, Matsui K. Endometriosis of the appendix resulting in perforated appendicitis. *Case Rep Gastroenterol* 2007;1(1):27–31.

18. Sakaguchi N, Ito M, Sano K, Baba T, Koyama M, Hotchi M. Intussusception of the appendix: A report of three cases with different clinical and pathologic features. *Pathol Int* 1995;45(10):757–61.

19. Bazot M, Lafont C, Rouzier R, Roseau G, Thomassin-Naggara I, Darai E. Diagnostic accuracy of physical examination, transvaginal sonography, rectal endoscopic sonography, and magnetic resonance imaging to diagnose deep infiltrating endometriosis. *Fertil Steril* 2009;92(6):1825–33.

20. Hudelist G, English J, Thomas AE, Tinelli A, Singer CF, Keckstein J. Diagnostic accuracy of transvaginal ultrasound for non-invasive diagnosis of bowel endometriosis: Systematic review and meta-analysis. *Ultrasound Obstet Gynecol* 2011;37(3):257–63.

21. Piketty M, Chopin N, Dousset B et al. Preoperative work-up for patients with deeply infiltrating endometriosis: Transvaginal ultrasonography must definitely be the first-line imaging examination. *Hum Reprod* 2009;24(3):602–7.

22. Bazot M, Darai E. Sonography and MR imaging for the assessment of deep pelvic endometriosis. *J Minim Invasive Gynecol* 2005;12(2):178–85; quiz 7, 86.

23. Koga K, Osuga Y, Yano T et al. Characteristic images of deeply infiltrating rectosigmoid endometriosis on transvaginal and transrectal ultrasonography. *Hum Reprod* 2003;18(6):1328–33.

24. Morotti M, Ferrero S, Bogliolo S, Venturini PL, Remorgida V, Valenzano Menada M. Transvaginal ultrasonography with water-contrast in the rectum in the diagnosis of bowel endometriosis. *Minerva Ginecol* 2010;62(3):179–85.

25. Bazot M, Detchev R, Cortez A, Amouyal P, Uzan S, Darai E. Transvaginal sonography and rectal endoscopic sonography for the assessment of pelvic endometriosis: A preliminary comparison. *Hum Reprod* 2003;18(8):1686–92.

26. Abrao MS, Neme RM, Averbach M, Petta CA, Aldrighi JM. Rectal endoscopic ultrasound with a radial probe in the assessment of rectovaginal endometriosis. *J Am Assoc Gynecol Laparosc* 2004;11(1):50–4.

27. Chapron C, Vieira M, Chopin N et al. Accuracy of rectal endoscopic ultrasonography and magnetic resonance imaging in the diagnosis of rectal involvement for patients presenting with deeply infiltrating endometriosis. *Ultrasound Obstet Gynecol* 2004;24(2):175–9.

28. Faccioli N, Manfredi R, Mainardi P et al. Barium enema evaluation of colonic involvement in endometriosis. *Am J Roentgenol* 2008;190(4):1050–4.

29. Squifflet J, Feger C, Donnez J. Diagnosis and imaging of adenomyotic disease of the retroperitoneal space. *Gynecol Obstet Invest* 2002;54(Suppl 1):43–51.

30. Bazot M, Darai E, Hourani R et al. Deep pelvic endometriosis: MR imaging for diagnosis and prediction of extension of disease. *Radiology* 2004;232(2):379–89.

31. Loubeyre P, Petignat P, Jacob S, Egger JF, Dubuisson JB, Wenger JM. Anatomic distribution of posterior deeply infiltrating endometriosis on MRI after vaginal and rectal gel opacification. *Am J Roentgenol* 2009;192(6):1625–31.

32. Biscaldi E, Ferrero S, Remorgida V, Fulcheri E, Rollandi GA. Rectosigmoid endometriosis with unusual presentation at magnetic resonance imaging. *Fertil Steril* 2009;91(1): 278–80.

33. Biscaldi E, Ferrero S, Remorgida V, Rollandi GA. Bowel endometriosis: CT-enteroclysis. *Abdom Imaging* 2007;32(4):441–50.

34. Biscaldi E, Ferrero S, Fulcheri E, Ragni N, Remorgida V, Rollandi GA. Multislice CT enteroclysis in the diagnosis of bowel endometriosis. *Eur Radiol* 2007;17(1):211–9.

35. Haas D, Chvatal R, Habelsberger A, Wurm P, Schimetta W, Oppelt P. Comparison of revised American Fertility Society and ENZIAN staging: A critical evaluation of classifications of endometriosis on the basis of our patient population. *Fertil Steril* 2011; 95(5):1574–8.

36. Tuttlies F, Keckstein J, Ulrich U et al. ENZIAN-score, a classification of deep infiltrating endometriosis. *Zentralblatt fur Gynakologie* 2005;127(5):275–81.

37. Keckstein J, Wiesinger H. Deep endometriosis, including intestinal involvement—The interdisciplinary approach. *Minim Invasive Ther Allied Technol* 2005;14(3):160–6.

38. Ferrero S, Camerini G, Venturini PL, Biscaldi E, Remorgida V. Progression of bowel endometriosis during treatment with the oral contraceptive pill. *Gynecol Surg* 2011;8(3):311–3.

39. Ferrero S, Camerini G, Ragni N, Menada MV, Venturini PL, Remorgida V. Triptorelin improves intestinal symptoms among patients with colorectal endometriosis. *Int J Gynecol Obstet* 2010;108(3):250–1.

40. Ferrero S, Venturini PL, Ragni N, Camerini G, Remorgida V. Pharmacological treatment of endometriosis: Experience with aromatase inhibitors. *Drugs* 2009;69(8):943–52.

41. Bassi MA, Podgaec S, Dias JA Jr, D'Amico Filho N, Petta CA, Abrao MS. Quality of life after segmental resection of the rectosigmoid by laparoscopy in patients with deep infiltrating endometriosis with bowel involvement. *J Minim Invasive Gynecol* 2011;18(6): 730–3.

42. Thomassin I, Bazot M, Detchev R, Barranger E, Cortez A, Darai E. Symptoms before and after surgical removal of colorectal endometriosis that are assessed by magnetic resonance imaging and rectal endoscopic sonography. *Am J Obstet Gynecol* 2004; 190(5):1264–71.

43. Sibiude J, Santulli P, Marcellin L, Borghese B, Dousset B, Chapron C. Association of history of surgery for endometriosis with severity of deeply infiltrating endometriosis. *Obstet Gynecol* 2014;124(4):709–17.

44. Nirgianakis K, McKinnon B, Imboden S, Knabben L, Gloor B, Mueller MD. Laparoscopic management of bowel endometriosis: Resection margins as a predictor of recurrence. *Acta Obstet Gynecol Scand* 2014;93(12):1262–7.

45. Carmona F, Martinez-Zamora A, Gonzalez X, Gines A, Bunesch L, Balasch J. Does the learning curve of conservative laparoscopic surgery in women with rectovaginal endometriosis impair the recurrence rate? *Fertil Steril* 2009;92(3):868–75.

46. Varol N, Maher P, Healey M et al. Rectal surgery for endometriosis—should we be aggressive? *J Am Assoc Gynecol Laparosc* 2003;10(2):182–9.

47. Donnez J, Squifflet J. Complications, pregnancy and recurrence in a prospective series of 500 patients operated on by the shaving technique for deep rectovaginal endometriotic nodules. *Hum Reprod* 2010;25(8): 1949–58.

48. Fanfani F, Fagotti A, Gagliardi ML et al. Discoid or segmental rectosigmoid resection for deep infiltrating endometriosis: A case-control study. *Fertil Steril* 2010;94(2): 444–9.

49. Nezhat C, Nezhat F, Pennington E, Nezhat CH, Ambroze W. Laparoscopic disk excision and primary repair of the anterior rectal wall for the treatment of full-thickness bowel endometriosis. *Surg Endosc* 1994;8(6):682–5.

50. Abrao MS, Podgaec S, Dias JA Jr, Averbach M, Silva LF, Marino de Carvalho F. Endometriosis lesions that compromise the rectum deeper than the inner muscularis layer have more than 40% of the circumference of the rectum affected by the disease. *J Minim Invasive Gynecol* 2008;15(3):280–5.

51. Anaf V, Simon P, El Nakadi I et al. Relationship between endometriotic foci and nerves in rectovaginal endometriotic nodules. *Hum Reprod* 2000;15(8):1744–50.

52. Remorgida V, Ragni N, Ferrero S, Anserini P, Torelli P, Fulcheri E. How complete is full thickness disc resection of bowel endometriotic lesions? A prospective surgical and histological study. *Hum Reprod* 2005; 20(8):2317–20.

53. Darai E, Dubernard G, Coutant C, Frey C, Rouzier R, Ballester M. Randomized trial of laparoscopically assisted versus open colorectal resection for endometriosis: Morbidity, symptoms, quality of life, and fertility. *Ann Surg* 2010;251(6):1018–23.

54. Ruffo G, Scopelliti F, Scioscia M, Ceccaroni M, Mainardi P, Minelli L. Laparoscopic colorectal resection for deep infiltrating endometriosis: Analysis of 436 cases. *Surg Endosc* 2010;24(1):63–7.

55. Dousset B, Leconte M, Borghese B et al. Complete surgery for low rectal endometriosis: Long-term results of a 100-case prospective study. *Ann Surg* 2010;251(5): 887–95.

56. Zheng Y, Zhang N, Lu W et al. Rectovaginal fistula following surgery for deep infiltrating endometriosis: Does lesion size matter? *J Int Med Res* 2017;46(2):852–64.

57. Roman H, Vassilieff M, Tuech JJ et al. Postoperative digestive function after radical versus conservative surgical philosophy for deep endometriosis infiltrating the rectum. *Fertil Steril* 2013;99(6):1695–704.

58. Possover M, Quakernack J, Chiantera V. The LANN technique to reduce postoperative functional morbidity in laparoscopic radical pelvic surgery. *J Am Coll Surg* 2005; 201(6):913–7.

59. Gordon SJ, Maher PJ, Woods R. Use of the CEEA stapler to avoid ultra-low segmental resection of a full-thickness rectal endometriotic nodule. *J Am Assoc Gynecol Laparosc* 2001;8(2):312–6.

60. Woods RJ, Heriot AG, Chen FC. Anterior rectal wall excision for endometriosis using the circular stapler. *ANZ J Surg* 2003;73(8): 647–8.

61. Roman H, Tuech JJ. New disc excision procedure for low and mid rectal endometriosis nodules using combined transanal and laparoscopic approach. *Colorectal Dis* 2014; 16(7):O253–6.

62. Vercellini P, Somigliana E, Vigano P, De Matteis S, Barbara G, Fedele L. Post-operative endometriosis recurrence: A plea for prevention based on pathogenetic, epidemiological and clinical evidence. *Reprod Biomed Online* 2010;21(2):259–65.

63. Seracchioli R, Mabrouk M, Manuzzi L et al. Post-operative use of oral contraceptive pills for prevention of anatomical relapse or symptom-recurrence after conservative surgery for endometriosis. *Hum Reprod* 2009;24(11):2729–35.

64. Busacca M, Bianchi S, Agnoli B et al. Follow-up of laparoscopic treatment of stage III & IV endometriosis. *J Am Assoc Gynecol Laparosc* 1999;6(1):55–8.

65. De Ceglie A, Bilardi C, Blanchi S et al. Acute small bowel obstruction caused by endometriosis: A case report and review of the literature. *World J Gastroenterol* 2008;14(21):3430–4.

66. Chan DL, Chua D, Ravindran P, Perez Cerdeira M, Mor I. A case report of endometriosis presenting as an acute small bowel obstruction. *Int J Surg Case Rep* 2017;41: 17–9.

67. Koninckx PR, Ussia A, Adamyan L, Wattiez A, Donnez J. Deep endometriosis: Definition, diagnosis, and treatment. *Fertil Steril* 2012;98(3):564–71.

68. Urbach DR, Reedijk M, Richard CS, Lie KI, Ross TM. Bowel resection for intestinal endometriosis. *Dis Colon Rectum* 1998;41(9):1158–64.

69. Ferrero S, Anserini P, Abbamonte LH, Ragni N, Camerini G, Remorgida V. Fertility after bowel resection for endometriosis. *Fertil Steril* 2009;92(1):41–6.

70. Meuleman C, Tomassetti C, Wolthuis A et al. Clinical outcome after radical excision of moderate-severe endometriosis with or without bowel resection and reanastomosis: A prospective cohort study. *Ann Surg* 2014;259(3):522–31.

71. Vercellini P, Barbara G, Buggio L, Frattaruolo MP, Somigliana E, Fedele L. Effect of patient selection on estimate of reproductive success after surgery for rectovaginal endometriosis: Literature review. *Reprod Biomed Online* 2012;24(4):389–95.

72. De Cicco C, Corona R, Schonman R, Mailova K, Ussia A, Koninckx P. Bowel resection for deep endometriosis: A systematic review. *BJOG* 2011;118(3):285–91.

73. Bailey HR, Ott MT, Hartendorp P. Aggressive surgical management for advanced colorectal endometriosis. *Dis Colon Rectum* 1994;37(8):747–53.

74. Meuleman C, Tomassetti C, D'Hoore A et al. Surgical treatment of deeply infiltrating endometriosis with colorectal involvement. *Hum Reprod Update* 2011;17(3):311–26.

12

Adenomyosis and endometriosis

MINAKSHI ROHILLA

INTRODUCTION

Endometriosis is a common gynecological condition seen frequently in reproductive age women. Presence of endometrial glands outside the endometrium is defined as endometriosis, while occurrence of endometrial glands and stroma within the myometrium, associated with myohyperplasia and hypertrophy, is known as adenomyosis [1]. Adenomyosis was first described by Rokitansky in 1860 and von Recklinghausen in 1896 [2]. Adenomyosis is a disease of reproductive age women; however, it is more commonly seen in multiparous perimenopausal women [3]. The current definition of adenomyosis was provided in 1972 by Bird: the benign invasion of endometrium into the myometrium, producing a diffusely enlarged uterus which microscopically exhibits ectopic non-neoplastic, endometrial glands and stroma (connective or supporting tissue of the endometrial cell) surrounded by hypertrophic and hyperplastic myometrium [4].

ETIOPATHOGENESIS

The exact etiology of adenomyosis is still unknown while it is supposed that it may be as a result of injury to the endometrial basal layer secondary to childbirth or dilatation and curettage, causing invasion of endometrial glands into the myometrium. Hyperestrogenism and genetic and immunological factors may also play a part in the etiopathogenesis of adenomyosis.

HISTOPATHOLOGY

A histopathological criterion of more than 2.5 mm depth of endometrial glands below the endometrial interface had been supported by literature; absence of endometrial submucosa is another characteristic feature of adenomyosis [5]. Ectopic endometrial glands undergo hormonal changes throughout the menstrual cycle and cause dysmenorrhea. Adenomyosis can be diffuse in whole myometrium or it may be a localized form resembling leiomyoma, hence known as adenomyoma; however, it cannot be enucleated because of the absence of capsule. Prevalence of adenomyosis in a histopathologically confirmed specimen has been estimated at around 5%–70%; in 6%–24% of women, pelvic endometriosis is associated with other pathologies such as leiomyoma and hyperplasia, and adenocarcinoma, and rarely, has also been found in hysterectomy specimens of adenomyosis [6].

SYMPTOMS AND SIGNS

Approximately 35% of women with adenomyosis are asymptomatic, while 70%–80% of women with adenomyosis present in the fourth and fifth decades of life. Further, 5%–25% of adenomyosis cases may be seen in patients younger than 39 years, and only 5%–10% occur in elderly women more than 60 years of age. Diagnosis is usually made in symptomatic women in the forties and fifties age groups; however, it may be found incidentally in younger women undergoing evaluation for infertility or who have abnormal uterine bleeding and dysmenorrhea. Common clinical presentations are menorrhagia, dysmenorrhea, dyspareunia, and chronic pelvic pain, while some women may rarely present with metrorrhagia or dyschesia. Menorrhagia may happen due to dysfunctional contractility of the myometrium, anovulatory cycles, or hyperplasia of the endometrium. There is a positive association of adenomyosis with age, parity, spontaneous miscarriages, infertility. and surgical termination of pregnancy. Advances in imaging and delayed age of marriage and pregnancy are possibly contributing factors to diagnosis of more cases of adenomyosis in infertile couples. Structural abnormality of the endomyometrial interface, exaggerated immune response, and increased association with endometriosis have been proposed as possible etiologies in infertile couples [7]. Use of tamoxifen in postmenopausal women has also been found to be associated with adenomyosis, possibly because of reactivation of the ectopic endometrial glands. Symptoms may vary depending upon the extent and depth of the disease. Pelvic examination may disclose a tender globular uterus. Specificity of clinical presentation only, is poor, ranging from 2.6% to 26% [2].

CLASSIFICATION

Adenomyosis has been classified according to the extent of endometrial penetration into the myometrium.

Siegler et al. suggested the following numeric grading according to adenomyotic involvement of the myometrium [8]:

- Grade 1: Inner third of myometrium
- Grade 2: Two-thirds of myometrium
- Grade 3: Entire myometrium

Hulka et al. classified the disease by mild and diffuse/severe [9]:

- Mild: Microscopic foci of adenomyosis/inner third of myometrium is involved
- Severe or diffuse: Spread to outer two-thirds of myometrium/entire uterus is involved

A universal grading system would be helpful in better understanding the extent of the disease and to provide prognosis and response to the treatment.

Histologic criteria of adenomyosis should include four parameters [1]:

1. Presence of ectopic endometrium >2.5 mm away from endo myometrial junction
2. Penetration of ectopic endometrium within the myometrium
   I. Mild: One-third
   II. Moderate: Between one-third and two-thirds
   III. Severe: More than two-thirds
3. Degree of spread (number of foci per low-power field)
   I. Grade 1: Less than 3 islets
   II. Grade 2: 4–10 islets
   III. Grade 3: >10 islets
4. Configuration of lesions
   I. Diffuse
   II. Nodular

DIAGNOSIS

Initial workup of menorrhagia and dysmenorrhea should be the same as for any women in that specific age group. Endometrial evaluation after excluding pregnancy and local pathological cause, along with evaluation for any thyroid dysfunction or bleeding disorder, is a must for any perimenopausal woman presenting with abnormal bleeding. Diagnosis of adenomyosis is largely based on the clinical presentation; there is no dependable sensitive and diagnostic test available at present. Honeycomb appearance in hysterosalpingography was used in the past as an imaging modality for diagnosis. Transvaginal ultrasonography (TVS) and MRI of the pelvis have recently emerged as the best possible diagnostic modalities. Findings of TVS may be symmetrical uterine enlargement without any mass effect, unequal enlarged anterior and posterior wall of the uterus, absence of subendometrial anechoic layer, poorly defined hyperechoic areas, and presence of anechoic cyst or lacunae in the myometrium. Sensitivity and specificity of transvaginal ultrasound ranges between 53%–89% and 50%–99% [5]. Increased diffuse or localized thickening of the junctional zone on T2-weighted sagittal images on MRI is suggestive of adenomyosis; normal endomyometrial junctional zone thickness varies from 2 to 8 mm. High-intensity foci of the endometrium normally seen at the endometrial zone may be seen within the myometrium. Literature supports comparable efficacy of TVS and MRI of the pelvis for the diagnosis of adenomyosis uterus; however, MRI may be more useful in cases of diagnostic dilemma between leiomyoma uterus and adenomyosis [2]. MRI is particularly advantageous to know the accurate location and spread of the uterine adenomyosis so that the exact site, direction, and depth of the incision can be decided preoperatively [11]. High cost and low availability still limit the use of MRI routinely.

TREATMENT

Hysterectomy is the mainstay of treatment for women who have completed their families; however, diagnosis of adenomyosis is rarely made with certainty before surgery, and this invites many options of medical therapy. Diagnostic challenges limit well-designed studies targeting treatment of adenomyosis; hence, most therapies are targeted to symptomatic relief only.

Medical therapy

Nonsteroidal anti-inflammatory drugs and tranexamic acid, which is an antifibrinolytic, are effective for relief of symptoms such as dysmenorrhea and in cases of menorrhagia, respectively. Suppression of hypothalamic-pituitary–ovarian axis is the main aim of hormone therapy; hormone therapy in the form of progesterone, oral contraceptive pills (OCPs), levonorgestrel-releasing intrauterine device (LNG-IUD) or danazol-secreting intrauterine device, and gonadotropin-releasing hormone (GnRH) analogues are being used to keep endometriotic implants inactive. Recent literature suggests the use of selective estrogen receptor modulators (SERMs), selective progesterone receptor modulators (SPRMs), and aromatase inhibitors (AIs).

OCPs and high-dose progesterone are used to create a pseudopregnancy-like condition as a result of decidualization and subsequent atrophy of the endometriotic implants. Low-dose OCPs have shown better safety, adequate efficacy, and significant long-term symptomatic relief in women with adenomyosis/endometriosis [12].

Although LNG-IUD is not FDA approved for use in pain related to dysmenorrhea, it has been shown to decrease the severity of dysmenorrhea and has been recommended as a treatment option to reduce the amount of heavy menstrual bleeding and uterine volume often secondary to adenomyosis [13,14]. Irregular menstrual bleeding for the first 3–4 months remains the main complaint of women.

GnRH analogues are known to cause medical menopause and hence lead to atrophy of adenomyoma and ectopic implants, resulting in relief in dysmenorrhea and menstrual bleeding; however they cannot be used for more than 6 months in view of the resultant decrease in bone mineral density and postmenopausal symptoms. GnRH analogues have been found to be very effective in women with infertility and pain secondary to adenomyosis and have resulted in successful deliveries [15]. In a randomized controlled trial, there was no difference in reduction of the Visual Analogue Scale (VAS) for pain related to endometriosis/adenomyosis when GnRH analogues versus LNG-IUD were used for 6 months [16].

Use of danazol has been largely outdated because of serious side effects such as hot flushes, mood instability, and genital atrophy; however, a recently manufactured intrauterine device impregnated with danazol has shown some relief in the symptoms without the same androgenic side effects as with oral danazol [17,18].

Recently, selective estrogen receptor modulators and aromatase inhibitors (AIs) have been introduced as newer medical therapies for endometriosis/adenomyosis. SERMs (e.g., clomiphene, tamoxifen, toremifene, and raloxifene) have a tissue-specific estrogen agonist and antagonist action. Stratton and colleagues experimented with the effectiveness of SERMs in treating chronic pelvic pain associated with endometriosis, but the study had to be terminated early when the SERM group experienced more pain and underwent second surgeries significantly earlier than the controls. However, an exact cause–effect relationship could not be established, and probably, other factors were also implicated in the pelvic pain [19]. The ideal SERM for treatment of adenomyosis would have estrogen-antagonist activity selectively on the endometrium and agonist on other tissues of the body.

Aromatase is an enzyme required for conversion of androgens to estrogens; increased expression of aromatase P450 enzyme receptors [20] in adenomyotic nodules has attracted attention of researchers for a long time for the use of aromatase inhibitors in women with endometriosis and/or adenomyosis. In a systematic review of 10 studies and 250 women by Ferrero et al. in which the effectiveness of AIs in reducing endometriosis-related pain was analyzed, there was improved quality of life with significant reduction in severity of pain when an AI was used in combination with other medical therapies; however, there were increased side effects and recurrence of symptoms on discontinuation of medication in some studies [21].

Surgical therapy

Medical therapy on the whole gives symptomatic temporary relief only; hence, surgical excision of adenomyotic tissue still remains as a mainstay of treatment, especially for young women presenting with severe symptoms or infertility. For a long time, there has been a lack of agreement in the literature regarding an association of adenomyosis with infertility and, hence, the need for conservative surgery in women desirous of preserving the uterus. However, in a recent review and meta-analysis by Vercellini et al., reproductive results in women with or without adenomyosis were compared, and it was found that women with adenomyosis had decreased implantation rates, less clinical pregnancy rates and less live birth rates than women without adenomyosis [22].

Since it is almost impossible to remove adenomyosis completely without hysterectomy, conservative surgery for adenomyosis and complexity of removal of adenomyotic tissue has always been a matter of discussion. Various methods of uterus-preserving surgical techniques in patients with symptomatic adenomyosis have been tried since 1992, initially laparotomy, and later on, various laparoscopic techniques have developed for excision of adenomyosis (Tables 12.1 and 12.2).

Table 12.1 Partial adenomyosis excision (laparotomy/laparoscopic)

No.	Surgical method	Approach	Technique	Results
1.	Classical hysteroplasty/ metroplasty [23,24]	Laparotomy	Classical V-shaped resection of adenomyosis [25]	One successful live birth [24]
2.	Wedge resection of the uterine wall [26]	Laparotomy/ Laparoscopy	Removal of parts of the uterine serosa and adenomyoma via wedge resection	Less effective and high recurrence
3.	Modified reduction surgery [25]	Laparotomy/ Laparoscopy	Cutting of adenomyosis tissue in to thin slices	50.5% live births, 38.8% abortions
4.	Transverse H incision of the uterine wall [27]	Laparotomy	Removal of adenomyoma tissue after wide separation of serosa from myometrium through transverse H incision on body of uterus and closure with subserosal interrupted suture	22.5% live births, 16.1% miscarriages
5.	Wedge-shaped uterine wall removal [28]	Laparotomy	Wedge resection after sagittal incision in the uterus with lamination of layers on endometrial and serosal side; serosal closure-baseball stitch	22.8% live births

Table 12.2 Complete adenomyosis excision

No.	Surgical technique	Details	Results
1.	Double-flap method [25,29]	Complete extraction of adenomyosis without opening the uterine cavity; uterine wall is formed by superimposing the uterine muscle flaps from serosal sides; open surgery and delicate suturing is mandatory. Serosa of first seromuscular flap was stripped before stitching second flap. Laparotomy is preferred; laparoscopic assisted adenomyomectomy can also be performed [29]. Effective for diffuse and nodular adenomyosis.	Symptomatic improvement in all except one at 3 months, hysterectomy in one woman (27 months postsurgery)
2.	Triple-flap method [30]	Complete extraction of adenomyosis under palpation after opening the uterine cavity; uterine wall strengthened by one endometrial muscle and two serosal muscle flaps. Effective for diffuse and nodular adenomyosis via laparotomy.	Return of normal blood flow in 81%. 51% live births by elective cesarean
3.	Asymmetric dissection method [31,25]	Asymmetric, longitudinal dissection of the uterus to divide inside and outside. After opening uterine cavity, adenomyosis was excised leaving >5 mm over endometrial and serosal side as well. Uterine wall constructed with left-side flap overlapping the right side of uterus. Designed for diffuse adenomyosis via laparotomy.	Two pregnancies, postoperative spontaneous rupture of uterus in five cases

LAPAROSCOPIC SURGERY FOR ADENOMYOSIS

Tissue of adenomyosis is fibrotic, hard, and devoid of any capsule or boundary with the normal myometrium; hence, it is best excised when palpated during open surgery. In addition to this, the limited movement of surgical instruments in minimally invasive laparoscopic surgery, until now, makes the laparotomy one of the most judicious methods to resect adenomyosis. Optimum laparoscopic resection can be achieved with localized, nodular adenomyosis; however, diffuse adenomyosis requires extensive dissection with an advanced endosuturing technique to prevent immediate and long-term postoperative complications. Meticulous suturing of the uterine wall is the basis of prevention of rupture of the uterus during future pregnancy. Laparoscopic resection of adenomyosis includes the following steps [25]:

1. Careful inspection of whole abdominal cavity to see and treat endometriosis anywhere else in the pelvis or peritoneal cavity.

2. Ensure adenomyosis versus leiomyoma and operability once again.
3. Incision on the uterus along the adenomyoma–longitudinal or transverse using monopolar needle or harmonic scalpel.
4. Resection of adenomyoma with use of bipolar coagulation judiciously.
5. Suturing of endometrial cavity opened for diffuse endometriosis.
6. Suturing of uterine wall defect space in 2–3 layers.
7. Reinforce uterine wall by double flap method of seromuscular layer.
8. Retrieval of adenomyotic tissue by morcellator or endobag.
9. Laparoscopic-assisted adenomyomectomy can be done by small suprapubic incision for removal of tissue and optimal suturing of uterine wall [29].

Depending upon the skill of the surgeon, the same steps of laparotomy can be followed in laparoscopic surgery as well; however, use of energy sources for coagulation of tissue should be minimized.

Postsurgery results

Postsurgery, there are inconsistent results in the literature regarding improvement in dysmenorrhea, menorrhagia, and fertility rate; pregnancy rate varied from 17% to 72% depending upon the use of assisted reproductive technology. To date, more than 2300 adenomyomectomies have been reported worldwide; out of these, 80% were performed in Japan. Approximately 500 pregnancies had been confirmed and 80% had delivered, including two cases of stillbirths [25]. Twenty-three cases of rupture of the uterus were reported post-adenomyomectomy; there is certainly a higher risk of uterine rupture post-adenomyomectmy than those without history of surgery. Total risk of uterine rupture after adenomyosis is 6%, however it is more than 1% risk due to pregnancy after surgery of adenomyosis than 0.26% in pregnancies after myomectomy [32]. Most of the reports of uterine rupture are post-laparoscopic adenomyomectomies and were unpredictable and silent [33,25].

RUPTURE OF THE UTERUS

All factors linked to poor wound healing of the uterine scar, such as excessive use of electrocoagulation, inadequate reinforcement of the uterine wall leading to improper hemostasis and hematoma formation, postoperative wound infection, and short interval between surgery and future pregnancy may cause rupture of the uterus. Overuse of electrocautery may impair wound healing and dehiscence secondary to tissue necrosis and scarring; there are more reports of histological delay of wound healing with electrocautery than with the use of cold knife or surgical blade [34,35]. Out of all 23 cases of uterine rupture following surgery for adenomyosis, monopolar cautery, laser knife, and other energy sources were used in 17 cases; however, there were no reports of rupture of the uterus following use of cold knife/surgical scalpel only. A maximum 3–12 months of contraceptive advice was offered to the women seeking conception; most of the uterine ruptures postsurgery have been reported with a surgery to pregnancy interval of less than a year. However, a few cases of uterine rupture have been published even after a year of contraception [33,25]. Resumption of blood flow in the resected area of the uterine wall was one of the criteria to allow pregnancy by many authors [30]. Laparoscopic-assisted adenomyomectomy had been reported as a safe substitute to laparotomy which allows better closure of the uterine wall through pfannensteil incision [36].

ENDOMETRIOSIS AND ADENOMYOSIS

Both conditions have similar symptoms such as menorrhagia, dysmenorrhea, and dyspareunia; in adenomyosis, the pain comes about during menstruation, while in endometriosis it may be present pre- and postmenstrual, depending upon the extent of the disease. Endometriosis may present with ovarian endometriomas whereas adenomyosis is usually associated with a tender and enlarged uterus. There is a strong association between adenomyosis and endometriosis; hence, it is a must to thoroughly evaluate at the time of surgery; in order to avoid suboptimal treatment of infertility and incomplete symptomatic relief, it is important to see and treat for any other areas of endometriosis along with adenomyosis in the abdomen and pelvic cavity [10].

CONCLUSION

Adenomyosis is an enigmatic gynecological condition; its diagnosis and management remain a great challenge to physicians. After completion of childbearing, hysterectomy is the only definitive treatment for adenomyosis; however, conservative treatment is also required for women desirous to conceive and in need of symptomatic relief. The plan of management needs to be individualized depending upon the symptoms and desire for further conception; many newer medical treatment modalities and conservative surgical approaches are currently being practiced. Conservative surgical treatment for adenomyosis may be an efficacious alternative for infertile women who fail to conceive after adequate treatment of infertility; however, literature supporting this is still suboptimal.

REFERENCES

1. Vercellini P, Viganò P, Somigliana E, Daguati R, Abbiati A, Fedele L. Adenomyosis: Epidemiological factors. *Best Pract Res Clin Obstet Gynaecol* 2006;20:465–77.
2. Mehasseb MK, Habiba MA. Adenomyosis uteri: An update. *Obstet Gynaecol* 2009;11: 41–7.

3. Levy G, Dehaene A, Laurent N et al. An update on adenomyosis. *Diagn Intervent Imag* 2013;94:3–25.

4. Bird CC, McElin TW, Manalo-Estrella P. The elusive adenomyosis of the uterus - revisited. *Am J Obstet Gynaecol* 1972;112:583–93.

5. Uduwela AS, Perera MA, Aiqing L, Fraser IS. Endometrial–myometrial interface: Relationship to adenomyosis and changes in pregnancy. *Obstet Gynecol Surv* 2000;55: 390–400.

6. Hong SC, Khoo CK. An update on adenomyosis uteri. *Gynecol Minim Invasive Ther* 2016;5:106–8.

7. Nagandla K, Idris N, Nalliah S, Sreeramareddy CT, George SRK, Kanagasabai S. Hormonal treatment for uterine adenomyosis. *Cochrane Database Syst Rev.* 2014;(11). Art. No.: CD011372. doi: 10.1002/14651858.CD011372.

8. Siegler AM, Camilien L. Adenomyosis *J Reprod Med.* 1994 Nov;39(11):841–53.

9. Hulka CA, Hall DA, McCarthy K, Simeone J. Sonographic findings in patients with adenomyosis: Can sonography assist in predicting extent of disease? *AJR Am J Roentgenol.* 2002 Aug;179(2):379–83.

10. Nezhat C, Li A, Abed S, Balassiano E, Soliemannjad R, Nezhat A. Strong association between endometriosis and symptomatic leiomyomas. *JSLS.* 2016;20, e2016.00053.

11. Dueholm M, Lundorf E, Sørensen JS, Ledertoug S, Olesen F, Laursen H. Reproducibility of evaluation of the uterus by transvaginal sonography, hysterosonographic examination, hysteroscopy and magnetic resonance imaging. *Hum Reprod.* 2002;17:195–200.

12. Vercellini P, Vigano P, Somigliana E, Fedele L. Endometriosis: Pathogenesis and treatment. *Nat Rev Endocrinol* 2013;10:261–75.

13. Kauffman RP. Review: Levonorgestrel IU system, OCPs, and antifibrinolytics each reduce bleeding in endometrial dysfunction. *Ann Intern Med* 2013;159:JC10.

14. Farquhar C, Brosens I. Medical and surgical management of adenomyosis. *Best Pract Res Clin Obstet Gynaecol.* 2006;20:603–16.

15. Lin J, Sun C, Zheng H. Gonadotropin-releasing hormone agonists and laparoscopy in the treatment of adenomyosis with infertility. *Chin Med J (Engl)* 2000;113:442–5.

16. Petta CA, Ferriani RA, Abrao MS et al. Randomized clinical trial of a levonorgestrel-releasing intrauterine system and a depot GnRH analogue for the treatment of chronic pelvic pain in women with endometriosis. *Hum Reprod* 2005;20:1993–8.

17. Igarashi M, Abe Y, Fukuda M, Ando A, Miyasaka M, Yoshida M. Novel conservative medical therapy for uterine adenomyosis with a danazol-loaded intrauterine device. *Fertil Steril* 2000;74:412–13.

18. Liu X, Yu S, Guo SW. A pilot study on the use of andrographolide to treat symptomatic adenomyosis. *Gynecol Minim Invasive Ther* 2014;3:119–26.

19. Stratton P, Sinaii N, Segars J et al. Return of chronic pelvic pain from endometriosis after raloxifene treatment: A randomized controlled trial. *Obstet Gynecol* 2008;111: 88–e96.

20. Tsui K-H, Lee W-L, Chen C-Y et al. Medical treatment for adenomyosis and/or adenomyoma. *Taiwanese J Obste Gynecol.* 2014;53: 459–65.

21. Ferrero S, Gillott DJ, Venturini PL, Remorgida V. Use of aromatase inhibitors to treat endometriosis-related pain symptoms: A systematic review. *Reprod Biol Endocrinol.* 2011;9:89.

22. Vercellini P, Consonni D, Dridi D, Bracco B, Frattaruolo MP, Somigliana E. Uterine adenomyosis and *in vitro* fertilization outcome: A systematic review and meta-analysis. *Hum Reprod* 2014;29:964–77.

23. Hyams LL. Adenomyosis, its conservative surgical treatment (hysteroplasty) in young women. *NY State J Med* 1952;52:2778–84.

24. Van Praagh I. Conservative surgical treatment for adenomyosis uteri in young women: Local excision and metroplasty. *Can Med Assoc J* 1965;93:1174–5.

25. Osada H. Uterine adenomyosis and adenomyoma: The surgical approach. *Fertil Steril.* March 2018;109(3):0015–282.

26. Sun AJ, Luo M, Wang W, Chen R, Lang JH. Characteristics and efficacy of modified adenomyomectomy in the treatment of uterine adenomyoma. *Chin Med J (Engl)* 2011;124:1322–6.

27. Fujishita A, Hiraki K, Kitajima M et al. Shikyusenkinsho to shikyu no onzon-chiryo.

[Uterine adenomyosis and uterine preservation treatment.] *J Obstet Gynecol Prac (Tokyo)* 2010;59:769–76.

28. Saremi AT, Bahrami H, Salehian P, Hakak N, Poolad A. Treatment of adenomyomectomy in women with severe uterine adenomyosis using a novel technique. *Reprod Biomed Online.* 2014;28:753–60.

29. Kim J-K, Shin C-S, Ko Y-B, Nam S-Y, Yim H-S, Lee K-H. Laparoscopic assisted adenomyomectomy using double flap method. *Obstet Gynecol Sci* 2014;57(2):128–35.

30. Osada H, Nagaishi M, Teramoto S. Shikyukin furappuho niyoru shikyu-senkinsho tekishutsujutsu: Rinshoteki choki-yogo oyobi shikyuharetsuyobokoka no kento. [Adenomyomectomy by uterine muscle flap method: Clinical outcome and investigation of the preventive effect on uterine rupture.] *Obstet Gynecol (Tokyo)* 2017;84:1303–15.

31. Nishida M, Takano K, Arai Y, Ozone H, Ichikawa R. Conservative surgical management for diffuse uterine adenomyosis. *Fertil Steril* 2010;94:715–9.

32. Sizzi O, Rossetti A, Malzoni M et al. Italian multicenter study on complications of laparoscopic myomectomy. *J Minim Invasive Gynecol* 2007;14:453–62.

33. Iwahashi H, Miyamoto M, Masuyama H et al. Ninshin nijuni-shu ni shikyuharetsu sita shikyusenkinsho kakushutsujutsu go ninshin no ichi-rei. [A case of uterine rupture caused by pregnancy at week 22 of gestation after adenomyomectomy.] *Acta Obstet Gybaecol Jpn* 2017;69:741.

34. Rosin RD, Exarchakos G, Ellis H. An experimental study of gastric healing of following scalpel and diathermy incisions. *Surgery* 1976;79:555–9.

35. Cobellis L, Pecori E, Cobellis G. Comparison of intramural myomectomy scar after laparotomy or laparoscopy. *Int J Gynaecol Obstet* 2004;84:87–8.

36. Nezhat C, Nezhat F, Bess O, Nezhat CH, Mashiach R. Laparoscopically assisted myomectomy: A report of a new technique in 57 cases. *Int J Fertil Menopausal Stud* 1994;39:39–44.

13

Helping a woman afflicted with endometriosis to conceive

SEEMA CHOPRA AND SHALINI GAINDER

Endometriosis is one of the important known causes of infertility. If managed properly in expert hands, the affected women can still hope to conceive. As reported in the literature, infertility in 75% of the couples is a result of anovulation, tubal pathology, or male factor abnormalities. In the remaining 25%, infertility is either unexplained or is due to endometriosis (in up to 40% of these cases). Compared with the general population, the prevalence of endometriosis in infertile women increases up to 50% [1]. Also, the fecundity rate in this subset of the population is quite low, 2%–10% per month in comparison with 15%–20% in fertile couples [2].

A cause-and-effect relationship between endometriosis and infertility is yet to be proved. Still, it is considered an important entity responsible for the inability to conceive. The mechanisms leading to infertility because of endometriosis appear to correlate well with the severity of disease, although the exact mechanism is not well delineated.

STAGE-WISE PROBABLE MECHANISM OF INFERTILITY IN ENDOMETRIOSIS

Mild or minimal endometriosis

In stage 1 endometriosis, the ovaries and fallopian tubes are usually not affected. Therefore, other local factors may be responsible for reproductive failure in these women. These can be: proinflammatory substances secreted by endometriotic implants such as cytokines (IL-1β, IL-8, IL-6, and TNF-α), estradiol, and progesterone, which attract macrophages, vascular endothelial growth factors (VEGFs), and interleukin-8 [3]. The adverse effect of these inflammatory toxins inhibiting natural conception is mainly on the developing follicle, the oocyte, and the fertilized zygote. These also have an effect on tubal motility to some extent. In women with endometriosis undergoing ART, fertilization rates are decreased probably because of oocyte quality, and endometrial receptivity for the embryo is altered, thus leading to a failed ART cycle.

Moderate to severe disease and reproduction

As the disease severity worsens, in addition to all the above factors, pelvic adhesions as a consequence of severe disease inhibit ovulation from ovarian endometrioma, and tubal transport of the ovum and sperm is impaired because of its altered motility.

TREATMENT MODALITIES

Taking into consideration the various factors that cause infertility in women with endometriosis, treatment options include medical management, surgical methods, combined medical and surgical procedures, or assisted reproduction techniques (ARTs). The choice of modality depends upon the stage of disease and patient preference. The baseline factors affecting treatment include age of the woman, duration of infertility, ovarian reserve, semen parameters, and prior surgery for endometriosis.

After initial workup of infertility to correct the underlying causes, if any, the following options can be considered for achieving a successful conception and live birth in women with endometriosis. For women with no or correctable causes, in case of inability to conceive after taking care of these causes, the stage of endometriosis guides the subsequent fertility treatment. In those women with irreversible causes of infertility, one can offer the option to proceed directly to ART [5].

Treatment options can be planned keeping in mind the following factors: age of the woman, stage of disease, objective assessment of ovarian reserve, presence of endometrioma, prior surgery for endometriosis, tubal factor, and ART.

Is it logical to wait for spontaneous conception in women with endometriosis?

For women with an incidental diagnosis of asymptomatic ovarian endometrioma and feature excluding the possibility of malignancy on the basis of imaging and biochemical markers in young women who are planning pregnancy and don't have any menstrual irregularity, they should be encouraged for trial of natural conception before seeking fertility treatment. The ovulation rates remain the same in the affected ovary when compared to the healthy ovary (49.7% vs. 50.3%). Also, the number, size laterality of the endometrioma, or the presence of deep endometriosis had no bearing on ovulation rates. At the same time, waiting for natural conception versus outright fertility treatment and the need of surgery should be revaluated in women with decreased ovarian reserve [6].

Age of the woman and need for treatment

A younger (less than 35 years of age) infertile woman diagnosed with endometriosis can be allowed a period of at least 6 months to try for natural conception with timed mid-cycle intercourse. If she doesn't conceive, ovulation induction with clomiphene + intrauterine insemination (IUI) is a viable, low-cost option with good chances of conception and low incidence of associated risks. This will help enhance follicular development, ovulation, and luteal phase progesterone support and facilitate fertilization after insemination with good-quality sperm. COH (controlled ovarian hyperstimulation) + IUI has a cumulative pregnancy rate of nearly 40% [7]. This treatment plan can be individualized for another woman with the same profile as per her preference and affordability. She may proceed directly for IVF in order to have the maximum chance of a live birth.

Patients over 35 years of age are more likely to be offered assisted conception in view of decreased ovarian reserve with aging. Again, they can plan for ovulation induction if cost is a hindrance. The advantage of proceeding with ART as the first option is better as it reduces the time to pregnancy (median time to pregnancy of 8 and 11 months, respectively) [8]. As an additional benefit, ART offers the option of cryopreservation of excess embryos for use in subsequent ART cycles.

Still, ovulation induction with gonadotropin + IUI is the less preferred option because of the increased rate of multiple gestations, including a 20% rate of twin pregnancy [9]. This can be prevented in ART as the number of embryos transferred is controlled by the clinician.

For couples who do not desire or are unable to proceed with ART, we offer three to five cycles of CC (clomiphene citrate) or an aromatase inhibitor such as letrozole, as per clinical indication, along with IUI.

Stage of disease

In infertile women with laparoscopically confirmed and staged endometriosis as the only cause of infertility, the incidence of spontaneous conception without any intervention is only 30% in moderate endometriosis and nil in cases of severe phenotypes [11]. In minimal to mild endometriosis, use of medical agents such as danazol, GnRH analogues, and OCP for suppression of ovarian function is not effective and is therefore not indicated to improve fertility by increasing rates of ovulation after stopping these agents [12]. The benefit of operative laparoscopy and adhesiolysis is associated with a higher number of pregnancies/live births compared with only diagnostic laparoscopy in this subset of women [13]. Comparison of efficacy of different surgical techniques in terms of postoperative cumulative pregnancy rate after 36 months of procedure was shown to be 87% with CO_2 laser vaporization with or without resection of endometriosis and 71% with monopolar electrocoagulation [14].

The beneficial effect of surgery in mild endometriosis is not of significance, as is also reported in the literature. In order to achieve one additional live birth in women with minimal or mild endometriosis, 12 patients need to undergo surgical treatment, that is, an absolute gain of 8.6% in favor of surgical intervention [15]. Laparoscopic surgery is effective for the treatment of infertility associated with moderate to severe endometriosis. The crude pregnancy rate is 48% and the cumulative spontaneous pregnancy rate within 3 years after surgery varies between 46% and 77% for moderate and 44% and 74% for severe endometriosis [16].

Endometrioma

The presence of ovarian endometrioma is usually classified as rASRM staging of moderate or severe disease. As of now, there is no randomized controlled trial favoring excision of endometrioma to improve spontaneous pregnancy rates. Observational studies have reported a pregnancy rate of 30%–67% one year after surgery. An absolute benefit increase of 25% over background pregnancy rate is expected after considering other confounding factors and publication bias [15].

While deciding on the route of surgical modality of treatment, laparoscopy is preferred over laparotomy as the former offers advantages such as magnified view of operative field, minimal tissue damage, early recovery, and shorter hospital stay [17]. Spontaneous conception rates are best immediately after the first surgery as later on, severe peri-ovarian adhesions are formed which hinder ovum pick up at the fimbrial end. Therefore, fecundability doesn't improve with repeated surgery for endometriosis as was shown in a systematic review that demonstrated a 50% decrease in pregnancy rate after reoperation (i.e., 22% vs. 40% after primary surgery) [18].

Regarding the extent of surgery, according to the ESHRE Guideline 2013 [19], in infertile women with ovarian endometrioma of >3 cm in size, excision of endometrioma capsule increases the spontaneous postoperative pregnancy rate more than ablative surgery, which includes drainage of cyst and electrocoagulation of its wall [20]. For excision of endometrioma, the cyst wall is opened with cold scissors or a laser electrosurgical energy source. The plane of cleavage between the cyst wall and ovarian tissue is identified and the cyst wall is stripped away by applying the principle of traction and counter traction. There is a potential risk of decrease in the ovarian reserve with either technique, secondary to unintentional removal of normal ovarian tissue during excision or due to thermal damage to the ovarian cortex during ablation. This can be explained by the fact that ovarian endometrioma does not have a true capsule and cyst wall thickness is 1.4 ± 0.6 mm. Therefore, removal of some healthy ovarian cortex is inevitable during surgical excision of endometrioma. It has been confirmed that more than 80% of specimens of excised endometrioma show the presence of healthy ovarian tissue on histopathological examination [21,22]. Further, the response to ovarian stimulation is decreased after surgery. Most likely this is not attributable to surgery, as supported by the results of a meta-analysis, which showed that affected ovaries had lower antral follicle counts (AFCs) than contralateral healthy ovaries, both before and after surgery [23].

Also, COH does not predispose to increase in growth or rupture of endometrioma. With respect to oocyte retrieval in the presence of endometrioma, a theoretical increased risk of abscess formation has not been proved [24]. Still, antibiotic prophylaxis may be used by some, although the risk of abscess is negligible [19].

The ESHRE guideline group [19] discussed the importance of women being properly informed about the risk of reduced ovarian function following surgical intervention and even the possible risk of an oophorectomy, according to intraoperative findings at the time of surgery. Another important but controversial aspect of a surgical approach in such patients is that before proceeding for endometrioma surgery, especially if bilateral, the woman should also be informed about the possibility of preoperative oocyte cryopreservation for future fertility treatment [25].

Deep infiltrating endometriosis and infertility treatment

In women with infertility having rectovaginal endometriosis, no advantage of surgery could be demonstrated with respect to reproductive outcome compared to expectant management for 24 months, as the cumulative pregnancy rate was similar in the two groups (44.9% vs. 46.8%) [26]. A few reports in the literature did show postoperative pregnancy rates of 23%–57% after surgical resection of deep endometriosis with colorectal involvement [27]. The effect of treating rectovaginal disease on spontaneous fertility is not well understood as the results may be confounded by simultaneous treatment of other endometriotic lesions as well [12]. It is also possible that relief of dyspareunia after surgery in such women may have a positive contribution in terms of spontaneous conception rates. On the other hand, it should not be forgotten that surgery for deep endometriosis is associated with a high postoperative complication rate of 13.9% and impact of these complications on reproductive performance is not very clear [18].

Endometriosis Fertility Index for prognostication of fertility after surgical staging of endometriosis

The Endometriosis Fertility Index (EFI) [28] is a simple, robust, and validated clinical tool developed after analyzing more than two decades of clinical data; the EFI predicts an infertile endometriosis patient's probability of pregnancy with standard, non-IVF treatment in those women who have undergone surgical staging. It takes into account the surgical least function score, historical factors, and the American Fertility Society (AFS) Score. The total EFI score ranges from 0 to 10, 0 being predictive of no chances of conception. The

postoperative least function score is of importance to predict the pregnancy. It correlates with the AFS scores as the relationship between adhesions and the least function score persists, and the perspectives that adhesions hinder with tubal function leading to infertility and that dense adhesions, especially ovarian, cul-de-sac obliteration, and ovarian endometrioma are also contributors toward preventing conception.

Assisted reproductive techniques (ARTs) and endometriosis

To address the need of assisted reproduction over expectant management in women with mild or minimal endometriosis, and no other detectable cause, surgical reduction of the disease followed by 3–6 cycles of Superovulation (SO) + IUI is likely to give the best chance of live birth without the need for IVF [5]. This was supported by the results of a randomized controlled trial that showed superovulation with gonadotropins and intrauterine insemination has an odds ratio of 5.6 (95% CI, 1.8–17.4) for live birth [5,24].

Another meta-analysis regarding IVF in women with endometriosis compared to controls found that in stage I/II endometriosis, there was a 7% reduction in fertilization rate and no difference in implantation rate and clinical pregnancies compared to controls. The outcome was not favorable in stage III/IV endometriosis, as there was no difference in fertilization rate, and even worse, there was a 21% decrease in the implantation rate as well as clinical pregnancies. Live birth rates were, for all stages of endometriosis, not different [29].

Discussing the role of medical treatment before IVF in women with endometriosis-positive results are seen in terms of more than fourfold increases in the odds of clinical pregnancy rates following ovarian suppression for 3–6 months before IVF with estrogen-progestin pills [30] and a GnRH agonist [31].

Surgery before ART

There are no data to suggest that surgery for an endometrioma prior to IVF will facilitate oocyte retrieval as well as prevent adhesion reformation in the pelvis. The negligible risks of infection of an endometrioma (0%–1.9%) and contamination of follicular fluid with endometrioma contents during oocyte retrieval (2.8%–6.1%) do not justify surgery for the same before IVF treatment [32]. Another worry is the effect of ART treatment protocols on recurrence rates of endometriosis, which has not been confirmed in the literature as there is very much lower possibility of disease progression in terms of pelvic endometriosis and ovarian endometrioma secondary to IVF treatment [19,32]. According to ESHRE guidelines [19], it is recommended to opt for ovarian cystectomy for endometrioma prior to ART, only with the aim to improve chronic pelvic pain or the accessibility of follicles if technically not feasible or if there is suspicion of malignancy.

Hence, in a nutshell, various prognostic factors, which have a bearing on success of an ART cycle include age of the woman, ovarian reserve status, laterality of the disease, number and size of the cysts, symptoms indicating severe disease, any suspicious radiological features, presence of extraovarian disease, and prior history of ovarian surgery [33]. Any such factors that might have a negative influence on the reproductive outcome in infertile women with endometriosis make the woman eligible for IVF treatment directly rather than waiting for spontaneous conception. The guidelines also concluded that cystectomy for an endometrioma larger than 3 cm does not improve pregnancy rates prior to IVF treatment, and surgery should not be considered for this indication alone [19].

Ovarian reserve and endometriosis

Anti-Müllerian hormone (AMH) is a dimeric glycoprotein, which is a member of the transforming growth factor family, exclusively secreted by granulosa cells of primary, preantral, and small antral follicles (4–6 mm) [4], making it an ideal marker of the ovarian reserve. Its values decrease with age. Bentzen and co-workers reported an AMH level decline of 5.6% per year with increasing age [35]. Therefore, four confounders, including age (<40), cyst diameter (>5 cm), baseline serum AMH (≥3.1 ng/mL), and cyst laterality were taken into account for comparison with pre- and postoperative outcome of at least 3-month follow-up after surgery. The initial analysis revealed a marked decline of 1.14 ng/mL, about 38% from baseline, which was sustained for up to 6 months. Therefore, there is a significant 38% decline in AMH after surgery which can have a negative impact on fertility [36].

PREGNANCY AND ENDOMETRIOSIS

It is long-established that pregnancy has a favorable effect on endometriosis and its symptoms such as chronic pelvic pain, primarily by inhibition of ovulation and thus preventing hemorrhage in ectopic endometrial implants. Pregnancy may also lead to altered endocrine, immune-mediated, and angiogenetic changes in these implants. With advances in research, there are studies showing further evidence supporting the effect of endometriosis on pregnancy and its outcomes and vice versa [37]. Symptomatology of endometriosis improves during pregnancy, both due to regression in cyst size as well as an increase in placental estrogen secretion, which helps modulate pain through changes in the peripheral nervous system that sensitize the central response through neuropathic mechanisms (i.e., the nociceptive responses in functional pain syndromes) [38].

During pregnancy after diagnosed endometriosis, as a result of various alterations in hormonal environment, placentation may be abnormally deep into the myometrium and ectopic endometriotic tissue will be incompletely decidualized [39]. These effects have multifactorial etiology, but a progesterone-receptor defect leads to resistance to its actions, thereby causing defective endometriotic stromal cell differentiation and decidualization. Alterations at the molecular level are mainly responsible for this progesterone resistance in endometriosis [40].

Another diagnostic, as well as therapeutic, dilemma is the presence of ovarian endometriomas during pregnancy because of changes in their size and sonological features. It was observed by Ueda and colleagues that pregnancy may lead to decrease in dimensions in 52%, no change in 28%, and there was an increase in 20% of cases [41]. Another study also reported disappearance of endometrioma in 46%, the number remained the same in a significant 33%, decreased in 13%, and increased in 8% [42]. These changes may be secondary to amenorrhea during pregnancy.

Differential diagnosis entertained for decidualized endometriomas during pregnancy are borderline ovarian neoplasms, or benign cystadenofibromas because of the similarities in the sonographic features of these adnexal masses. Although transvaginal ultrasound is considered the gold standard for evaluation of ovarian endometrioma, even this modality has a low sensitivity and specificity during pregnancy [43]. A typical decidualized endometrioma has ground glass or low-level echogenic contents in a unilocular or multiseptated mass along with vascularized papillary projections with smooth outline. These papillations are a feature of malignancy and are present in borderline masses as well as endometriomas with malignant degeneration, but with irregular contour [44]. This differentiation from decidualized endometrioma of pregnancy is important in order to avoid unwarranted surgery. Noncontrast MRI as a diagnostic tool in the case of inconclusive findings on ultrasonography is a safe option in pregnancy [45].

In order to differentiate malignant adnexal masses from endometriosis, biomarkers are not very helpful in pregnancy as CA-125 levels are physiologically raised in pregnancy. Still, high values of 1000 U/mL after 12 weeks of gestation are considered to be of diagnostic significance in such situations [46]. Combined assessment of human epididymis protein 4 (HE4) levels along with CA-125 may be of help as HE4 levels in pregnancy are significantly less than in the nonpregnant premenopausal cohort, especially in women with endometriosis [47].

Addressing the recurrence rates after pregnancy, endometriomas diagnosed prior to IVF conception were not seen on imaging in 40% of such women on postpartum follow-up of up to 18 months [42]. The limitation for studying the recurrence is the fact that the chances of pregnancy depend upon the stage of disease from the beginning [19]. Hence, in surgically staged endometriosis, recurrence is lower in those who conceive than those with infertility, as observed over a period of 2–6 years [37].

COMPLICATIONS DURING PREGNANCY DUE TO ENDOMETRIOSIS

Spontaneous hemoperitoneum (SH)

SH is a rare complication during pregnancy endangering the life of a woman who conceives with the diagnosis of endometriosis. Analysis of 20 such cases of SH due to ruptured utero-ovarian vessels demonstrated bleeding from the uterine surface in 70%, from vessels in the parametrium in 15%,

and from those over the uterosacral ligament in 5%. Decidualization of endometriosis could be confirmed on histopathology of specimens in one-third cases. There was no maternal mortality reported, but a high perinatal mortality rate of 36% was associated with this complication [38].

Infected endometrioma/rupture of endometrioma

These are extremely rarely reported events, but should be considered in women who develop pelvic pain during pregnancy with prior diagnosis of ovarian endometriosis. Once diagnosed, it usually requires surgical intervention followed by drainage of the abscess [41]. Sometimes ruptured endometrioma presents as acute abdomen itself implies pain. This is encountered in 30% of cases, mostly in pregnancies after ART with a history of interventional procedures during the IVF cycle [37].

Uterine rupture

Very rarely, antepartum hemorrhage is due to acute uterine rupture related to endometriosis [48].

Extrapelvic endometriosis

Spread of endometriosis, though rare, is still possible to a location away from the pelvis by any route (i.e., hematogenous, lymphatic, or direct dissemination). This can lead to spontaneous pneumothorax during pregnancy, as has been reported by different authors. It usually presents as respiratory distress and chest pain and can occur in any trimester of pregnancy. One or the other intervention such as thoracoscopy, removal of multiple pleural cysts, pleurodesis, and thoracostomy drainage was carried out in these cases. The presence of decidualized endometriosis tissues was confirmed on histology. Sometimes it may involve the thoracic aorta [37].

Endometriosis and pregnancy outcomes

Because of paucity of data from well-designed prospective trials regarding the effect of endometriosis on the physiology pregnancy, robust clinical evidence is needed to determine the potential association between endometriosis and pregnancy outcome.

Abortion

In an analysis of the results of seven retrospective studies, including those with ART procedures, only two of them could find an association between abortion and endometriosis [37].

Preeclampsia

In a retrospective case control study by the American College of Obstetricians and Gynecologists (ACOG), it was demonstrated that the incidence of preeclampsia was significantly less (0.8%) in women with endometriosis compared with the control group (5.8%). This study had data based on recall, thus the reliability is questionable. Hence, the association between preeclampsia and endometriosis is debatable until we have further evidence in this direction [49].

Preterm labor

As endometriosis is associated with inflammation at the site of ectopic implants as its hallmark, the same inflammatory factors may influence the interaction between decidua/trophoblast and thus lead to alterations in endometrial physiology. The resulting derangements could be responsible for the possible pathogenic event and, therefore, preterm birth. The literature is inconclusive regarding any such definitive association because of heterogeneity in study design and population, disease severity, and its phenotype [50].

Placenta previa

Incidence of abnormal placentation is not increased in women with endometriosis, as was seen in a small case control study, matched for parity and ART procedures.

Gestational diabetes mellitus (GDM)

There is no consistent association between GDM and endometriosis as seen in literature, except one study showing such association [37].

OPERATIVE DELIVERY

Multiple episodes of indeterminate antepartum hemorrhage in women may be the contributor to a two-time increase in cesarean delivery in women with endometriosis. In another study in women who conceived after surgery for endometriosis, 65.4% of women had vaginal birth and 112 (34.6%) underwent cesarean section. The operative delivery rates were higher in women with ovarian endometrioma and peritoneal involvement (40.4%) and rectovaginal endometriosis (42.9%) than in those with less severe disease such as ovarian (20.5%) or peritoneal endometriosis only (31.8%). Cesarean section was mostly for nonrecurrent indications [51].

In a recent study regarding pregnancy after surgically confirmed endometriosis, which included follow-up of 8710 such women for a period of 1–30 years, women with endometriosis compared to those without endometriosis were likely to have worse outcomes beyond 24 weeks of pregnancy. There was significantly higher risk of placenta previa, indeterminate antepartum hemorrhage, postpartum hemorrhage, instrumental vaginal delivery delivery/operative delivery, and preterm birth. While correlation with hypertensive disorders of pregnancy, placental abruption, low birth weight, and neonatal death were not significant [52]. A similar outcome was seen in another meta-analysis from 24 studies, which included 1,924,114 women [53].

FETAL EFFECTS

Data regarding a potential association between endometriosis and increased risk of a small for gestational age (SGA) baby are still controversial. The results from various studies, mostly involving ART populations supporting the association [50], as well as refuting it [42], are available. An Italian study [51] and a large Swedish retrospective cohort study [54] also showed the same result denying an association between endometriosis and SGA babies. In a study [51] comparing spontaneous conception, singleton pregnancy following surgical treatment for endometriosis, the risk of SGA and low birth weight babies as the outcome was similar in the different phenotypes of endometriosis and was equivalent to their national population-based statistics.

CONCLUSION

In conclusion, although endometriosis is a known cause of infertility, still various treatment options are available for such infertile couples. Multimodality management helps the patient to conceive and achieve live birth. Relevant guidelines are there, which should be followed to have a successful fertility outcome. The effect of endometriosis on pregnancy, and of the pregnancy on evolution of disease, is debatable.

REFERENCES

1. D'Hooge T, Debrock S, Hill J, Meuleman C. Endometriosis and subfertility: Is relationship resolved? *Semin Reprod Med* 2003;21:243–54.
2. The Practice Committee of the American Society for Reproductive Medicine. Endometriosis and fertility. *Fertil Steril* 2004;81:1441–6.
3. Piva M, Horrowitz G, Sharpe-Timms KL. Interleukin-6 differentially stimulates haptoglobin production by peritoneal and endometriotic cells in vitro: A model for endometrial peritoneal interaction in endometriosis. *J Clin Endocrino IMetab* 2001;86:2553–61.
4. Burney R, Talbi S, Hamilton A. Gene expression analysis of endometrium reveals progesterone resistance and candidate susceptibility genes in women with endometriosis. *Endocrinology* 2007;148:3814–26.
5. Mavrelos D, Saridogan E. Treatment of Endometriosis in Women Desiring Fertility. *J Obstet Gynecol India* 2015;65(1):11–6, 8–24. doi: 10.1007/s13224-014-0652-y. [Epub 2015 Jan 22. Review]
6. Leone Roberti Maggiore U, Scala C, Venturini PL, Remorgida V, Ferrero S. Endometriotic ovarian cysts do not negatively affect the rate of spontaneous ovulation. *Hum Reprod* 2015;30:299–307.
7. Dickey RP, Taylor SN, Lu PY, Sartor BM, Rye PH, Pyrzak R. Effect of diagnosis, age, sperm quality, and number of preovulatory follicles on the outcome of multiple cycles of clomiphene citrate-intrauterine insemination. *Fertil Steril* 2002;78(5):1088.
8. Reindollar RH, Regan MM, Neumann PJ et al. A randomized clinical trial to evaluate optimal treatment for unexplained infertility: The fast track and standard treatment (FASTT) trial. *Fertil Steril* 2010;94:888.
9. Guzick DS, Carson SA, Coutifaris C et al. Efficacy of superovulation and intrauterine insemination in the treatment of infertility. National Cooperative Reproductive Medicine Network. *N Engl J Med* 1999;340:177.
10. Hornstein MD, Gibbons WE. Treatment of infertility in women with endometriosis. In: Barbieri RL, Eckler K, eds. *Up To Date*. August 2019.
11. Olive DL, Stohs GF, Metzger DA, Franklin RR. Expectant management and hydrotubations in the treatment of endometriosis-associated infertility. *Fertil Steril* 1985;44:35–41.
12. Hughes E, Brown J, Collins JJ, Farquhar C, Fedorkow DM, Vandekerckhove P. Ovulation suppression for endometriosis for women with subfertility. *Cochrane Database Syst Rev* 2007;(3):CD000155. [Review. PMID: 17636607.]
13. Jacobson TZ, Duffy JM, Barlow D, Farquhar C, Koninckx PR, Olive D. Laparoscopic surgery for subfertility associated with endometriosis. *Cochrane Database Syst Rev* 2010;(1):CD001398. doi:10.1002/14651858. CD001398.pub2.
14. Chang FH, Chou HH, Soong YK, Chang MY, Lee CL, Lai YM. Efficacy of isotopic 13CO2 laser laparoscopic evaporation in the treatment of infertile patients with minimal and mild endometriosis: A life table cumulative pregnancy rates study. *J Am Assoc Gynecol Laparosc* 1997;4:219–23.
15. Vercellini P, Somigliana E, Viganò P et al. Surgery for endometriosis-associated infertility: A pragmatic approach. *Hum Reprod (Oxford, England)*. 2009;24:254–69.
16. Vercellini P, Fedele L, Aimi G, De Giorgi O, Consonni D, Crosignani PG. Reproductive performance, pain recurrence and disease relapse after conservative surgical treatment for endometriosis: The predictive value of the current classification system. *Hum Reprod* 2006a;21:2679–85.
17. Royal College of Obstetricians and Gynaecologists. *Green-Top Guideline No. 24: Endometriosis, Investigation and Management*. London: Royal College of Obstetricians and Gynaecologists, 2006.
18. Vercellini P, Somigliana E, Daguati R, Barbara G, Abbiati A, Fedele L. The second time around: Reproductive performance after repetitive versus primary surgery for endometriosis. *Fertil Steril* 2009;92:1253–5.
19. Dunselman GA, Vermeulen N, Becker C et al. ESHRE guideline: Management of women with endometriosis. *Hum Reprod* 2014;29:400–12.

20. Hart RJ, Hickey M, Maouris P, Buckett W. Excisional surgery versus ablative surgery for ovarian endometriomata. *Cochrane Database Syst Rev* 2008;(2):CD004992. [Edited (no change to conclusions), published in Issue 5, 2011.]

21. Muzii L, Bianchi A, Bellati F et al. Histologic analysis of endometriomas: What the surgeon needs to know. *Fertil Steril.* 2007;87:362–6.

22. Donnez J, Squifflet J, Jadoul P, Lousse JC, Dolmans MM, Donnez O. Fertility preservation in women with ovarian endometriosis. *Front Biosci (Elite Ed)* 2012;4:1654–62.

23. Muzii L, Di Tucci C, Di Feliciantonio M et al. The effect of surgery for endometrioma on ovarian reserve evaluated by antral follicle count: A systematic review and meta-analysis. *Hum Reprod.* 2014;29(10):2190–8. doi:10.1093/humrep/deu199.

24. Koch J, Rowan K, Rombauts L, Yazdani A, Chapman M, Johnson N. Endometriosis and fertility – a consensus statement from a ACCEPT. *Aust N Z J Obstet Gynaecol* 2012;52:513–22.

25. Somigliana E, Berlanda N, Benaglia L, Vigano P, Vercellini P, Fedele L. Surgical excision of endometriomas and ovarian reserve: A systematic review on serum anti-Müllerian hormone level modifications. *Fertil Steril* 2012;98:1531–8.

26. Vercellini P, Pietropaolo G, De Giorgi O, Daguati R, Pasin R, Crosignani PG. Reproductive performance in infertile women with rectovaginal endometriosis: Is surgery worthwhile? *Am J Obstet Gynecol* 2006;195:1303–10.

27. Meuleman C, Tomassetti C, D'Hoore A et al. Surgical treatment of deeply infiltrating endometriosis with colorectal involvement. *Hum Reprod Update.* 2011;17:311–26.

28. Adamson GD, Pasta DJ. Endometriosis Fertility Index: The new, validated endometriosis staging system. *Fertil Steril* 2010; 94:1609–15. 2010 by American Society for Reproductive Medicine.)

29. Harb HM, Gallos ID, Harb M, Coomarasamy A. The effect of endometriosis on in vitro fertilization outcome: A systematic review and meta-analysis. *BJOG* 2013;120(11):1308–20.

30. de Ziegler D, Gayet V, Aubriot FX et al. Use of oral contraceptives in women with endometriosis before assisted reproduction treatment improves outcomes. *Fertil Steril* 2010;94:2796–9.

31. Sallam HN, Garcia-Velasco JA, Dias S, Arici A, Abou-Setta AM. Long-term pituitary down-regulation before in vitro fertilization (IVF) for women with endometriosis. *Cochrane Database Syst Rev* 2006;(1):CD004635.

32. Jayaprakasan K, Becker C, Mittal M on behalf of the Royal College of Obstetricians and Gynaecologists. The Effect of Surgery for Endometriomas on Fertility. Scientific Impact Paper No. 55. *BJOG* 2017;125:e19–28.

33. Alborzi S, Keramati P, Younesi M, Samsami A, Dadras N. The impact of laparoscopic cystectomy on ovarian reserve in patients with unilateral and bilateral endometriomas. *Fertil Steril* 2014;101:427–34.

34. Weenen C, Laven JS, von Bergh AR et al. Anti-Müllerian hormone expression pattern in the human ovary: Potential implications for initial and cyclic follicle recruitment. *Mol Hum Reprod* 2004;10:77–83

35. Bentzen AJG, Forman JL, Johannsen TH, Pinborg A, Larsen EC, Andersen AN. Ovarian antral follicle subclasses and anti-Müllerian hormone during normal reproductive. *J Clin Endocrinol Metab* 2013;98:1602–11.

36. Mohamed AA, Al-Hussaini TK, Fathalla MM, El Shamy TT, Abdelaal II, Amer SA. The impact of excision of benign nonendometriotic ovarian cysts on ovarian reserve: A systematic review. *Am J Obstet Gynecol.* 2016 Aug;215(2):169–76.

37. Maggiore ULR, Ferrero S, Mangili G, Bergamini A, Inversetti A, Giorgione V, Viganò P, Candiani M. A systematic review on endometriosis during pregnancy: Diagnosis, misdiagnosis, complications and outcomes, *Human Reproduction Update* January/February 2016;22(1):70–103, https://doi.org/10.1093/humupd/dmv045

38. Craft RM. Modulation of pain by estrogens. *Pain* 2007;132:S3–12.

39. Brosens I, Brosens JJ, Fusi L, Al-Sabbagh M, Kuroda K, Benagiano G. Risks of adverse pregnancy outcome in endometriosis. *Fertil Steril* 2012a;98:30–5.

40. Bulun SE, Cheng YH, Yin P, Imir G, Utsunomiya H, Attar E, Innes J, Julie Kim J. Progesterone resistance in endometriosis: Link to failure to metabolize estradiol. *Mol Cell Endocrinol* 2006;248:94–103.

41. Ueda Y, Enomoto T, Miyatake T, Fujita M, Yamamoto R, Kanagawa T, Shimizu H, Kimura T. A retrospective analysis of ovarian endometriosis during pregnancy. *Fertil Steril* 2010;94:78–84.

42. Benaglia L, Bermejo A, Somigliana E, Scarduelli C, Ragni G, Fedele L, Garcia-Velasco Juan A. Pregnancy outcome in women with endometriomas achieving pregnancy through IVF. *Hum Reprod* 2012;27:1663–7.

43. Barbieri M, Somigliana E, Oneda S, Wally Ossola M, Acaia B, Fedele L. Decidualized ovarian endometriosis in pregnancy: A challenging diagnostic entity. *Hum Reprod* 2009;8:1818–24.

44. Testa AC, Timmerman D, Van Holsbeke C et al. Ovarian cancer arising in endometrioid cysts: Ultrasound findings. *Ultrasound Obstet Gynecol* 2011;38:99–106.

45. Morisawa N, Kido A, Kataoka M, Minamiguchi S, Konishi I, Togashi K. Magnetic resonance imaging manifestations of decidualized endometriotic cysts: Comparative study with ovarian cancers associated with endometriotic cysts. *J Comput Assist Tomogr* 2014;38:879–84.

46. Goh W, Bohrer J, Zalud I. Management of the adnexal mass in pregnancy. *Curr Opin Obstet Gynecol* 2014;26:49–53.

47. Moore RG, Miller MC, Eklund EE, Lu KH, Bast RC Jr, Lambert-Messerlian G. Serum levels of the ovarian cancer biomarker HE4 are decreased in pregnancy and increase with age. *Am J Obstet Gynecol* 2012;206:349. e1–349.e7.

48. Chen ZHY, Chen M, Tsai H-D, Wu C-H. Intrapartum uterine rupture associated with a scarred cervix because of a previous rupture of cystic cervical endometriosis. *Taiwan J Obstet Gynecol* 2011;50:95–7.

49. American College of Obstetricians and Gynecologists. Hypertension in pregnancy. *Obstet Gynecol* 2013a;122:1122–31.

50. Conti N, Cevenini G, Vannuccini S, Orlandini C, Valensise H, Gervasi MT, Ghezz i F, Di Tommaso M, Severi FM, Petraglia F. Women with endometriosis at first pregnancy have an increased risk of adverse obstetric outcome. *J Matern Fetal Neonatal Med* 2014;9:1–4.

51. Vercellini P, Parazzini F, Pietropaolo G, Cipriani S, Frattaruolo M, Fedele L. Pregnancy outcome in women with peritoneal, ovarian and rectovaginal endometriosis: A retrospective cohort study. *BJOG* 2012;119:1538–43.

52. Saraswat L, Ayansina DT, Cooper KG, Bhattacharya S, Miligkos D, Horne AW, Bhattacharya S. Pregnancy outcomes in women with endometriosis: A national record linkage study. *BJOG* 2017;124:444–52. 1 ratio.

53. Zullo F, Spagnolo E, Saccone G, Acunzo M, Xodo S, Ceccaroni M, Berghella V. Endometriosis and obstetrics complications: A systematic review and meta-analysis. *Fertility and Sterility*, 2017;108(4):667–672.e5 doi: 10.1016/j.fertnstert.2017.07.019. [Epub 2017 Sep 2. Review. PMID: 28874260]

54. Stephansson O, Kieler H, Granath F, Falconer H. Endometriosis, assisted reproduction technology, and risk of adverse pregnancy outcome. *Hum Reprod* 2009; 24:2341–7.

14

Alternative medicine for endometriosis: Diet and nutrition

NANCY SAHNI

INTRODUCTION

Endometrial tissue that normally lines the uterus sometimes grows outside the uterus inside the abdominal cavity over the peritoneum, which lines the other reproductive organs such as the ovaries, the bladder, the fallopian tubes, and the intestines. These abnormal adhesions as a response to backflow of menstrual blood into the peritoneal cavity, in addition to altered proactive process, induce inflammation and trigger endometriosis due to atypical immune cell behavior. Pain in the pelvic area, obstruction of the bowl, and infertility are some of the effects of atypical adhesions which cumulate as symptoms of endometriosis [1].

Despite best medical and surgical treatment of this disease, there is no foolproof remedy that promises non-recurrence of the same since all these treatments fail to address the cause of the disease, the side effects of the treatment, and quality-of-life outcomes of the patient. More natural treatments need to be explored and researched. "We are what we eat" is an age-old saying that has been scientifically proven in keeping at bay so many diseases and even curing some of them. This adage needs to be explored and researched as far as endometriosis is concerned, since therapeutic dietary modifications have proven to be a boon for such patients [2].

"Let food be your medicine" is a proverb that somewhat holds true for treating painful symptoms related to endometriosis to a great extent. Changes in diet based on scientific knowledge can reduce painful symptoms of cramps and inflammation by reducing bloating and estrogen levels, as well as balancing hormones. Eating natural foods without any additives and preservatives reduces toxic load and therefore helps in relieving symptoms [3].

A well-balanced diet sufficient in macro- and micronutrients naturally helps to improve energy levels as well as boosts immunity. Having a strong immune system means that the gut is healthy and the digestive tract is producing sufficient good bacteria and certain micronutrients that help fight the disease.

Endometriosis can be tackled to a great extent by targeting specific nutrients that help in reducing inflammation. Diet needs to be followed as a therapy to eliminate or alleviate painful symptoms of endometriosis, since these symptoms relate very well to the chemical changes taking place inside the body because of the type of food ingested. The food ingested provides us with macro- and micronutrients as well as encourages or discourages hormone and enzyme production. This very basic function of food is the core of the endometriosis-managing diet plan. By selecting particular food groups targeting specific hormones, enzymes, as well as macro- and micronutrient supply, the bodily discomfort related to endometriosis can be highly dealt with.

The following points need some attention for successful medico-nutritional therapy for endometriosis:

- *Food allergies and food sensitivity*: "We are what we eat" holds true when we look at the way our digestive system works. It takes almost two days for food remnants to pass through the entire digestive tract. While this is being done, nutrients are absorbed in the stomach and small intestines. Digestion is facilitated by number of important enzymes and hormones. It all appears to be a pleasant experience for our body when it receives final nutrients for every organ to function properly, but what if the food is not real food? If the food one eats is artificial food (additives, preservatives, pesticide sprays, hormone-induced food, etc.), our body cannot recognize it and, in the process, becomes confused about its metabolism [4].

  Overindulgence of carbohydrates, caffeine, and alcohol, as well as lack of dietary fiber, etc., all causes a lot of digestive issues that are unpleasant and may trigger endometriosis pain.

  Avoiding food allergies, sensitivities, and artificial foods may reduce endometriosis pain to "0" on a scale of "0–10" for pain severity. This was reported in two cases [5]. The study presents the case of two infertile women severely inflicted with endometriosis pain. After unsuccessful attempts to treat them with surgical and medical management, diet modification was attempted for neutralizing reported food allergies which was highly successful as reported above. These allergies included cane sugar, baker's yeast, wheat, barley malt, rye, and onions in one of the cases and corn, cane sugar, baker's yeast, eggs, milk, peanuts, potatoes, and tomatoes in the second case. It is noteworthy that sugar can be an inflammatory trigger since it causes an acidic environment in body. Therefore it's very important to identify food intolerances and eliminate trigger foods.

- *Trans fats and refined sugars*: A diet high in trans fats may elevate the risk of having endometriosis. In a large sampled study, it was confirmed that women consuming the highest quantities of trans fats were 48% more at risk of having endometriosis [6]. Estrogen is stored in body fat and acts as a fodder for endometriosis. Switching from a high-fat diet to a low-fat diet and from refined carbohydrates to complex carbohydrates has been successful in lowering estrogen levels in women without adjusting the calorie content of the diet. Sugar (a refined carbohydrate) causes an inflammatory reaction and increases inflammation by producing an acidic environment [7]. All bakery items like confectionaries, doughnuts, cakes, biscuits, and pastries are rich in refined sugars as well as trans fats (Figure 14.1).

- *Red meat*: Inflammation is associated with endometriosis, and red meat is associated with elevating inflammation. Higher consumption of red meat is linked to higher inflammatory plasma biomarkers [8]. Some studies point to an association between higher consumption of red meat with increased levels of estrogen, which in turn increases the risk of having endometriosis.

- *Alcoholic and caffeinated beverages*: Data suggest that taking too much alcohol and caffeine-laden drinks such as coffee, tea, soft drinks, energy drinks, and so on, might increase the risk of endometriosis since these elevate the level of estrogen in the body, which is a boost for endometriosis. Therefore, it's better to play it safe by eliminating the same or reducing/restricting the amount. Alcohol weakens the

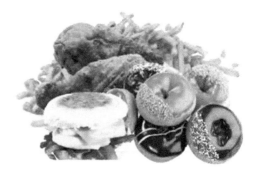

Figure 14.1 Sources of trans fats and refined carbohydrates. Bakery items, fried food.

liver since it consumes vitamin B stored in the liver. A healthy liver helps the body to eliminate excess estrogen (Figure 14.2) [9].

- *Fresh unprocessed food consumption*: Research evidence states that eating enough natural, unprocessed foods like fruits, vegetables, and whole grains free of pesticides and other chemicals (i.e., organic is best; peel and wash fruits and vegetables to minimize toxic chemicals if not organic produce), boosts fiber as well as antioxidant intake, which is linked with a lower risk of endometriosis and even relieves the painful symptoms of women with endometriosis. Antioxidants help fight painful symptoms as well as oxidative stress and optimum fiber intake decreases circulating estrogens. Soluble fiber found in fruit and vegetables (green vegetables, dark green leafy vegetables) are the best option. Grains and pulses provide insoluble fiber. Balance between the two fibers should be maintained.
- *Avoidance of toxins inside and outside your body*: Toxins are found in additives, preservatives, pesticides, insecticides, and so on. It is always advisable to be close to nature and avoid going overboard on convenience foods and preserved, processed foods (imported cold-stored fruits and vegetables) and food packaging (soft plastic wraps, stored or microwaved in plastic), as all these are proinflammatory and increase estrogen load through xeno-estrogens (chemical-based estrogens). Even xeno-estrogens found in toiletries and cosmetics need to be checked and minimized since studies show endometriosis may be linked to excess xeno-estrogen exposure [10].
- *Artificial sweeteners*: Thanks to the "low calorie" notion, nowadays, all "sweet" foods have to be checked twice for the type of sweetener used since use of artificial sweeteners is rampant in packed foods such as cakes, cookies,

and so on, and beverages like colas, juices, and squashes. These sweeteners have been linked with increasing gut motility as the microbial environment in the gastrointestinal (GI) tract is affected by chemicals in artificial sweeteners. Women suffering from endometriosis already face lots of GI issues such as bloating, loose motions, flatulence, and so on. Therefore, use of artificial sweeteners might trigger the already existing GI disturbance. One study has shown a link with the use of artificial sweeteners and elevated estrogen and inflammation [11], which can act as a booster to endometriosis.

DIETARY NUTRIENTS AND THEIR ROLE IN ENDOMETRIOSIS

- *Omega-3 fatty acids*: Omega-3 fatty acids act as anti-inflammatory substances in the body opposite to omega-6 fatty acids, which promote inflammation. Since endometriosis is associated with increased pain and inflammation, eating foods rich in omega-3 fatty acids or precursors of omega-3 fatty acids over omega-6 fatty acids can be beneficial for women suffering from the disease. These are polyunsaturated fatty acids. For a normal metabolism, omega-3 fatty acids are very important. Synthesis of these fatty acids in mammals is impaired; however, mammals can get shorter-chain fatty acids, ALA (alpha linolenic acid), from the food they eat which can be utilized to synthesize omega-3 fatty acids like EPA (eicosapentaenoic acid) and DHA (docosahexaenoic acid). In certain studies, it has been proved that a higher ratio of omega-3 fatty acids over omega-6 fatty acids inhibits the implantation of endometrial cells. Research also states that women consuming higher amounts of omega-3 fatty acids have a lower chance of encountering endometriosis compared with women having lower amounts of the same [12]. The ratio of omega-6 to omega-3 in an ideal diet is 3:1. The richest sources of omega-3 fatty acids include oily fish, fish oil, walnuts, sunflower seeds, flax seeds, chia seeds, pumpkin seeds, and dark green leafy vegetables (Figure 14.3).
- *Micronutrients*: Patients with endometriosis have elevated markers of lipid peroxidation, i.e., higher oxidized lipoproteins and lower antioxidants

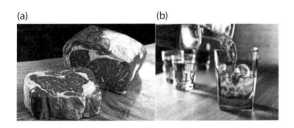

(a)   (b)

Figure 14.2 **(a)** Red meat. **(b)** Alcohol.

(a) (b) (c)

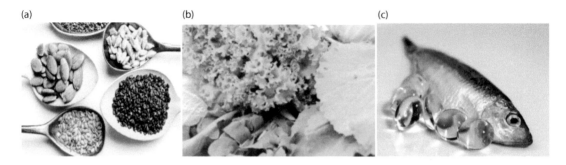

Figure 14.3 Sources of omega-3 fatty acids. (a) Seeds: pumpkin, sunflower, chia, flax. (b) Green leafy vegetables. (c) Oily fish and fish oil supplements.

in peritoneal fluid. There is an enhancement in generation of reactive oxygen species (ROS) by peritoneal fluid macrophages. In one study, patients were administered 1200 IU of vitamin E and 100 mg of vitamin C for a period of 8 weeks, which resulted in a considerable decrease in inflammatory markers and significantly reduced pelvic pain [13]. This indicates that the diet should be rich in micronutrients.

Vitamin C can be easily incorporated in the diet by simply squeezing some lemon juice on daily

(a) (b)

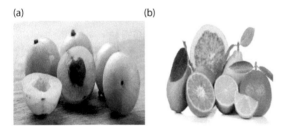

Figure 14.4 Sources of vitamin C. (a) Indian gooseberry. (b) Citrus fruits: orange, grapefruit, lemon, sweet lime.

vegetables and pulses as well as on salads and in soups. Incorporate fruits in a daily diet. Citrus fruits provide approximately 50 mg of vitamin C/100 g. Other fruits like guava also provide a good amount of vitamin C. Uncooked greens like broccoli and leafy vegetables provide approximately 100 mg/100 g. Indian gooseberry (amla) alone provides approximately 600 mg/100 g (Figure 14.4) [14].

Vitamin E–rich sources are nuts and oil seeds, for example, sunflower seeds (35 mg/100 g), almonds (26 mg/100 g), hazelnuts (15 mg/100 g), peanuts (9 mg/100 g), pumpkin seeds (2.2 mg/100 g), and so on. A handful of nuts and seeds should be a part of daily diet. Certain oils are very rich in vitamin E. Wheat germ oil provides approximately 150 mg/100 g, sunflower oil and almond oil—40 mg/100 g, cotton seed oil and safflower oil—35 mg/100 g, rice bran oil—32 mg/100 g, and canola oil—18 mg/100 g (Figure 14.5) [15].

- *Zinc:* Zinc has long been known for its role in boosting antioxidant reactions and curtailing oxidative stress. It interferes with the biological processes like inflammation, which is a base of

(a) (b) (c) (d)

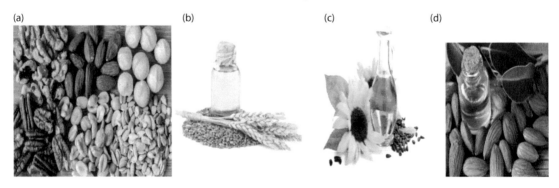

Figure 14.5 Sources of vitamin E. (a) Nuts and seeds: walnuts, peanuts, hazelnuts, sunflower seeds, pumpkin seeds, almonds, pecans. (b) Wheat germ oil. (c) Sunflower oil. (d) Almond oil.

(a)   (b)   (c)   (d)

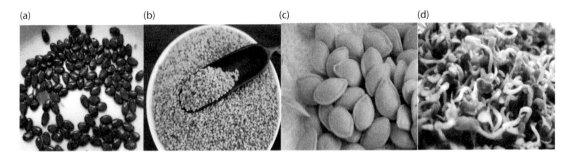

Figure 14.6 Sources of zinc. (a) Watermelon seeds. (b) Sesame seeds. (c) Squash seeds. (d) Sprouts.

development for lesions. Studies also indicate that endometriosis-afflicted women have lower serum zinc levels [16].

One should try to fulfill the zinc requirements from natural sources, that is, dietary intake. A significant amount of zinc with good bioavailability is available in pumpkin seeds, watermelon seeds, sesame seeds, squash seeds, and nuts like cashew nuts (Figure 14.6) [15]. Zinc is found in grains as well but is not so much available to the body due to the presence of phytates. Some processes such as fermentation and sprouting of grains improve the bioavailability of zinc from grains. Other rich sources like seafood and oysters are not accessible everywhere.

Judicious combinations in the diet can fulfill the daily requirement with convenience. Knowledge about how to do so is a must.

FUNCTIONAL FOODS HELP IN TACKLING ENDOMETRIOSIS WHEN INCORPORATED DAILY IN DIET

- *Turmeric*: Turmeric has a naturally occurring phytochemical called curcumin. This phytochemical is a potent anti-inflammatory, antineoplastic, and is rich in antioxidants. It has been studied by several researchers for its benefit in dealing with endometriosis since it has been found that curcumin suppresses the proliferation of endometrial cells by reducing the E_2 value [17].

  Approximate curcumin content in turmeric is 2%. Along with curcumin, it also contains the curcuminoids demethoxcurcumin and bisdemethoxy curcumin. Seven grams of turmeric powder contains approximately 140 mg of curcumin. Bioavailability of curcumin is increased by 2000% if it is combined with piperine (black pepper) powder and then administered [18].

- *Green tea*: Green tea has 30%–40% of its dry weight of polyphenols, particularly catechins. It contains more catechin concentration than black tea or oolong tea due to the minimal oxidation during processing [19]. Like most polyphenols, catechins and procyandins possess antioxidant activity. Green tea is an immunity booster and expels dioxins (PCBs and PPBs, chemical versions of estrogen) from the body. Cytokines in green tea mediate the regulation of inflammatory responses.

  A potential connection exists between exposure to organochlorine chemicals and the increasing prevalence of endometriosis. Research has proved that catechins in green tea protect or regenerate α-tocopherol in human low-density lipoprotein (LDL), which functions as a major antioxidant in human LDL [20]. Green tea polyphenols can significantly reduce endothelial cell proliferation in a dose-dependent manner and cause the accumulation of cells in the G1 phase without affecting cell viability (Figure 14.7).

SPECIAL DIETS FOR ENDOMETRIOSIS

- *FODMAP restricted diet*: It has been documented that patients suffering from painful endometriosis experience higher visceral sensitivity as compared to irritable bowel syndrome (IBS) patients. This explains the reason for even stage 1 or 2 endometriosis-afflicted patients suffering from severe symptoms, which do not match the stage of the disease [21]. Therefore, following a low FODMAP diet, which is designed to relieve painful symptoms in the intestines, will work

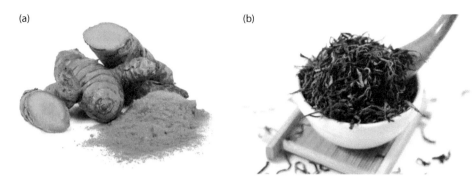

Figure 14.7 Functional foods. (a) Turmeric root powder. (b) Green tea leaves.

for endometriosis-related pain as well. This diet includes avoiding fermentable oligo, di- and monosaccharides, and polyols (found in wheat, barley, onions, garlic, pulses, and beans) since the gut bacteria ferment FODMAPs, which results in gas formation, discomfort, and pain. Research findings reveal that 72% of women having both endometriosis and IBS reported relief after following a low FODMAP diet as compared to 49% of women reporting relief having only IBS [22].

- *Gluten-free diet*: Excluding wheat from the diet has not only proved to be a boon for women that have endometriosis with celiac disease, but also in women without celiac disease [23]. Gluten-free diets have been successful in alleviating symptoms such as inflammation, pain, and bloating. According to a few studies, inflammation caused by celiac disease may also trigger endometriosis. Besides being sensitive to gluten, other factors in wheat, such as phytic acid and phytoestrogens, are also eliminated when excluding wheat from diet. Xeno-estrogens and pesticides present in wheat (related to modified ways of wheat production nowadays due to genetic research changing the amino acid sequence in it) are eliminated as well with a gluten-free diet. Other reasons might be consuming wheat produced from which gliadin protein has been removed or removal of wheat germ that might trigger inflammation [24]. Therefore, by following a wheat-free diet, the food becomes free of all these factors which might trigger painful symptoms of endometriosis.

Last but not least, a word about prostaglandins, which are complex natural fatty acids and are of two types: one act as vasodilators that are involved in inflammation and prevent clot formation, while others act as vasoconstrictors that aid clot formation. PGE2 prostaglandin (elevated levels by consuming saturated fats, red meat, animal fats, fried foods) is found in excess in women suffering from endometriosis which causes pain, inflammation, and contractions of the uterus [25]. Good prostaglandins are found in omega-3 rich fatty acid containing foods (oily fish, walnuts, pumpkin seeds, dark green leafy vegetables). The above-mentioned foods and food groups in this chapter, which have a positive effect on reducing endometriosis, are the ones which increase good prostaglandins as well.

The latest medical and surgical treatments focus more on the symptoms of the disease rather than the disease itself and unfortunately have many side effects. Following a healthy diet plan will also help in hormone rebalancing since natural plant sterols or phyto-estrogens found in certain foods (herbs like parsley, fennel, etc; green vegetables; red and purple berries; nuts and seeds) block estrogen receptors, thereby rejecting excess estrogen.

DIET SUMMARY

Based on the above brief discussion about various nutrients and dietary modifications as a part of medico-nutritional therapy for endometriosis, a summary of food items that should be a part of daily meals include:

- *Green/green leafy vegetables*: 4–5 servings (1 serving = 1/2 cup cooked vegetable) (prefer zucchini, gourds, pumpkin, tomato, red bell pepper, spinach, turnip, potato, mint, carrot, basil, eggplant; avoid cabbage, garlic, onions, mushrooms, green peas, beetroot, lettuce if following a low FODMAP diet plan)

- *Seasonal fruits*: 4 servings (1 serving = 1/2 cup cut fruit or 1/2 cup berries) (prefer citrus fruits, kiwi, pineapple, banana, grapefruit, grapes, lemon, pomegranate, berries; avoid apple, apricot, cherry, plum, peach, mango, pear if following a low FODMAP diet plan)
- *Nuts*: A handful (approximately 1 oz) (almonds, walnuts, pecans, macadamia nuts, peanuts; avoid high FODMAP pistachios)
- *Seeds*: A handful of mixed (approximately 1 oz) (sunflower/pumpkin/melon/sesame)
- *Lentils/pulses*: 1 serving (1 serving = 1/2 cup) (can be consumed in heat-treated sprouts form)
- Cereal: 2–3 servings (1 serving = 1 cup cooked cereal) (choose gluten free—quinoa, rice, buckwheat flour, sorghum flour, millet flour, teff flour, arrowroot flour, brown rice flour, corn flour, maize flour, chickpea flour, tapioca flour, cassava flour—these flours are low FODMAP as well)
- *Fish/poultry/egg* (avoid red meat): 150–200 g/1–2 OR
- *Curd/cottage cheese*: 200 g/50 g
  (For a lactose-free in diet, use almond milk/rice milk/coconut milk—freshly made)
- *Green tea*: 3–5 cups (prefer with basil leaves infused)
- *Chia seeds*: 2 tsp
- *Flax seeds*: 1–2 tsp
- *Turmeric root powder*: 1–3 tsp
- *Lemon*: 1–2
- Limit use of sugar, honey (should be certified organic honey if used) and stay away from artificial sweeteners

The above food items approximately fulfill the macro- and micronutrient requirements along with special nutrients such as omega-3 fatty acids, vitamin C, zinc, curcumin, polyphenols, and catechins. The above diet is also low FODMAP and can be made gluten free by choosing appropriate gluten-free cereals.

Activity: Brisk walking, swimming, badminton, gym, power yoga, etc. (45 minutes to 1 hour twice a day for at least 5 days/week.)

CONCLUSION

"All diseases begin in the gut" is an age-old saying and is very true. Our body gives us many signals that all is not well when one has frequent headaches, regurgitation, flatulence, bloating, nausea, stomachache, loose stools, constipation, and so on; but we are so wrapped up in our day-to-day stresses that we tend to ignore the root cause and take a pill and move on. Too much stress, fasting or feasting, too much sugars and fats, eating on the run, too much of processed foods, and so on, all lead to unhealthy gut. If we look closely, all these are the dietary factors triggering symptoms of endometriosis which millions of women worldwide suffer from. Three important steps are remove, repair, and restore. Remove the offending foods and habits which lead to triggers of the disease; repair the gut by eating healthy, natural, unprocessed, anti-inflammatory foods; and finally restore the gut bacterial flora through all pre- and probiotic via healthy eating habits and lifestyle. This will help in diminishing negative prostaglandins, which are derived from the diet. There is a dire need to conduct nutritional clinical intervention trials to explore and learn the mechanisms of action of certain nutrients in foods on endometriosis and its symptoms.

REFERENCES

1. Herington JL, Bruner-Tran KL, Lucas JA, Osteen KG. Immune interactions in endometriosis. *Expert Rev Clin Immunol* 2011;7:611–26.
2. Francesco S, Adalgisa P, Talia CPB, Silvia P, Maria Rosa B, Emilio P. Hormonal suppression treatment or dietary therapy versus placebo in the control of painful symptoms after conservative surgery for endometriosis stage III–IV - A randomised comparative trial. *Fertil Steril* 2007;88(6):1541–7.
3. Ibarreta D, Daxenberger A, Meyer HHD. Possible health impact of phytoestrogens and xenoestrogens in food. *APMIS* 2001;109(3):161–84.
4. Shin HJ, Cho E, Lee HJ, Fung TT, Rimm E, Rosner B, Manson JE, Wheelan K, Hu FB. Instant noodle intake and dietary patterns are associated with distinct cardiometabolic risk factors in Korea. *J Nutr* 2014;144(12):2094
5. Mason R. 2008. A diet for treating food allergies, sensitivities, and detoxification: An interview with Jeffrey A. Morrison, M.D., C.N.S. *Altern Complement Ther* 2008;14(2):85–90.

6. Missmer SA, Chavarro JE, Malspeis S, Bertone-Johnson ER, Hornstein MD, Spiegelman D, Barbieri RL, Willett WC, Hankinson SE. A prospective study of dietary fat consumption and endometriosis risk. *Hum Reprod* 2010;25(6):1528–35.

7. Monroe BR, James B, David P R, Stephen I, John H, Nathan P. Effects of a high-complex-carbohydrate, low-fat, low-cholesterol diet on levels of serum lipids and estradiol. *Am J Med* 1985;78(1):23–7.

8. Ley SH, Sun Q, Willett WC, Eliassen AH, Wu K, Pan A, Grodstein F, Hu FB. Associations between red meat intake and biomarkers of inflammation and glucose metabolism in women. *Am J ClinNutr.* 2014;99(2):352–60.

9. Bode C, Bode JC. Alcohol's role in the gastrointestinal tract disorders. *Alcohol Health Res World* 1997;21(1):76–83.

10. Keyhan H, Bidgoli SA, Kashi AM. Increased risk of endometriosis by long term exposure to xenoestrogens: A case control study in Iranian women. *JPHS* 2016;4:79–86.

11. Twigg HL. Humoral immune defence (antibodies) recent advances. *Proc Am Thorac Soc* 2005;2:417–21.

12. Parazzini F, Viganò P, Candiani M, Fedele L. Diet and endometriosis risk: A literature review. *Reproductive Biomedicine Online* 2013;26(4):323–36.

13. Santanam N, Kavtaradze N, Murphy A, Dominguez C, Parthasarathy S. Antioxidant supplementation reduces endometriosis-related pelvic pain in human. *Transl Res* 2013;161(3):189–95.

14. Gopalan C, Rama Sastri BV, Balasubramanian SC. *Nutritive value of Indian Foods. Revised and updated by NarasingaRao, DeosthaleY.G, Pant K.C. National Institute of Nutrition.* ICMR 1989;60–4.

15. U.S. Department of Agriculture, Agricultural Research Service. 2011. USDA National Nutrient Database for Standard Reference, Release 24. Nutrient Data Laboratory Home Page, http://www.ars.usda.gov/ba/bhnrc/ndl

16. Messalli EM, Schettino MT, Mainini G, Ercolano S, Fuschillo G, Falcone F, Esposito E, Di Donna MC, De Franciscis P, Torella M. The possible role of zinc in the etiopathogenesis of endometriosis. *Clin Exp Obstet Gynecol* 2014;41(5):541–6.

17. Zhang Y, Cao H, Yu Z, Peng H-Y, Zhang C-J. Curcumin inhibits endometriosis endometrial cells by reducing estradiol production. *Iran J Reprod Med.* 2013;11(5):415–22.

18. Shoba G, Joy D, Joseph T, Majeed M, Rajendran R, Srinivas PS. Influence of piperine on the pharmacokinetics of curcumin in animals and human volunteers. *Planta Med* 1998;64:353–6.

19. Mejia EG, Mares MVR, Puangpraphant S. Bioactive components of tea: Cancer, inflammation and behaviorBrain, *Behavior, and Immunity.* 2009;23(6):721–31.

20. Zhu QY, Huang Y, Tsang D, Chen Z-Y. Regeneration of α-tocopherol in human low-density lipoprotein by green tea catechin. *J Agric Food Chem* 1999;47(5):2020–5.

21. Issa B, Onon TS, Agrawal A, Shekhar C, Morris J, Hamdy S. Visceral hypersensitivity in endometriosis: A new target for treatment? *Gut* 2012;61(3):367–72.

22. Judith SM, Gibson PR, Perry RE, Burgell RE. Endometriosis in patients with irritable bowel syndrome: Specific symptomatic and demographic profile, and response to the low FODMAP diet. *ANZJOG* 2017;57(2):201–5.

23. Caserta D, Matteucci E, Ralli E, Bordi G, Moscarini M. Celiac disease and endometriosis: An insidious and worrisome association hard to diagnose: A case report. *Clin Exp Obstet Gynecol* 2014;41(3):346–8.

24. Monica D, Anne W, Giuditta P, Stefano B, Francesco S. Ancient wheat species and human health: Biochemical and clinical implications. *J Nutr Biochem* 2018;52:1–9.

25. Lethaby A, Duckitt K, Farquhar C. Non-steroidal anti-inflammatory drugs for heavy menstrual bleeding. *Cochrane Database Syst Rev* 2013;(1). Art. No.: CD000400. DOI: 10.1002/14651858.CD000400.pub3

Novel treatment modalities

SEEMA CHOPRA

Endometriosis is a challenging medical condition with debilitating effects on the quality of life of women, as well as their mental and emotional health. More so, it remains a diagnostic dilemma as the symptoms are atypical or sometimes even asymptomatic. The classic triad of dysmenorrhea, dyschezia, and dyspareunia can make one suspicious of the disease entity. The incidence is reported to be 6%–10% in reproductive age, with a much higher prevalence in women with infertility (20%–50%) and is 30%–80% in women with chronic pelvic pain [1,2].

These endometriotic lesions are hormonally active, have excess production of estrogen locally, and exhibit progesterone resistance. The ectopic endometrial implants are estrogen dependent for their growth and persistence. EP-2 leads to activation of cyclic AMP and increases the expression of key steroidogenic genes and aromatase activity, eventually leading to increased intrinsic estradiol production. Also, estradiol produced from ovary and peripheral fat contributes to the progression of endometriotic implants [3].

Also, it is well known that these implants have increased production of proinflammatory cytokines, prostaglandins (PGs), and metalloproteinases which impair the molecular and immunologic functions leading to pain and a failure of the immune system to suppress and clear the inflammatory response [4]. These cytokines, especially IL-1b and angiogenic factors such as vascular endothelial growth factor (VEGF), induce COX-2 expression and increase PG production in endometriotic implants.

There is low progesterone receptor level in these implants and therefore decreased conversion of estradiol to less biologically active estrone. As a result, increased production of estradiol and its decreased clearance is responsible for the growth of endometriosis [5,6]. Hence, these can be suppressed by altering the hormonal milieu as is done in medical management.

The lesions are found primarily on the ovaries, intestines, and pelvic peritoneum and may occasionally involve the pericardium, pleura, lung parenchyma, and brain. The treatment objectives include the relief of pain and the prevention of recurrence. These agents should suppress the synthesis of estrogen, reduce the bleeding, and induce atrophy of the endometriotic implants, thus creating a "pseudo-pregnancy" or "pseudo-menopause" status [7,8]. Although all agents are clinically effective, they differ in their mechanism of action, route of administration, length of therapy, and their side effects. First-line treatment includes oral contraceptives pills and progesterones, which have significant limitations. Thus, it is essential to develop effective and well-tolerated therapies that are optimal for long-term use.

Despite medical, surgical, and combined medical and surgical modalities, the recurrence of endometriosis is estimated to be 21.5% at 2 years and 40%–50% at 5 years [9]. Current hormonal therapies used to treat endometriosis have no role in improving endometriosis-related infertility, and they aim only to alleviate pain symptoms. Thus, these therapies do not definitively "cure" the disease, which may not only persist but may also progress. The effort is to find an ideal treatment option for this recurrent disease entity. For the benefit to the patient, the therapeutic agent should be able to prevent the development of new lesions while inhibiting further growth of already-existing lesions of all endometriosis phenotypes including superficial disease, endometrioma, deep infiltrating endometriosis, and extrapelvic endometriosis, as well as adenomyosis. It should also be able to cure the disease rather than suppress it and treat pain and fertility simultaneously. The drug should be noncontraceptive in nature as the prevalence of endometriosis is high in infertile women and it shouldn't interfere with spontaneous ovulation, and it should not cause teratogenesis if conception occurs while on treatment. The drug should be affordable for its users, safe, and with an acceptable side effect profile as the treatment of endometriosis is long term.

The current treatment with hormone therapy for relief of endometriosis-associated pain is mediated by blocking the hypothalamopituitary-ovarian axis and suppression of ovulation, thereby inducing amenorrhea. On the contrary, the embryo implantation is hindered by associated endometrial atrophy, which is not desirous in patient of infertility. A systematic review of 25 trials [10] failed to show any evidence of benefit with the use of ovulation suppression in women with endometriosis who wished to conceive. As of now, NSAIDs are the only medical option for treatment of chronic pelvic pain in subfertile women with endometriosis, along with the maintenance of fertility.

While current literature indicates that current medical therapy does not resolve endometriomas, symptomatic medical management of ovarian endometriomas is therefore aimed at decreasing their size, preventing rupture, torsion, or development of malignancy [11]. Aggressive disease phenotypes are another risk factor for failure of medical treatment. Consequently, these patients require a multidisciplinary, multimodality approach. Surgical removal of endometrioma laparoscopically usually follows one or the other medical therapy.

TREATMENT MODALITIES

Surgical excision of endometriosis as a primary treatment modality significantly ameliorates pain, with the limitations that it may be associated with the inherent risk of complications due to the procedure and the recurrence of disease and, hence, pain even after surgery [3]. There always is a concern regarding decrease in ovarian reserve after any surgery for ovarian endometrioma. Surgery affects ovarian reserve in women planning pregnancy as shown by a statistically significant postoperative fall of AMH concentration [12]. Hence, endometriosis being a chronic disease, with recurrence over a period of time even after surgery, makes medical therapy of importance in the long-term treatment of this disease entity. Estradiol (E2) is of paramount importance in the maintenance of endometriosis. Hormonal therapies currently used to treat endometriosis-related pain primarily act by suppressing ovulation and, thus, inducing a relatively hypoestrogenic state, and aim only to alleviate pain. Thus, these suppress and do not "cure" the disease. Consequently, when hormonal treatment is discontinued either because of the side effects or the woman's desire to conceive, pain usually recurs [13,14]. First-line hormonal therapies used to treat pain in women with endometriosis are combined oral contraceptives (COCs) and progestins. The current guidelines recommend an accurate diagnostic workup of women with endometriosis prior to administering second-line hormonal agents, namely-GnRH antagonists and agonists, SPRMs, SERMs, and aromatase inhibitors. Other treatments are nonhormonal.

GnRH ANTAGONISTS

GnRH antagonists act by causing direct suppression of gonadotropin release from the pituitary in a dose-dependent manner; this leads to an immediate decrease in the circulating levels of gonadal steroid hormones [15], thus creating a hypoestrogenic environment to treat ectopic endometriotic implants. As compared to GnRH agonists, GnRH antagonists immediately downregulate gonadotropin secretion by competing with the endogenous GnRH for its pituitary receptors. The advantage is avoidance of initial flare usually encountered with agonist use which may improve the compliance of the patients for long-term use. Another advantage over agonists is that circulating estradiol levels in a woman on an antagonist are in a range that is sufficient to avoid menopausal symptoms because of estrogen deprivation. Available preparations include injectables (ganirelix, cetrorelix) and oral nonpeptide forms (elagolix, abarelix, ozarelix, TAK-385) [16]. Cetrorelix (3 mg subcutaneously every week for 2 months) was used in 15 patients after laparoscopic surgery of endometriosis [17]. All patients were symptom-free during the treatment; the serum level of E2 oscillated around a mean concentration of 50 pg/mL, and there was almost complete lack of adverse events related to hypoestrogenism. A minority experienced headache (20%) and irregular bleeding (20%).

Elagolix

Elagolix is a gonadotropin-releasing hormone (GnRH) antagonist rapidly bioavailable after oral administration, which causes the swift decrease of gonadotropins and E2 concentrations [18]. Recently, the U.S. FDA has approved the drug elagolix (Orilissa) for its use in endometriosis, specifically for managing pain in human beings. Safety and efficacy of elagolix for treating endometriosis-associated pain was studied in a phase 2, multicenter, double-blind, RCT that included 155 women [19]. There was no adverse event of estrogen withdrawal with elagolix (150 mg every day or 75 mg twice a day) as compared with subcutaneous depot medroxyprogesterone acetate (MPA) (104 mg/0.65 mL subcutaneously at weeks 1 and 12) for 24 weeks. It caused minimal mean changes from baseline in bone mineral density (BMD) and in blood concentrations of N-telopeptide (a biomarker used to measure the rate of bone turnover) [20]. Recently, double-blind, phase 3, RCTs (Elaris Endometriosis I and Elaris Endometriosis II) assessed the efficacy of elagolix in two different dosages (150 mg once daily and 200 mg twice daily) for treating

endometriosis-related pain symptoms [21]. The recommended dose and duration of use of elagolix is 150 mg, once daily, for up to 24 months and for up to 6 months for the 200 mg, twice-daily therapy. It was shown to significantly reduce the chronic pelvic pain associated with endometriosis, including menstrual as well as nonmenstrual pelvic pain and dyspareunia [19]. In the phase 2 studies, women with endometriosis-associated pain were randomized with either different doses of elagolix (75, 150, or 250 mg) or placebo or depot MPA. The primary and secondary outcomes included the daily assessment of dysmenorrhea, nonmenstrual pelvic pain, and dyspareunia using a modified Biberoglu-Behrman (B&B) Scale, Visual Analogue Scale (VAS), and percentage change in BMD, respectively. The outcome measures were assessed at different time periods of 6, 12, and 24 months. Elagolix showed comparable efficacy for endometriosis-related pain symptoms toward the end of treatment and had minimal impact on BMD. However, there were certain adverse events associated with elagolix such as headache, nausea, and nasopharyngitis [19]. Besides elagolix, phase 2 studies have also assessed the safety and efficacy of cetrorelix, TAK-385 (Relugolix), KLH-2109 (OBE-2109), and ASP1707 in comparison with placebo/other standard drugs for endometriosis treatment. The severity of pain, safety, tolerability, and pharmacokinetics of the drug molecules were studied as outcome measures [22]. The drug was tested in phase 3 trials in two 6-month, randomized, double-blind, placebo-controlled trials in women with moderate to severe endometriosis pain that compared a total of 952 adult women 18–49 years of age with 734 women treated with placebo. It significantly reduced menstrual pain in about 45% of women at a low dose and 75% given a high dose, compared with about 20% with placebo. It caused side effects in around 5% because of hypoestrogenism, such as hot flashes, headaches, and bone thinning. Elagolix is not recommended for women who are planning to conceive or may be pregnant, have osteoporosis, have severe liver disease, or are on OATP1B1 inhibitors.

Sequential weekly administration of cetrorelix in a 3 mg dosage over 8 weeks was shown to be a feasible option to treat endometriosis-associated pain and regression of implants in 60% of patients. Serum estradiol oscillated around a mean concentration of 50 pg/mL during therapy.

Relugolix (TAK-385) is a new oral GnRH-antagonist. A phase 2, open-label, RCT including 397 women with endometriosis-associated pain showed that Relugolix (10 mg, 20 mg, and 40 mg orally once daily) and Leuprolide (LEU) for 24 weeks are equally effective in treating pain symptoms [23]. An ongoing double-blind, placebo-controlled, phase 3 RCT is testing the efficacy and safety of Relugolix (40 mg once daily) co-administered with either 12 or 24 weeks of low-dose E2 (1 mg) and NETA (0.5 mg) in women with endometriosis-associated pain (NCT03204318) [24].

GnRH AGONIST

Used as a second-line therapy, GnRH analogues for the treatment of endometriosis include injectable depot formulations of GnRH-as, which are decapeptides that differ from the endogenous GnRH by the substitution of one or several amino acids. These drugs act by suppressing the production and release of gonadotropins by down regulating the pituitary GnRH receptors and, thus, inhibiting the ovarian production of estrogen. This hypoestrogenism and the subsequent status of amenorrhea induce the regression of endometriotic lesions. However, GnRH-as may also cause several adverse events such as the alteration of lipid profile, depression, hot flushes, urogenital atrophy, and loss of BMD; this of course limits their long-term use. A Cochrane review including 27 studies comparing GnRH-as versus danazol in patients with endometriosis showed no significant difference between the two treatments in improving dysmenorrhea, deep dyspareunia, and noncyclic pelvic pain [25].

GnRH agonists are available in both nasal and injectable forms and offer high rates of pain relief and a longer symptom-free period for up to 12 months. Leuprolide acetate 3.75 mg monthly injection or 11.25 mg used every 3 months; goserelin and nafarelin are the most commonly used preparations. Studies have shown that GnRH agonists cause significant reduction in pelvic pain in women with endometriosis; however, they are approved for continuous use for only up to 6 months due to concerns of side effects secondary to hypoestrogenism, such as bone loss, vaginal atrophy and dryness, hot flashes, and abnormalities in lipid profiles [26]. The addition of add-back therapy provides symptomatic relief and decreases the rate of bone loss. Norethindrone acetate, a progestin, is the only FDA-approved add-back therapy, but low-dose estrogen and a combination of estrogen and progesterone have also been used [27]. The combination of GnRH agonists and norethindrone acetate are only approved for use for a duration of 12 months, as the data beyond that duration are not available. Another limitation of the use of GnRH agonists is that they suppress ovulation and cannot be used in women desiring fertility.

The FDA has approved the use of norethindrone (5 mg daily) as add-back therapy in conjunction with a GnRH agonist. In women who cannot tolerate high-dose norethindrone, a daily combination of transdermal estradiol (25 mcg) and oral medroxyprogesterone acetate (2.5 mg) can be used. However, this regimen may not completely prevent bone mineral loss, and it has not been approved by the FDA. Calcium supplementation (1000 mg daily) is recommended for women taking add-back therapy [28].

Progestins

Although estrogens are the main hormone responsible for growth and progression of ectopic endometrial implants, local progesterone resistance is an important part of pathogenesis of endometriosis. Exogenous progestins decrease the secretion of follicle stimulating hormone and luteinizing hormone by decreasing the frequency and increasing the amplitude of pulsatile GnRH in the hypothalamus.

Various progestins available for the treatment of endometriosis include NETA, CPA, MPA, DSG, ETG, LNG, and dienogest (DNG). These can be administered by different routes: orally, by depot subcutaneous injection, by subdermal implant, or by intrauterine device. Currently, the FDA has approved only depot MPA and NETA as monotherapies for the treatment of endometriosis [28]. The advantage of progestin alone over combination with estrogen is the lower thrombotic risk. Moreover, progestins are better tolerated than COCs in patients suffering migraine with aura and to those suffering migraine without aura in patients of less than 35 years of age, where COC are a relative contraindication [29]. Also progestins have a good tolerability profile with long-term use while spotting, breakthrough bleeding, depression, breast tenderness, and fluid retention are the most frequently encountered adverse events [24,29]. On comparing with other modalities, only MPA in a high dose (100 mg daily) was found to be more efficacious than the placebo. With respect to the route of administration, depot administration of progestins was not found to be superior to other treatments (low-dose COCs or LEU) in improving symptoms [30].

Dienogest

Dienogest (DNG) (17α-hydroxy-3-oxo-19-norpregna-4,9-diene-21-nitrile) is a of 19-nortestosterone [derivative 18], by replacing ethinyl group with cyanometalic group at position 17α. This confers DNG the dual advantage of 19-nortestosterone derivatives in terms of high bioavailability, short plasma half-life, favorable effect on the endometrium and, in addition, those of progesterone derivatives such as antiandrogenic activity and inhibition of gonadotropin secretion. The drug is 90% bound to albumin, and only 10% is present in plasma in the free form [31,32]. The drug does not bind to sex hormone–binding globulin (SHBG) or corticoid-binding globulin, and therefore has no effect on the plasma levels of these proteins. Thus serum levels of testosterone remain unchanged as it is not displaced from its binding protein, the SHBG, and thereby DNG is devoid of the undesirable androgenic effects. Drug interaction with cytochrome CYP3A4 inducers or inhibitor drugs alters the concentration at steady state, as DNG is metabolized primarily by this enzyme. The therapeutic efficacy of DNG is altered when administered in association with estradiol valerate and other enzymes, inducing drugs such as rifampin, carbamazepine, phenobarbital, and phenytoin, or drugs that inhibit CYP3A4 such as erythromycin, ketoconazole, itraconazole, nefazodone, ciprofloxacin, fluvoxamine, and grapefruit juice [33].

As compared to GnRH, DNG (2 mg/day) was found to be as effective as GnRH-as in reducing pelvic pain and growth of endometriotic lesions in a systematic review. Among the different progestins, in a 24-week, open-label, prospective study, the efficacy of DNG for women with rectovaginal endometriosis who had persisting pain symptoms during previous treatment with NETA, DNG was shown to be superior to NETA in improving pain and quality of life. DNG inhibits endometriotic lesions through different mechanisms on the ectopic endometrium. When used continuously, it gives rise to a hyperprogestogenic and hypoestrogenism environment, which leads to decidualization of the ectopic endometrium and, later on, its atrophy.

When DNG is given at a dose of 2 mg/ day, DNG causes only moderate estrogen suppression, the average serum concentrations of E2 remain in the range of 20–50 pg/mL, and this dose is considered sufficient to inhibit endometriotic lesion growth as well as it is adequate to prevent hypoestrogenic side effects [34,35].

DNG is metabolized in the liver; therefore its use is contraindicated in patients with hepatic insufficiency or acute or chronic diseases of the liver. DNG, when administered in a once daily dose starting in mid-cycle, can lead to changes in pituitary and ovarian function according to the time interval between day of administration and the LH surge. For initiation of therapy, administration of 2 mg DNG 48 hours prior to the expected time of ovulation prevents ovulation. If administered 1 day prior to ovulation (0.5 or 2 mg), it doesn't inhibit ovulation but results in a lower LH peak alteration in the function of the corpus luteum. The menstrual cycle remains unaltered when DNG is administered after ovulation. This anovulatory action is reversed after the drug is discontinued [33].

The use of DNG as maintenance therapy after the GnRH agonist to treat pelvic pain associated with endometriosis was studied by Kitawaki et al. [36]. The authors compared a GnRH agonist (leuprolide acetate or buserelin acetate [BA]) for 4–6 months and then DNG (1 mg/day for 12 months) versus only DNG (2 mg/day) for 12 months. Although there was no significant difference in pain reduction between the two groups, the authors concluded that DNG long-term therapy helps to maintain the relief in symptomatology of pelvic pain achieved with the GnRH agonist and also helps in decreasing the irregular vaginal bleeding seen with the DNG in the initial days of therapy.

The objective reduction of the lesions with DNG 1 mg b.i.d. for 24 weeks were observed on second laparoscopy in 66.7% of women. The most frequent adverse effects seen during long-term treatment (52 weeks) with DNG at 2 mg/day in 135 women were headache, constipation, nausea, hot flushes, weight gain, dizziness, and breast tenderness [37].

SELECTIVE PROGESTERONE RECEPTOR MODULATORS

Selective progesterone receptor modulators (SPRMs) bind to the progesterone receptor to block or modify its signaling downstream. They have pure agonist and antagonist, as well as mixed agonist/antagonist, activity. SPRMs seem to act by their anti-proliferative action on endometriotic tissue and decrease the prostaglandin production without risk of hypoestrogenic side effects or bone loss [38].

Mifepristone (RU486)

Being an antiprogestational agent, mifepristone is approved for medical termination of pregnancy. The mechanism of action in treatment of endometriosis is by causing amenorrhea, but doesn't lead to decrease in estrogen levels [39]. Still its use for medical management is restricted as its efficacy in comparison with other available therapeutic agents has not been proved in different trials.

Mifepristone at higher doses (5 and 10 mg daily) significantly improved the symptoms compared to mifepristone at a lower dose (2.5 mg) and to placebo. Moreover, 3.4% of the patients treated with mifepristone had a significant increase in transaminases. The authors concluded that mifepristone at 5 mg was safer and more effective than the other mifepristone doses and placebo. Another recent RCT including 150 patients with endometriosis compared oral gestrinone (2.5 mg twice weekly) and a combined treatment with oral gestrinone (2.5 mg twice weekly) and oral mifepristone (12.5 mg/time once daily). The combined treatment was more efficacious than gestrinone alone in improving dysmenorrhea, dyspareunia, and pelvic pain [40]. The prevalence of symptoms was significantly lower in the 5 mg and 10 mg groups after the treatment compared with the 2.5 mg and placebo group. The 5 mg group had fewer side effects in comparison with other groups [41].

Ulipristal acetate

In experimental studies, ulipristal acetate exhibited proapoptotic effects, thereby causing regression and atrophy of endometriotic lesions in rats. It helps in limiting the cell proliferation, as shown by a decrease in Ki-67 expression. Its anti-inflammatory effect was indicated by a decrease in cyclooxygenase-2 expression [42]. The clinical use of ulipristal acetate as a therapeutic agent for endometriosis is still under evaluation. It is approved as an emergency contraceptive in the United States. Europe and Canada allow ulipristal for the treatment of fibroids [43].

Asoprisnil

Another SPRM, asoprisnil significantly reduces nonmenstrual pelvic pain, which is a hallmark of the triad of chronic pelvic pain in women afflicted with endometriosis. Asoprisnil has been investigated for the treatment of endometriosis. In a randomized, placebo-controlled trial, this drug (5, 10, and 25 mg) caused a greater reduction of endometriosis-related dysmenorrhea compared with a placebo [43].

Tanaproget

Tanaproget is a newly developed SPRM. In vitro studies show this drug to be efficacious in down-regulation of endometrial matrix metalloproteinase expression. It showed regression of experimental endometriosis in in vivo studies in mice with disease established by tissues from patients with endometriosis with use of tanaproget [44]. Still, there is no recommendation for the use of tanaproget in humans.

The main concern with SPRMs is its long-term impact on the endometrial tissue, as these drugs permit an unopposed estrogenic effect on the endometrium that can predispose the patients theoretically to a risk of endometrial cancer. However, these effects are yet to be observed from long-term studies and, until these issues are clarified, there could be an obvious hesitation to use this drug for a period longer than 3 months.

SELECTIVE ESTROGEN RECEPTOR MODULATORS

Selective estrogen receptor modulators (SERMs) have tissue-selective actions, directly bind to estrogen receptor (ER)-α and/or ER-β in target cells, and act as an ER agonist in some tissues and an ER antagonist in other tissues.

An RCT comparing efficacy of 6-month treatment with raloxifene (180 mg daily) with a placebo in patients after laparoscopic excision of endometriosis was halted prematurely as the recurrence of symptoms necessitating surgery was earlier in the treatment group than in those receiving placebo. The partial agonistic activity of raloxifene on ER-α receptors could have been responsible for progression of endometriosis. On the molecular level, this drug has been shown to have agonistic activity to the G-protein-coupled ER (GPR30), which may be the reason for increased pain symptoms (i.e., hyperalgesia in comparison to placebo) [45].

Though in vitro and animal studies have shown that the tissue selective estrogen complex (TSEC) BZA-CEE is able to cause regression of endometriotic lesions [46], the effectiveness in the treatment of endometriosis-related pain in humans is yet to be investigated.

SR-16234 seems to be a purer ER-α antagonist and this characteristic may justify its evident effectiveness in the treatment of endometriosis [47].

NONHORMONAL TREATMENTS

NSAIDs

NSAIDs in varying formulations and dosages such as tolfenamic acid (200 mg three times per day) [48] and naproxen sodium (275 mg four times per day) [49] for the treatment of menstrual pain associated with endometriosis were considered superior to placebo. Although rofecoxib (25 mg per day) improved pelvic pain and dyspareunia secondary to endometriosis [50], the drug was reported to have an increased cardiovascular risk and was withdrawn from further use [51]. Thus, superiority of one drug over the other is not evident in the literature. At the same time, women on long-term prescription NSAIDs must be informed about the adverse events these drugs may be responsible for (such as peptic ulcers, risk of hypertension and cardiovascular events, and acute kidney injury).

HORMONAL THERAPY VERSUS DIET

It is well established that dysmenorrhea improved in patients treated with COCs. An RCT compared hormonal therapy with diet in women with American Society of Reproductive Medicine stage III-IV endometriosis; the study compared the 6-month therapy of COC (EE 0.03 mg and gestoden 0.75 mg) with dietary therapy (vitamins, minerals salts, lactic ferments, fish oil) with placebo and intramuscular triptorelin or leuprorelin (3.75 mg every month). On follow-up after 12 months, women receiving COC or GnRH-as had less severe dysmenorrhea than those receiving placebo or diet. However, efficacy of both hormonal therapies and dietary supplementation were comparable in decreasing the intensity of chronic pelvic pain and dyspareunia [52].

OTHER INVESTIGATIONAL HORMONAL THERAPIES

Aromatase inhibitors

Aromatase is expressed in certain human cells, including ovarian granulosa cells, placental syncytiotrophoblasts, testicular Leydig cells, and other extra glandular sites such as adipose tissue, the brain, and skin fibroblasts. The highest levels of aromatase are in the ovarian granulosa cells in premenopausal women. Women with endometriosis are likely to have underlying molecular abnormalities that allow the continued growth of these ectopic endometrial tissues. There is a direct correlation between local estrogen content of endometriotic lesion with the levels of enzyme aromatase cytochrome P450 responsible for steroidogenesis [4]. Also, levels of aromatase mRNA have been found to be elevated in extraovarian endometriotic lesions and ovarian endometrioma [53]. The primary substrate for aromatase activity as catalyst to give rise to estrone in endometriotic tissue are adrenal and ovarian androstenedione, which is further converted to the more active estradiol [54]. Additionally, ectopic endometriotic ovarian and peritoneal tissues express necessary genes needed to produce estradiol from cholesterol. In endometriosis, aromatase is regulated at the levels of transcriptional expression, protein expression, and enzyme activity [53]. The positive feedback loop because of aromatase favors expression of key genes that are responsible for steroidogenesis. Estrogen so produced in turn stimulates expression of the COX-2 enzyme, resulting in elevated levels of prostaglandin E2 (PGE2), which again is a potent stimulator of aromatase activity in endometriosis. This maintains continuous local production of E2 and PGE2 in endometriotic tissue [4]. There are three generations of aromatase inhibitors (AIs): first-generation inhibitor, glutethimide, induces a medical adrenalectomy, which not only has the desired effect on endometriotic implants, but also leads to side effects such as lethargy, skin rashes, and nausea. The second-generation inhibitors are more selective, include fadrozole and formestancel, and have comparatively fewer side effects. These are administered intramuscularly. The third-generation AIs, including letrozole, anastrazole, and examestane, are derivatives of triazole, ideal for clinical use as these are selective in action, reversible, and potent.

At a dose of 1–5 mg, letrozole and anastrazole inhibit estrogen levels by 97%–99%.

The main limiting factor for use of AIs is association with symptoms of hypoestrogenism such as hot flashes, weight gain, bone and joint pain, muscle aches, and sometimes mood swings, headache, vaginal spotting, fatigue, dizziness, depression, increased appetite, insomnia, rash, and decreased libido [55]. This affects the quality of life and therefore are not suitable for on long-term use for endometriosis and may only be considered in research settings when all other therapeutic options have been exhausted. To evaluate its use in combination with other therapeutic agents in order to decrease its dose and duration to decrease the side effects, a phase 4 RCT compared the combination of ATZ and LEU for prevention of recurrence of endometriosis with LEU as a monotherapy (NCT01769781). Similarly, an intravaginal ring releasing ATZ and LNG is being investigated for the treatment of endometriosis [56]. It has been shown in an RCT that use of an AI in combination with GnRHa for 6 months is more efficacious than GnRHa monotherapy in achieving a longer pain-free interval, as well as recurrence of symptoms, when used as a postoperative adjunctive therapy after conservative surgery for endometriosis [57].

Addition of progestins in combination with AIs was shown to be better than GnRHa in terms of symptomatic improvement and recurrence, as well as side effects. This was shown in an RCT in which women were treated with letrozole and were randomized to receive either oral norethisterone acetate or intramuscular injection of triptorelin; the administration of letrozole reduced the intensity of endometriosis-related pain symptoms, and the adverse events than the combination of letrozole and triptorelin [58]. Similar findings were reported in another nonrandomized trial in terms of improvement in chronic pelvic pain, but interruption of treatment resulted in recurrence of disease in both groups [59]. A prospective RCT compared the clinical efficacy and the adverse event profile of a cocktail regimen of anastrazole and goserelin versus goserelin alone. The recurrence rates in terms of pain were significantly lower in the anastrazole-goserelin group, but there was a greater BMD loss than in the goserelin only group [57]. Although AIs improve the quality of life, the safety of the molecule remains to be a point of concern because of more adverse effects (such as arthralgia and myalgia) [59].

Hence, while short-term treatment with AIs does appear to offer reasonable efficacy, there is not much literature regarding the effect of AI use in the long-term treatment of the disease. This is of relevance as endometriosis is a chronic disease and treatment duration is usually much longer than 6 months. Additionally, long-term therapy of endometriosis with an AI could suppress the aromatase activity within the osteoblasts, leading to increased osteoclastic activity and loss of BMD. While AIs are undoubtedly a valuable option in those failing to respond to conventional therapies, it is essential that the challenges associated with these drugs are addressed in further studies.

INVESTIGATIONAL NONHORMONAL THERAPIES: ANTI-ANGIOGENIC DRUGS

Dopamine receptor-2-agonists

The peritoneal fluid of women with endometriosis consists of pro-angiogenic factors such as vascular endothelial growth factor (VEGF), interleukin (IL)-8, and placenta growth factor. VEGF is a signaling protein produced by cells that stimulates the process of angiogenesis and vasculogenesis and thus plays a vital role in endometriosis. The amount of VEGF present in the peritoneal fluids positively correlates with the severity of disease. Thus, dopamine receptor-2-agonists such as cabergoline and quinagolide have been studied in several animal models [60]. It was observed that both the treatments equally inhibited angiogenesis and reduced the lesion size. In an RCT that compared cabergoline with triptorelin for the treatment of endometrioma, there was a significant decrease in the size of the lesion at the end of treatment in the cabergoline arm (6 4.7% vs. 21.7%) [61]. However, this study did not reveal if cabergoline offered relief of pelvic pain. Besides cabergoline, quinagolide has also shown encouraging results from nonrandomized and preclinical studies.

Statins

In a study by Esfandiari et al., statins were found to be effective in inhibiting the mechanisms of angiogenesis and cell proliferation involved in the development of endometriosis-like tissue. In vivo studies have exhibited that atorvastatin and simvastatin have been effective in decreasing the number and size of experimentally induced endometriotic implants [62].

However, only one RCT has been published that evaluated the effect of statins on endometriosis. This study compared the effectiveness of simvastatin with that of the GnRH agonist triptorelin after surgery for endometriosis; however, no significant difference in severity of dyspareunia, dysmenorrhea, and pelvic pain was observed between the two groups [63]. Thus, it is doubtful whether or not statins could be a potential therapeutic agent for endometriosis, and further investigations are required.

DANAZOL

Danazol, a derivative of 17 a-ethinyltestosterone, is an androgenic agent that inhibits the LH surge and decreases ovarian steroidogenesis by direct inhibition of the ovarian enzymes and is usually given in divided doses of 400–800 mg/d for 6 months. Side effects include acne, hirsutism, deepening of voice, weight gain, muscle cramps, liver dysfunction, and an abnormal lipid profile. As the side effects are mostly associated with oral administration, alternative routes such as a danazol vaginal ring and intrauterine devices are currently undergoing research, and studies have shown improvement in pain symptoms with better tolerability [64].

None of these drugs can eradicate the disease and, in some cases, the substantial side effects limit the long-term use of these therapies. Current medical therapies for endometriosis result in delayed conception and have not been shown to provide any fertility benefit subsequent to treatment.

For these reasons, new drugs that aim at new targets are under development. These include the levonorgestrel-releasing intrauterine device (LNG-IUD), GnRH antagonists, aromatase inhibitors, selective estrogen receptor modulators, progesterone antagonists, selective progesterone receptor modulators, angiogenesis inhibitors, and immunomodulator drugs [1].

IMPLANTS

There is an emerging role for the levonorgestrel-containing intrauterine device in the treatment of endometriosis. Although the exact mechanism of action of the LNG-IUD is unclear, recent evidence shows that the LNG-IUD delivers significant amounts of LNG into the peritoneal fluids, most probably inducing decidualization, which may be mediated through estrogen and progesterone receptor on the endometriotic implants. In the pilot studies in patients with surgically proven peritoneal, as well as rectovaginal, endometriosis, LNG-IUD has promising results as shown by improvement in pain control as well as a reduction in size of the rectovaginal nodules on ultrasonography. There was a significant reduction in symptoms, as well as staging of the disease, as documented in 34 women with laparoscopically confirmed, minimal to moderate endometriosis over a period of 6 months of its use [65]. As peritoneal fluid levels of LNG were closely related to the levels in serum, a Cochrane systematic review evaluated postoperative use of an LNG-IUD in women with endometriosis. It was shown that postoperative use of the LNG-IUD reduces the recurrence of dysmenorrhea in these women. The great advantage is LNG-IUD is that it is a low-cost therapy in the long term with usually fewer side effects than other progestogenic agents as it has local action and requires only one medical intervention in the form of insertion. Still, well-designed studies are required to recommend it as a therapeutic approach in endometriosis.

Subcutaneous implants are commonly marketed as Implanon and Nexplanon and are inserted intradermally. The therapeutic efficacy of depot medroxyprogesterone acetate and incidence of pain relief was compared with the implant by Walch et al. [66], and it was found that both groups had similar side effect profiles and degrees of satisfaction with either modality. Commonly reported side effects include irregular menstrual bleeding, weight gain, nausea, headache, breast tenderness, and acne and are similar to depot medroxyprogesterone acetate. In carefully selected women who do not desire fertility, an etonogestrel implant could be another option for treatment of endometriosis.

FUTURE THERAPIES

Other future therapies include TNF-α (tumor necrosis factor), PPAR-γ (peroxisome proliferator-activated receptor γ) ligands, and pentoxifylline.

TNF-α blockers

TNF-α is a proinflammatory cytokine and its levels have been found to be elevated in the peritoneal fluid of women with endometriosis with a direct correlation with the stage of the disease. Infliximab, a monoclonal antibody against TNF-α and etanercept, a fusion protein with the ability to neutralize TNF-α, are being actively studied in the treatment of endometriosis. In animal models, treatment with these agents has been shown to reduce the size and number of the endometriotic implants along with a decrease in the levels of inflammatory cytokines [67].

PPAR-γ ligands

PPARs are ligand-activated nuclear receptors with a suggested role in inflammation and lipid and glucose metabolism. PPAR-γ ligands have anti-inflammatory properties and reduce estrogen biosynthesis by inhibiting the aromatase enzyme. In experimental models, they have been shown to inhibit cell proliferation, increase apoptosis, and inhibit the growth of the endometriotic lesions by an effect on the angiogenic factor VEGF. There are concerns about the possible risk of myocardial infarction and cardiovascular side effects of rosiglitazone.

Pentoxifylline

Another agent that has been studied lately in the treatment of endometriosis is pentoxifylline. Currently used in the treatment of intermittent claudication, it helps in improving the vascular supply in stenotic arteries by inhibiting the phosphodiesterase enzyme. It also has TNF-α-blocking properties, suppressing the release of inflammatory mediators. Human studies are limited and a recent meta-analysis showed that there was no significant improvement in pelvic pain or clinical pregnancy rates in women treated with pentoxifylline [68].

CONCLUSION

To conclude, medical management of endometriosis is an area of interest for the gynecologist as the disease is known to follow a chronic indolent course. It is known to recur with whichever modality of treatment is used, surgical or medical. Infertility is another concern in this population, and hence, choice of therapeutic agent is a concern.

As research is ongoing to discover the exact etiology of the disease, so is the need for an ideal therapeutic agent to treat women from adolescence to menopause.

REFERENCES

1. Missmer SA, Hankinson SE, Spiegelman D et al. Incidence of laparoscopically confirmed endometriosis by demographic, anthropometric, and lifestyle factors. Am J Epidemiol 2004;160:784–796.
2. Spaczynski RZ, Duleba AJ. Diagnosis of endometriosis. Semin Reprod Med 2003;21: 193–208.
3. Zhao H, Zhou L, Shangguan AJ et al. Aromatase expression and regulation in breast and endometrial cancer. J Mol Endocrinol 2016;57:R19–R33.
4. Bulun SE. Endometriosis. N Engl J Med 2009;360:268–279.
5. Attia GR, Zeitoun K, Edwards D et al. Progesterone receptor isoform A but not B is expressed in endometriosis. J Clin Endocrinol Metab 2000;85:2897–2902.
6. Bulun SE, Cheng YH, Yin P et al. Progesterone resistance in endometriosis: Link to failure to metabolize estradiol. Mol Cell Endocrinol 2006; 248:94–103.
7. Yuan P, Huang Y, Cheng B, Zhang J, Xin X. Induction of a local pseudo-pregnancy for the treatment of endometriosis. Med Hypotheses 2010 Jan;74(1):56–8.
8. Mehedintu C, Plotogea MN, Ionescu S, Antonovici M. Endometriosis still a challenge. J Med Life 2014 Sep 15;7(3):349–57.
9. Guo SW. Recurrence of endometriosis and its control. Hum Reprod Update 2009;15:441–61.
10. Hughes E, Brown J, Collins JJ, Farquhar C, Fedorkow DM, Vanderkerchove P. Ovulation suppression for endometriosis for women with subfertility. Cochrane Database Syst Rev 2007:CD000155.
11. Practice Committee of the American Society for Reproductive Medicine. Treatment of pelvic pain associated with endometriosis: A committee opinion. Fertil Steril 2014;101:927–35.
12. Raffi F, Metwally M, Amer S. The impact of excision of ovarian endometrioma on ovarian reserve: A systematic review and meta-analysis. J Clin Endocrino LMetab 2012;97:3146–54.
13. Ferrero S, Alessandri F, Racca A et al. Treatment of pain associated with deep endometriosis: Alternatives and evidence. Fertil Steril 2015 Oct;104(4):771–792. PubMed PMID: 26363387.

14. Tafi E, Leone Roberti Maggiore U, Alessandri F et al. Advances in pharmacotherapy for treating endometriosis. *Expert Opin Pharmacother* 2015 Nov;16(16):2465–2483. PubMed PMID: 26569155.

15. Cetel NS, Rivier J, Vale W et al. The dynamics of gonadotropin inhibition in women induced by an antagonistic analog of gonadotropin-releasing hormone. *J Clin Endocrinol Metab* 1983 Jul;57(1):62–65.

16. Melis GB, Neri M, Corda V et al. Overview of elagolix for the treatment of endometriosis. *Expert Opin Drug Metab Toxicol* 2016;12:581–8.

17. Kupker W, Felberbaum RE, Krapp M et al. Use of GnRH antagonists in the treatment of endometriosis. *Reprod Biomed Online* 2002 Jul-Aug;5(1):12–16.

18. Struthers RS, Chen T, Campbell B et al. Suppression of serum luteinizing hormone in postmenopausal women by an orally administered nonpeptide antagonist of the gonadotropin-releasing hormone receptor (NBI-42902). *J Clin Endocrinol Metab* 2006 Oct;91(10):3903–3907.

19. Diamond MP, Carr B, Dmowski WP, Koltun W, O'Brien C, Jiang P, Chwalisz K. Elagolix treatment for endometriosis-associated pain: Results from a phase 2, randomized, double-blind, placebo-controlled study. *Reproductive Sciences* 2014;21(3), 363–371.

20. Carr B, Dmowski WP, O'Brien C et al. Elagolix, an oral GnRH antagonist, versus subcutaneous depot medroxyprogesterone acetate for the treatment of endometriosis: Effects on bone mineral density. *Reprod Sci* 2014;21:1341–51. medscape;

21. Taylor HS, Giudice LC, Lessey BA et al. Treatment of endometriosis associated pain with elagolix, an oral GnRH antagonist. *N Engl J Med* 2017 Jul 6;377(1):28–40.

22. Carr B, Giudice L, Dmowski WP et al. Elagolix, an oral GnRH antagonist for endometriosis associated pain: A randomized controlled study. *J Endometriosis Pelvic Pain Disord* 2013;5(3):105–115.

23. Osuga Y, Seki Y, Tanimoto M et al., editors Relugolix, an oral gonadotropin-releasing hormone (GnRH) receptor antagonist, in women with endometriosis (EM)-associated pain: Phase 2 safety and efficacy 24-week results. *19th European Congress of Endocrinology*; Lisbon, Portugal: Bioscientifica; 2017.

24. Ferrero S, Evangelisti G, Barra F. Current and emerging treatment options for endometriosis, *Expert Opinion on Pharmacotherapy* 2018;19(10):1109-1125.

25. Brown J, Pan A, Hart RJ. Gonadotrophin-releasing hormone analogues for pain associated with endometriosis. *Cochrane Database Syst Rev* 2010;(12):CD008475. PubMed PMID: 21154398. DOI:10.1002/14651858. CD008475.pub2.

26. Prentice A, Deary AJ, Goldbeck-Wood S et al. Gonadotrophin-releasing hormone analogues for pain associated with endometriosis. *Cochrane Database Syst Rev* 2000;2:CD000346.

27. Hornstein MD, Surrey ES, Weisberg GW et al. Leuprolide acetate depot and hormonal add-back in endometriosis: A 12-month study. Lupron Add-Back Study Group. *Obstet Gynecol* 1998;91:16–24.

28. ACOG 2011 Practice Bulletin No. 114: Management of Endometriosis. Published in. Obstetrics & Gynecology, July 2010. DOI, 10.1097/aog.0b013e3181e8b073. Pubmed ID.

29. Barra F, Scala C, Ferrero S. Current understanding on pharmacokinetics, clinical efficacy and safety of progestins for treating pain associated to endometriosis. *Expert Opin Drug Metab Toxicol* 2018 Apr;4. PubMed PMID: 29617576. DOI:10.1080/ 17425255.2018.1461840.

30. Brown J, Kives S, Akhtar M. Progestagens and anti-progestagens for pain associated with endometriosis. *Cochrane Database Syst Rev* 2012 Mar 14;(3):CD002122. PubMed PMID: 22419284. DOI:10.1002/14651858. CD002122.pub2.

31. Oettel M, Breitbarth H, Elger W et al. The pharmacological profile of dienogest. *Eur J Contracept Reprod Health Care* 1999;4:2-13 20. Foster RH, Wilde MI. Dienogest. Drugs 1998;56:825–33

32. Sasagawa S, Shimizu Y, Kami H et al. Dienogest is a selective progesterone receptor agonist in transactivation analysis with potent oral endometrial activity due to its efficient pharmacokinetic profile. *Steroids* 2008;73:222–31.

33. Bizzarri N, Remorgida V, Leone Roberti Maggiore U et al. Dienogest in the treatment of endometriosis. *Expert Opin Pharmac Other* 2014;15(13):1889–1902.

34. Klipping C, Duijkers I, Faustmann TA et al. Pharmacodynamic study of four oral dosages of dienogest. *Fertil Steril* 2010;94:S181.

35. Strowitzki T, Marr J, Gerlinger C et al. Dienogest is as effective as leuprolide acetate in treating the painful symptoms of endometriosis: A 24-week, randomized, multicentre, open-label trial. *Hum Reprod* 2010;25:633–41.

36. Kitawaki J, Kusuki I, Yamanaka K, Suganuma I. Maintenance therapy with dienogest following gonadotropin releasing hormone agonist treatment for endometriosis-associated pelvic pain. *Eur J Obstet Gynecol Reprod Biol* 2011;157(2):212–16.

37. Momoeda M, Harada T, Terakawa N et al. Long-term use of dienogest for the treatment of endometriosis. *J Obstet Gynaecol Res* 2009;35:1069–76.

38. Chwalisz K, Perez MC, DeManno D, Elger W. *Endocr Rev* 1 May 2005;26(3):423–438.

39. Kettel LM, Murphy AA, Morales AJ, Yen SS. Preliminary report on the treatment of endometriosis with low-dose mifepristone (RU 486). *Am J Obstet Gynecol* 1998;178:1151–6.

40. Xue HL, Yu N, Wang J et al. Therapeutic effects of mifepristone combined with gestrinone on patients with endometriosis. *Pak J Med Sci* 2016 Sep-Oct;32(5):1268–1272.

41. Carbonell JL, Riverón AM, Leonard Y, González J, Heredia B, Sánchez C. Mifepristone 2.5, 5, 10 mg versus placebo in the treatment of endometriosis. *J Reprod Health Med* January–June 2016;2(1):17-25.

42. Huniadi CA, Pop OL, Antal TA, Stamatian F. The effects of ulipristal onBax/ Bcl-2, cytochrome c, Ki-67 andcyclooxygenase-2 expression in a rat model with surgically induced endometriosis. *Eur J Obstet Gynecol Reprod Biol* 2013;169:360–5.

43. Chwalisz K, Perez MC, Demanno D et al. Selective progesterone receptor modulator development and use in the treatment of leiomyomata and endometriosis. *Endocr Rev* 2005 May;26(3):423–438.

44. Bruner-Tran KL, Zhang Z, Eisenberg E, Winneker RC, Osteen KG. Downregulation of endometrial matrix metalloproteinase-3 and -7 expression *in vitro* and therapeutic regression of experimental endometriosis *in vivo* by a novel nonsteroidal progesterone receptor agonist, tanaproget. *J Clin Endocrinol Metab* 2006;91:1554–60.

45. Alvarez P, Bogen O, Levine JD. Role of nociceptor estrogen receptor GPR30 in a rat model of endometriosis pain. *Pain* 2014 Dec;155(12):2680–2686.

46. Sakr S, Naqvi H, Komm B et al. Endometriosis impairs bone marrow-derived stem cell recruitment to the uterus whereas bazedoxifene treatment leads to endometriosis regression and improved uterine stem cell engraftment. *Endocrinology* 2014 Apr;155(4):1489–1497.

47. Harada T, Ohta I, Endo Y et al. SR-16234, a novel selective estrogen receptor modulator for pain symptoms with endometriosis: An open-label clinical trial. *Yonago Acta Med* 2017 Dec;60(4):227–233.

48. Kauppila A, Puolakka J, Ylikorkala O. Prostaglandin biosynthesis inhibitors and endometriosis. *Prostaglandins* 1979 Oct;18(4): 655–661.

49. Kauppila A, Ronnberg L. Naproxen sodium in dysmenorrhea secondary to endometriosis. *Obstet Gynecol* 1985 Mar;65(3):379–383.

50. Cobellis L, Razzi S, De Simone S et al. The treatment with a COX-2 specific inhibitor is effective in the management of pain related to endometriosis. *Eur J Obstet Gynecol Reprod Biol* 2004 Sep 10;116(1):100–102.

51. Bresalier RS, Sandler RS, Quan H et al. Cardiovascular events associated with rofecoxib in a colorectal adenoma chemoprevention trial. *N Engl J Med* 2005 Mar;352(11):1092–1102.

52. Sesti F, Pietropolli A, Capozzolo T et al. Hormonal suppression treatment or dietary therapy versus placebo in the control of painful symptoms after conservative surgery for endometriosis stage III-IV. A randomized comparative trial. *Fertil Steril* 2007 Dec;88(6):1541–1547.

53. Attar E, Tokunaga H, Imir G et al. Prostaglandin E2 via steroidogenic factor-1 coordinately regulates transcription of steroidogenic genes necessary for estrogen synthesis in endometriosis. *J Clin Endocrinol Metab* 2009;94:623–31.

54. Bulun SE. Aromatase deficiency and estrogen resistance: From molecular genetics to clinic. *Semin Reprod Med* 2000;18:31–9.

55. Ferrero S, Venturini PL, Ragni N, Camerini G, Remorgida V. Pharmacological treatment of endometriosis: Experience with aromatase inhibitors. *Drugs* 2009;69:943–52.

56. Schultze-Mosgau MH, Waellnitz K, Nave R et al. Pharmacokinetics, pharmacodynamics, safety and tolerability of an intravaginal ring releasing anastrozole and levonorgestrel in healthy premenopausal women: A Phase 1 randomized controlled trial. *Hum Reprod* 2016 Jun 19. PubMed PMID: 27390369. DOI:10.1093/humrep/dew145

57. Soysal S, Soysal ME, Ozer S et al. The effects of post-surgical administration of goserelin plus anastrozole compared to goserelin alone in patients with severe endometriosis: A prospective randomized trial. *Hum Reprod* 2004 Jan;19(1):160–167.

58. Ferrero S, Venturini PL, Gillott DJ, Remorgida V. Letrozole and norethisterone acetate versus letrozole and triptorelin in the treatment of endometriosis related pain symptoms: A randomized controlled trial. *Reprod Biol Endocrinol* 2011 Jun 21;9:88. doi: 10.1186/1477-7827-9-88.

59. Ferrero S, Camerini G, Seracchioli R, Ragni N, Venturini PL, Remorgida V. Letrozole combined with norethisterone acetate compared with norethisterone acetate alone in the treatment of pain symptoms caused by endometriosis. *Hum Reprod* December 2009;24(12):3033–3041.

60. Novella-Maestre E, Carda C, Noguera I, Ruiz-Saurí A, García-Velasco JA, Simón C, Pellicer A. Dopamine agonist administration causes a reduction in endometrial implants through modulation of angiogenesis in experimentally induced endometriosis. *Hum Reprod* May 2009;24(5):1025–1035.

61. Hamid AMSA, Madkour WAI, Moawad A et al. Does Cabergoline help in decreasing endometrioma size compared to LHRH agonist? A prospective randomized study. *Arch Gynecol Obstet* 2014;290:677.

62. Yilmaz B, Ozat M, Kilic S et al. Atorvastatin causes regression of endometriotic implants in a rat model. *Reprod Biomed Online* 2010;20(2):291–299.

63. Almassinokiani F, Mehdizadeh A, Sariri E et al. Effects of sim vastatin in prevention of pain recurrences after surgery for endometriosis. *Med Sci Monit Int Med J Exp Clin Res* 2013;19:534–539.

64. Igarashi M, Abe Y, Fukuda M et al. Novel conservative medical therapy for uterine adenomyosis with a danazol-loaded intrauterine device. *Fertil Steril* 2000;74:412–413.

65. Lockhat FB, Emembolu JO, Konje JC. The evaluation of the effectiveness of an intrauterine-administered progestogen (levo-norgestrel) in the symptomatic treatment of endometriosis and in the staging of the disease. *Hum Reprod* 2004;19:179–84.

66. Walch K, Unfried G, Huber J et al. Implanon versus medroxyprogesterone acetate: Effects on pain scores in patients with symptomatic endometriosis—A pilot study. *Contraception* 2009;79:29–34.

67. Koninckx PR, Craessaerts M, Timmerman D et al. Anti-TNF-alpha treatment for deep endometriosis- associated pain: A randomized placebo-controlled trial. *Hum Reprod* 2008;23:2017–2023.

68. Lu D, Song H, Li Y et al. Pentoxifylline for endometriosis. *Cochrane Database Syst Rev* 2012;1:CD007677.

16

Long-term complications associated with endometriosis

BHARTI JOSHI

Endometriosis, an enigmatic entity with considerable economic burden, affects 15% of reproductive aged women [1]. Since its conception, more and more cases are being identified because of awareness and advanced imaging techniques. Nonetheless, despite extensive research, clinicians still face challenges in management of endometriosis with chronic complications.

DEEP INFILTRATING ENDOMETRIOSIS

There are mainly three types of endometriosis identified apart from the AFS (American Fertility Society) classification. Superficial endometriosis involving mainly the peritoneum and/or ovary, ovarian endometriomas, and deeply infiltrating endometriosis (DIE). The latter involves the uterosacral ligament, the urinary system, the gastrointestinal system, and the upper vagina [2]. The histological findings of DIE include involvement of muscularis and depth of endometriotic implants

more than 5 mm below the peritoneum [3]. This entity presents with chronic pelvic pain refractory to medical treatment and occurs in 30%–40% of women with endometriosis. Long-standing endometriosis may lead to adhesions formation, internal scarring, and bowel and ureter obstruction [4]. Endometriomas may get complicated by superadded infection resulting in abscess formation.

This entity is responsible for refractory pelvic pain, of which the intensity is correlated with the depth of infiltration, and occurs in 30%–40% of the patients with endometriosis [5]. According to the neurological hypothesis, infiltration of nerves along the bowel or other ectopic sites cause persistent pain and irritation [6]. Various mechanisms like retrograde menstruation, coelomic metaplasia, migration through lymphatics, and embryonic rest theory explain the growth of ectopic endometriotic implants. These implants are histologically similar to adenomyosis of the uterus [7]. These women respond poorly to medical treatment and therefore are surgically treated. Preoperative workup should include detailed history, clinical examinations and relevant imaging to find out the extent and exact location of lesions or if there is multifocal involvement of abdominopelvic system as in deep infiltrating endometriosis. The chances of recurrence is around 30% due to the residual disease, as the lesions responsible for symptomatology are only excised [5,8].

BOWEL ENDOMETRIOSIS

The incidence of bowel endometriosis is reported to be 5%–12%, with rectosigmoid being the most common site [9]. Most of bowel endometriosis is secondary to pelvic endometriosis. Progressive invasion of muscularis propria of the bowel may result in obstruction, fibrosis, or stricture formation [10]. In its early stages, bowel endometriosis may be misdiagnosed due to nonspecific symptoms. The patients may complain of bloating, dyspepsia, abdominal pain and distension, tenesmus, and altered bowel habits [7]. There can be a history of rectal bleeding, and bowel endometriosis may mimic malignancy, ischemic colitis, or irritable bowel syndrome [11] (Figure 16.1).

A young woman presenting with abdominal pain and signs of obstruction should raise suspicion of bowel endometriosis [12]. The specificity and sensitivity of clinical examination is low. One can feel rectovaginal nodule during per rectal examination. This may be further confirmed on

endorectal ultrasound, which has good sensitivity in diagnosing rectal endometriosis. Magnetic resonance imaging has an accuracy of 72%–90% in enteric endometriosis [13]. The laparoscopy is considered a very good tool for diagnosing and managing such lesions. There is no doubt that complete excision is the treatment of choice to achieve maximum relief, but in the case of rectal endometriosis, as a rule, less is better [14]. Sometimes, the need for bowel resection may arise if obstruction is not relieved on conservative management and there is high suspicion of malignancy [11,12]. The complications after surgery for endometriosis are rectovaginal fistula, leak from colorectal anastomoses, bowel and bladder dysfunction, and pelvic abscess [14,15]. A multidisciplinary team involving a gynecologist, a gastroenterologist, and a urologist in the management of deep infiltrating endometriosis helps in optimizing outcomes with minimal morbidities and complications [7,14,15].

ABDOMINAL WALL ENDOMETRIOSIS

The entity is defined as the presence of endometriotic tissue in the abdominal wall. This is reported in 0.03% to 1.08% of women having a previous gynecological procedure. Abdominal wall endometriosis may manifest a long time after surgery and is seen in association with

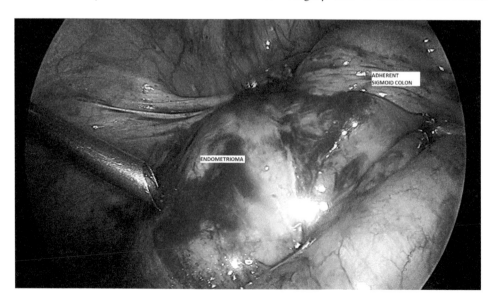

Figure 16.1 Endometrioma with adherent sigmoid colon.

pelvic endometriosis in 2.5% to 25% of cases [16]. Various theories such as direct implantation of tissue during surgery, hematogenous and lymphatic spread, and coelomic metaplasia explain the pathophysiology of this entity [16]. The incidence of malignant transformation is very low in abdominal wall endometriosis. If a mass associated with cyclical abdominal pain appears at the cesarean scar site or any other gynecological procedure site, diagnosis of abdominal wall endometriosis has to be entertained. Sometimes, there may be no history of cyclical pain or any gynecological procedure. In such cases, higher imaging, such as computed tomography (CT) or magnetic resonance imaging (MRI), or fine-needle biopsy may confirm the diagnosis [16]. Treatment involves a wide excision with 1 cm healthy margin and placement of mesh in case of large defect. Adjuvant hormonal therapy is to be considered to prevent recurrence and to suppress residual disease [16]. The suggestions to prevent occurrence of abdominal wall endometriosis are to use different suture material for uterine and abdominal closure, not to exteriorize the uterus for suturing, to use a wound edge protector, and to avoid swabbing of the uterine cavity.

URINARY TRACT ENDOMETRIOSIS

Of all women with endometriosis, urinary tract involvement is found in 0.3% to 5%, with the bladder being the most common, followed by the ureter and kidneys [17].

BLADDER ENDOMETRIOSIS

Vesical or bladder endometriosis may be seen in 11% of women suffering from deep infiltrating endometriosis. The proposed etiopathogenesis include development from Müllerian tissue and retrograde implantation of menstrual blood or directly from adjacent ovaries or uterus; presenting complaints include dysuria, frequency, hematuria, or chronic pelvic pain [18]. Symptoms may show cyclic variation due to more congestion in menstruation. Any postmenopausal woman on hormonal treatment with refractory cystitis should be evaluated for bladder endometriosis. One may feel a nodule anteriorly during pelvic examination, and transvaginal ultrasound can confirm the diagnosis. Cystoscopy and higher imaging can

complement the diagnosis in difficult situations and helps to differentiate from malignant conditions [18]. Isolated bladder endometriosis is seen in only 36% of cases, the rest are associated with pelvic or intestinal lesions [19].

Treatment modalities are medical and surgical. Cystoscopy helps in identifying the margin of implants and the level of resection. Transurethral, along with laparoscopic, excision of nodules may result in better outcome. Postoperative complications may include vesico-enteric or vesico-uterine fistula or intravesical hematoma [17–19]. Pang et al. managed a case of bladder endometriosis with a combined approach [20]. Recurrence may occur in up to 10% of the cases and depends upon the level of resection.

URETERAL ENDOMETRIOSIS

This is a rare entity with serious hazards (<0.3%). It commonly involves the left ureter and may result in loss of renal function [21]. Ureteral endometriosis is mainly localized to the lower third and is of two types. Intrinsic disease invades the muscularis and epithelium, while extrinsic involves the adventitia and surrounding tissue. Both can cause hydroureteronephrosis, compromising renal function. Many women may be asymptomatic at the beginning (56%). The diagnostic modalities include abdominal ultrasound, ureteroscopy, intravenous pyelography, and sometimes scintigraphy [22]. Ureterolysis is said to be an effective approach despite a reported recurrence rate [17].

RENAL ENDOMETRIOSIS

A rare condition with presenting symptoms of flank pain, hydronephrosis, hematuria, or a renal mass [23]. Most patients require nephrectomy in the absence of biopsy [24].

LIVER ENDOMETRIOSIS

Hepatic endometriosis is of rare occurrence. The majority of women have epigastric or abdominal pain. They may present with vomiting with bile sputum, jaundice, portal vein thrombosis, or hepatomegaly [25,26]. The lesion may be large, up to 20 cm, and is sometimes difficult to differentiate from malignancy; therefore, final diagnosis can be established on histology.

PANCREATIC ENDOMETRIOSIS

Women with pancreatic endometriosis have pain in the upper quadrant or presence of an abdominal mass. Higher imaging confirms the diagnosis and partial pancreatectomy is the treatment option.

OMENTAL ENDOMETRIOSIS

Omental endometriosis occurs by transperitoneal or lymphatic migration transmission of endometriotic tissue. Brown bloody ascites or dyspepsia are common presentations.

NERVOUS SYSTEM ENDOMETRIOSIS

Sciatic nerve endometriosis may present with root pain along with sensorimotor deficit. A similar presentation can be seen in obturator nerve involvement.

MASSIVE ASCITES IN ENDOMETRIOSIS

Massive bloody ascites in endometriosis is an extremely rare event with diagnostic conundrum. This presentation mimics malignant neoplasm. These women usually have ovarian endometrioma along with peritoneal deposits of endometriotic tissue [27]. Provoked inflammatory reaction causes exudation and ascites. Fine-needle biopsy helps in establishing the diagnosis by showing the presence of endometriotic implants.

SPONTANEOUS HEMOPERITONEUM IN PREGNANCY AND ENDOMETRIOSIS

This rare cause of hemoperitoneum in pregnancy is associated with high perinatal morbidity and mortality. The condition is seen mainly in the third trimester [28] and the possible mechanism is chronic inflammation of utero-ovarian vessels by endometriosis. Enlargement of the uterus puts these vessels under tension, thereby making it prone for rupture. At laparotomy, bleeding vessels are seen either in the parametrium or on the surface of the uterus. More cases will be seen in the future due to use of assisted reproductive techniques in infertile women with endometriosis [29].

MALIGNANCY

Malignant transformation is seen in 0.7%–1% of women with endometriosis with ovarian being the predominant one. The possible mechanisms are (1) transformation secondary to genetic mutations [30], (2) immunological changes causing uncontrolled proliferation [31], and (3) direct transition of atypical endometriosis to malignancy [32]. Endometrioid adenocarcinoma is the most common histologic type (23%–69.1%), followed by clear-cell carcinomas (13.5%–23%), and then sarcomas and other rare ones [31]. Tumors of extragonadal sites are mostly endometrioid. These tumors are low grade and confined to the site, and histology demonstrates endometrial stroma with endometrial glands [33]. The underlying risk factors for malignant transformation are poorly known and some have observed an association between unopposed estrogen and development of endometroid or clear-cell neoplasms. Increasing parity, prolonged use of contraceptive pills, and breastfeeding are said to have a protective effect. Any pelvic mass in postmenopausal woman with a history of endometriosis should raise suspicion of malignant transformation. The symptoms are usually specific to the organ involved, and biopsy from the tissue confirms the diagnosis. Immunohistochemistry helps in identifying the origin of the tumor. Surgery with complete resection of the tumor remains the mainstay of treatment. Most of these require adjuvant treatment in the form of chemotherapy or radiotherapy [31]. Malignant transformation confined to the site of origin has a better prognosis compared with disseminated disease.

CONCLUSION

Endometriosis is a chronic disease with multiple morbidities. A multidisciplinary approach is required for the management of extragonadal endometriosis. Despite advancement of imaging modalities, diagnosis may be missed due to unusual location and presentation. Therefore, one must maintain an index of suspicion. Malignant transformation, although rare, can cause severe morbidity and mortality.

REFERENCES

1. Hemmings R, Rivard M, Olive DL, Poliquin-Fleury J, Gagne D, Hugo P, Gosselin D. Evaluation of risk factors associated with endometriosis. *Fertil Steril* 2004;81:1513–21

2. Chapron C, Chopin N, Borghese B, Foulot H, Dousset B, Vacher-Lavenu MC, Vieira M, Hasan W, Bricou A. Deeply infiltrating endometriosis: Pathogenetic implications of the anatomical distribution. *Hum Reprod* 2006;21:1839–45

3. Chapron C, Pietin-Vialle C, Borghese B, Davy C, Foulot H, Chopin N. Associated ovarian endometriomas is a marker for greater severity of deeply infiltrating endometriosis. *Fertil Steril* 2009;92:453–7

4. Acosta S, Leandersson U, Svensson SE, Johnsen J. A case report. Endometriosis caused colonic ileus, ureteral obstruction and hypertension. A case report. Endometriosis caused colonic ileus, ureteral obstruction and hypertension. *Lakartidningen (in Swedish)* May 2001;98(18):2208–12

5. Chapron C, Fauconnier A, Vieira M, Barakat H, Dousset B, Pansini V, Vacher-Lavenu MC, Dubuisson JB. Anatomical distribution of deeply infiltrating endometriosis: Surgical implications and proposition for a classification. *Hum Reprod* 2003;18:760–6

6. Anaf V, El Nakadi I, Simon P, Van de Stadt J, Fayt I, Simonart T, Noel JC. Preferential infiltration of large bowel endometriosis along the nerves of the colon. *Hum Reprod* 2004;19:996–1002.

7. Brouwer R, Woods RJ. Rectal endometriosis: Results of radical excision and review of published work. *Aust N Z J Surg* 2007;77:562–71.

8. Vignali M, Bianchi S, Candiani M, Spadaccini G, Oggioni G, Busacca M. Surgical treatment of deep endometriosis and risk of recurrence. *J Minim Invasive Ginecol* 2005;12:508–13.

9. Wills HJ, Reid GD, Cooper MJ, Tsaltas J, Morgan M, Woods RJ. Bowel resection for severe endometriosis: An Australian series of 177 cases. *Aust N Z J Obstet Gynaecol* 2009;49:415–8.

10. Yantiss RK, Clement PB, Young RH. Endometriosis of the intestinal tract: A study of 44 cases of a disease that may cause diverse challenges in clinical and pathologic evaluation. *Am J Surg Pathol* 2001;25:445–54.

11. Bianchi A, Pulido L, Espin F, Hidalgo LA, Heredia A, Fantova MJ, Muns R, Suñol J. Intestinal endometriosis. Current status. *Cir Esp* 2007;81:170–6.

12. Del Rey Moreno A, Jiménez Martín JJ, Moreno Ruiz FJ, Hierro Martín I. Asociación de enteritis quística profunda, ileocolitis de Crohn y endometriosis como causa de obstrucción intestinal. *Cir Esp* 2008;83:271.

13. Kataoka ML, Togashi K, Yamaoka T, Koyama T, Ueda H, Kobayashi H, Rahman M, Higuchi T, Fujii S. Posterior cul-de-sac obliteration associated with endometriosis: MR imaging evaluation. *Radiology* 2005;234:815–23.

14. De Cicco C, Corona R, Schonman R, Mailova K, Ussia A, Koninckx PR. Bowel resection for deep endometriosis: A systematic review. *BJOG* 2011;118:285–91.

15. Dousset B, Leconte M, Borghese B, Millischer AE, Roseau G, Arkwright S, Chapron C. Complete surgery for low rectal endometriosis. Long-term of a 100-case prospective study. *Ann Surg* 2010;251:887–95.

16. Bektas H, Bilsel Y, Sari YS, Ersöz F, Koç O, Deniz M, Boran B, Huq GE. Abdominal wall endometrioma: A 10-year experience and brief review of the literature. *J Surg Res* 2010;164:77–81.

17. Mereu L, Gagliardi JL, Clarizia R, Mainardi P, Landi S, Minelli L. Laparoscopic management of ureteral endometriosis in case of moderate-severe hydroureteronephrosis. *Fertil Steril* 2010;93:46–51.

18. Le Tohic A, Chis C, Yazbeck C, Koskas M, Madelenat P, Panel P. Endométriose vésicale: Diagnostic et traitment. À propos d'une série de 24 patientes. *Gynecol Obstet Fertil* 2009;37:216–21.

19. Fedele L, Bianchi S, Zanconato G, Bergamini V, Berlanda N, Carmignani L. Long-term follow-up after conservative surgery for bladder endometriosis. *Fertil Steril* 2005b;83:1729–33.

20. Pang ST, Chao A, Wang CJ, Lin G, Lee CL. Transurethral partial cystectomy and laparoscopic reconstruction for the management of bladder endometriosis. *Fertil Steril* 2008;90:2014 e1–e3.

21. Li CY, Wang HQ, Liu HY, Lang JH. Management of ureteral endometriosis: A report of ten cases. *Chin Med Sci J* 2008;23:218–23.

22. Camanni M, Delpiano EM, Bonino L, Deltetto F. Laparoscopic conservative management of ureteral endometriosis. *Curr Opin Obstet Gynecol* 2010;22:309–14.

23. Dirim A, Celikkaya S, Aygun C, Caylak B. Renal endometriosis presenting with a giant subcapsular hematoma: Case report. *Fertil Steril* 2009;92:391 e5–e7.

24. Veeraswamy A, Lewis M, Mphil AM, Kotikela S, Hajhosseini B, Nezhat C. Extragenital Endometriosis. *Clin Obstet Gynecol* 2010;53:449–66.

25. Nezhat C, Kazerooni T, Berker B, Lashay N, Fernandez S, Marziali M. Laparoscopic management of hepatic endometriosis: Report of two cases and review of the literature. *J Minim Invasive Gynecol* 2005;12:196–200.

26. Schuld J, Justinger C, Wagner M, Bohle RM, Kollmar O, Schilling MK, Richter S. Bronchobiliary fistula: A rare complication of hepatic endometriosis. *Fertil Steril* 2011;804:e15–8.

27. Sait KH. Massive ascites as a presentation in a young woman with endometriosis: A case report. *Fertil Steril* 2008;90:2015 e17–e19.

28. Brosens IA, Fusi L, Brosens JJ. Endometriosis is a risk factor for spontaneous hemoperitoneum during pregnancy. *Fertil Steril* 2009;92:1243–5.

29. Grunewald C, Jördens A. Intra-abdominal hemorrhage due to previously unknown endometriosis in the third trimester of pregnancy with uneventful neonatal outcome: A case report. *Eur J Obstet Gynecol Reprod Biol* 2010;148:204–5.

30. Akahane T, Sekizawa A, Purwosunu Y, Nagatsuka M, Okai T. The role of p53 mutation in the carcinomas arising from endometriosis. *Int J Gynecol Pathol* 2007;26:345351.

31. Modesitt SC, Tortolero-Luna G, Robinson JB, Gershenson DM, Wolf JK. Ovarian and extraovarian endometriosis-associated cancer. *Obstet Gynecol* 2002;100:788–95.

32. Van Gorp T, Amant F, Neven P, Vergote I. Endometriosis and the development of malignant tumours of the pelvis. A review of literature. *Best Pract Res Clin Obstet Gynaecol* 2004;18:349–71.

33. Slavin RE, Krum R, Van Dinh T. Endometriosis-associated intestinal tumours: A clinical an pathological study of 6 cases with a review of the literature. *Hum Pathol* 2000;31:456–63

17

Recurrence of endometriosis

RAKHI RAI AND SEEMA CHOPRA

Recurrent endometriosis is a challenging task for the gynecologist. Endometriosis is a chronic disorder, mainly presenting as pain and infertility, affecting 6%–10% of reproductive age women; 87% of patients with chronic pelvic pain and 38% of infertile women have endometriosis [1]. Endometriosis is the result of retrograde menstruation by the peritoneal implantation of endometrial glands and stroma.

It is a debilitating disease. Recurrence occurs due to regrowth of residual endometriotic cells or growth of microscopic endometriotic lesions, which remained undetected at time of surgery, or due to development of de novo/fresh lesions, or combination of above. Recurrence rates vary between 6%–67% [2]. Recurrence rates differ according to the criteria used for the definition of recurrence (i.e., symptoms such as dysmenorrhea/dyspareunia, clinical features such as nodularity on examination or pelvic mass, or imaging features). Bussaca et al. [3] evaluated 1106 women and found recurrence in 144 women. A 4-year recurrence rate was found to be 24.6%, 17.8%, 30.6%, and 23.7% for ovarian, peritoneal, deep ovarian, and

peritoneal endometriosis, respectively. Recurrence rate increases as time passes; 8 years recurrence rates were 42%, 24.1%, 43.4%, and 30.9%, respectively. Vignali [4] found a recurrence rate of pain in 3- and 5-year periods as 20.5% and 43.5%, respectively. Parazzini et al. [5] found 2-year recurrence rate of stage I/II endometriosis as 5.7%, which rises to 14.3% for stage III/IV endometriosis.

RISK FACTORS FOR RECURRENCE

Various risk factors have been attributed to recurrence of endometriosis. Various studies have evaluated the different parameters, as shown in Table 17.1.

Koga et al. [9] found that previous medical management increases the risk of recurrence due to masking of endometriotic lesions during surgery by medical management. Also, medical treatment may alter genome processes of endometriotic cells, leading to suppression of normal eukaryotic cells and an increase in dyskaryotic cells in endometriotic implants.

Table 17.1 Showing various studies and risk factors studied

Study	Risk factors
Li et al. [6] (study on follow-up of 285 patients for a minimum 36 months after conservative surgery)	Young age Bilateral pelvic involvement on history by endometriosis Previous endometriotic surgery Tenderness Nodularity in cul-de-sac Left-sided endometrioma High revised American Fertility Society Score
Saleh and Tulandi [7]	Larger cysts Advanced stage of disease Previous endometriotic surgery
Porpora et al. [8]	Prior surgery Pelvic adhesions High rAFS
Vignali et al. [4]	Completeness of first surgery
Bussacca et al. [3]	Deep endometriosis Stage III/IV disease Young age

Pregnancy is a protective factor due to increased progesterone levels. Vercellium et al. [10] found that LNG-IUD reduces risk of recurrence after 1 year when compared to expectantly observed patients.

BIOMARKERS

Endometriosis is a major contributor to disability and compromised quality of life of women. Early diagnosis is the need of the hour that requires a specific and sensitive biomarker for diagnosing endometriosis nonsurgically, thereby preventing late sequelae of endometriosis. The gold standard for diagnosis of endometriosis is visualization of lesions directly on laparoscopy or laparotomy and confirmation by histopathology, but it is associated with various side effects of surgery such as infection, bleeding, or injury to adjacent organs. Noninvasive tests are required for the diagnosis of endometriosis in patients with pelvic pain with normal ultrasound reports to detect endometriosis at an early stage. Increased progesterone receptor isoform B (PRB) and decreased nuclear factor kappa B immunoreactivity are found in the recurrent group. Further studies are needed to determine immunoreactivity with a larger number of kappa B and PRB as biomarkers for recurrent endometriosis [11].

Plasma brain-derived neurotrophic factor is a noninvasive biomarker for patients with stage I/II endometriosis, as per Wessels et al. [12], with sensitivity of 91.7% and specificity of 69.4%.

An increased level of synuclein gamma, which is involved in cellular proliferation interacting with mitotic checkpoint kinase Bub RI in human endometriotic lesions, suggests its role in endometriosis pathogenesis [13].

GLYCOPROTEINS

CA-125 is the most extensively studied biomarker but is nonspecific as it is also raised in ovarian malignancy. In a meta-analysis by Mol et al. [14], sensitivity for stage I–IV endometriosis was 50%, which raised to 60% in stage III/IV. The various combinations of biomarkers have been studied but none have been validated [15,16]. The CA-125, surviving mRNA, CA19-9 combination showed a sensitivity of 87% with a 10% false positive rate [17]. CA-125, monocyte chemoattractant protein 1, chemokine receptor type 1 mRNA showed a specificity of 81.6% and a sensitivity of 92.2% for detection of endometriosis [18].

The CA-125, IL 8, TNF-α combination showed a sensitivity of 89.7% and a specificity of 71% [19]. The CA-125, laminin 1, syntaxin 5 combination was studied by Ozhan et al. [20] and found 90%

sensitivity and 70% specificity. A CA-125, CA 19-9, CA 15-3 panel was found to be increased in the endometrium and area under the curve was highest for CA-125 [21]. The panel of CA-125, annexin V, vascular endothelial growth factor, and soluble intercellular adhesion molecule (sICAM1) showed a specificity of 55%–75% and a sensitivity of 74%–99% but needs further prospective trials [22].

Zinc alpha 2 glycoprotein was identified by mass spectrophotometry and confirmed by ELISA to be differentially expressed in the endometrium as compared to controls but has a low sensitivity of 69.9% with 100% specificity [23].

Glycodelin A was found to be increased in women with endometriosis when being tested in serum in the follicular phase with a sensitivity of 82.1% and specificity of 78.4% [24].

IMMUNOLOGICAL AND INFLAMMATORY CYTOKINES

Interleukin 4 [25] was found to be increased in adolescents with endometriosis.

Raised copeptin, at a cutoff of 25.18 pg/mL, has a sensitivity of 65% and a specificity 58.35% in predicting endometriosis, with a positive correlation to severity of endometriosis [21]. Increased YK 40 is another inflammatory biomarker [26]. The CA-125, IL-8, TNF-α combination has a specificity of 89.7% and a sensitivity of 71.1% [19]. IL-8, MCP1, and RANTES were increased in 46.1%, 50%, and 75% of cases, respectively [27]. However, consensus has not yet been reached on the use of cytokines to discriminate endometriosis from other patients.

OXIDATIVE STRESS

There is increased oxidative stress in female patients with endometriosis. There is a decrease in HDL, paroxonase 1, and superoxide dismutase, with an increase in LDL, cholesterols, triglycerides, lipid peroxides, vitamin E, and heat shock protein 70b [28–30].

CELL ADHESION AND INVASION

SICAM-1 increases in early stages and decreases in stage III/IV endometriosis [31]. Osteopontin, a cell adhesion molecule, increases in all stages [32].

Matrix metalloproteinases (MMPs) facilitate invasion of the peritoneum by endometrial fragments. MMP-2, -9 are significantly higher in endometriosis cases [33–35].

ANGIOGENESIS

The role of VEGF as a biomarker of endometriosis is still not clear, with variable results in different studies [31,36]. Pigment epithelium derived factor, an angiogenesis inhibitor with anti-inflammatory properties, was found to be decreased in endometriosis patients by Chen et al. [37]. Fibroblast growth factor 2, angiogenin, and Flt 1 (VEGFR 1) have all been reported to be raised in the serum of women with endometriosis [31].

HORMONES

No consensus exists regarding steroid hormone levels as there are contrasting results [31].

AUTOANTIBODIES

Antiendometrial antibodies as a biomarker are a promising aspect [31].

Specific antibodies such as antibodies against carbonic anhydrase, α2-HS glycoprotein, transferrin, copper oxidized low-density lipoprotein, lipid peroxide modified rabbit serum albumin, laminin-I, cardiolipin, PDIK1L, and syntaxin 5 can be used as potential biomarkers [31,38,39].

MicroRNAs (miRNAs) are the short, noncoding sequences regulating gene expression at the posttranscriptional level [40]. The reduced proclivity of miRNA to degradation relative to mRNA [41] and strong correlation between tissue and serum miRNA expression evidenced in other disorders are favorable features of miRNA in the context of biomarker potential [42]. Fassbender et al. [43] suggested the role of miRNAs in blood as a biomarker of endometriosis. Increased levels of miR-16, 195, 191 [44] and decreased levels of miR-20a, 17-5p, and 22 have been seen in endometriosis [45].

METABOLOMICS

Stearic acid is decreased in endometriosis patients [46]. The combination of hydroxysphingomyelin C16:1 and the ratio between phosphatidylcholine

C36:2 to ether-phospholipid C34:2 has a specificity of 84.3% and a sensitivity of 90.0% for detecting endometriosis [47]. Further research is required to prove the role of metabolomics in the detection of endometriosis [48].

CIRCULATING CELL-FREE DNA

Circulating cell-free DNA levels are increased in endometriosis patients but this needs further studies [49].

CELL POPULATIONS

A subset of CD4 regulatory T cells, CD25 forkhead box 3 (FOXP3), has been found to be decreased in endometrioma patients compared with healthy controls [50].

URINE BIOMARKERS

Creatinine-corrected soluble fms-like tyrosine kinase (sFlt-1) was found to be significantly elevated in the urine of women with endometriosis using enzyme-linked immunosorbent assays (ELISA) [51]. Metalloproteinases MMP-9, MMP-2, and MMP-9/neutrophil gelaltinase-associated lipocalin was significantly higher in a cohort of 33 women who had endometriosis compared with 13 unaffected controls [52]. Cho et al. found 22 urine proteins including vitamin D–binding protein, enolase 1, prealbumin, and alpha1-antitrypsin, but none of them have high sensitivity and specificity for detection of endometriosis [53].

ENDOMETRIAL BIOMARKERS

Endometrial biomarkers, although more invasive as detection requires an endometrial biopsy, are more specific and can be done in the office setting [48].

ENDOMETRIAL TRANSCRIPTOME

Significant differences exist in the gene expression at the transcript level between eutopic endometrium and endometriosis. Studies have identified genes and pathways that may be involved in disease pathogenesis. Both array-based global and targeted gene expression reveal potential candidates for the development of an endometrial-based biomarker [54].

MicroRNAs

Endometrial miRNAs show a differential expression between the endometrium and ectopic endometrial tissue. miRNAs expression shows dynamic changes with the menstrual cycle. Differential expression of 22 miRNAs between eutopic and ectopic endometrium was found by Teague et al. [55]. Another recent study found differential expression of 156 miRNAs, including 12 miRNAs involved in fibrinolysis and angiogenesis [56]. In a study by Burney et al. [57], a miRNA-mRNA parallel array-based comparison done between the endometrium of four women with moderate to severe endometriosis and early secretory endometrium of three control women, 6 endometriosis-associated miRNA were found from miRNA 34 and miRNA 9 families [57]. This study is strengthened by the fact that it was done on surgically confirmed endometriosis, but the drawback was the presence of myoma in control patients, which could act as a confounding factor in delineating the endometriosis-specific miRNA differences. It also compared expression of miRNA between mild and severe endometriosis and found increased endometrial expression of miR 21 in mild and DICER, multidomain ribonuclease that processes double-stranded RNAs (dsRNAs) to 21-nt small interfering RNAs (siRNAs) during RNA interference and excises microRNAs (miRNAs) from precursor hairpins in advanced endometriosis [58]. Overexpression of miR 135a/b in different phases of the menstrual cycle and downregulation of HOXA10 has been found, which was further confirmed by luciferase assay in endometrial stromal cells [59].

Aberrant miRNA expression in eutopic endothelium in women with endometriosis seems to be a promising biomarker but needs further studies for validation of individual miRNA dysregulation.

ENDOMETRIAL PROTEOMES

Different proteomes have been found using the SELDI TOF MS platform in women with or without endometriosis [60]. In one of the largest studies involving 53 endometrial samples [61], endometriosis was diagnosed with 87.5% sensitivity and 86.2% specificity by a panel of three differentially expressed peptide peaks (15.128, 15.334, 16.069 m/z). Five peptide peaks were described in another study (1.949, 5.183, 8.650, 8.659, 13.910 m/z), with a specificity of 90% and a sensitivity of 89.5% [62]. Fassbender et al. found differential expression of five peptide peaks (2072, 2973, 3623, 3680, 21133 m/z) in the early secretory endometrial phase for diagnosing endometriosis with 80% specificity and 91% sensitivity [60]. These peptide peaks have not been validated in an independent study cohort so far. In most of the studies, menstrual cycle phase of endometrial samples has not been mentioned [48].

NEURONAL MARKER

Protein gene product (PGP) 9.5 stained nerve fibers were found in functional endometrium of women with endometriosis, confirmed surgically in sharp curettage and hysterectomy specimens [63]. The density of nerve fibers was 14 times higher in stage I/II endometriosis and a PGP 9.5, vasoactive intestinal peptide, and substance P combination was diagnostic of endometriosis with 95% sensitivity and 100% specificity [64]. Proper sampling and determination of the functional endometrial layer were the main points to be emphasized [65]. PGP 9.5 immunohistochemistry for detection of endometriosis could not be recapitulated in another study, maybe due to curette- not pipelle-based sampling, improper orientation of functional layer in curette samples, and inclusion of women on hormonal treatment [66]. Also, nerve fibers are detected in 29% of samples in women without endometriosis, raising questions about the efficacy of these assays [66]. Larger studies are required to validate the neuronal marker as a biomarker of endometriosis.

Standard operating procedures need to be developed for sample collection, processing, storage of samples, and data collection to minimize the inconsistencies in different studies [48].

In spite of number of studies, not a single biomarker or a panel of biomarkers has been validated for diagnosis of endometriosis with adequate sensitivity and specificity.

TREATMENT

Recurrence of endometriosis may be asymptomatic or may be associated with pain or infertility. Combined treatment postsurgery is recommended to prevent recurrence of endometriosis [67]. Prolonged oral contraceptive pill (OCP) use or progestins can be used to prevent recurrence. GnRH agonists can also be used postsurgery. Six cycles of GnRH agonists after surgery prevents recurrence better than three cycles of GnRH agonists [67,68]. Oral progestins such as medroxyprogesterone, dienogest, and danazol are effective in reducing pain and preventing growth of lesions. LNG-IUS insertion postsurgery helps to control symptoms and to decrease recurrence risk. It also protects against bone loss [67].

Recurrence of endometriosis can be managed either surgically or medically. According to ACOG updated guidelines [1], NSAIDs or combined OCPs can be used for pain management in women who wish to preserve fertility. Depot or oral medroxyprogesterone is also effective. A levonorgestrel-releasing intrauterine device (LNG-IUD) can also be used for pain relief. If the patient fails to respond to the above therapies, GnRH agonists or androgens can be tried. If GnRH agonist therapy is used, add-back therapy with progestogens is recommended to reduce bone loss. The most commonly recommended progestogen by the FDA is norethindrone 5 mg daily. For those who can't tolerate norethindrone, a daily combination of oral medroxyprogesterone acetate 2.5 mg and transdermal estradiol 25 ug can be used. Supplementation with 1000 mg calcium is also recommended. Dienogest [69,70] 2 mg per day can be used and is well-tolerated for recurrent endometrioma. It reduces the size of the cyst as well as the pain-free interval within 3 months of usage.

Surgical treatment in women with recurrent endometrioma should be considered on a case-by-case basis. Second surgery should be avoided in women who wish to conceive as it may lead to decreased or complete loss of ovarian function, thereby decreasing the number of oocytes retrieved during IVF [71,72]. There is increased risk of premature ovarian failure in the case of bilateral ovarian endometrioma resection. ART in the form in vitro fertilization (IVF) is preferred over repeat surgery in infertile women, as it has a negative impact on IVF outcome unless pain is still present.

Surgical management of recurrent endometrioma is usually not the management of choice due to the risk of loss of ovarian reserve, but on the other hand, recurrent endometrioma is associated with high risk of malignancy, especially in patients greater than 40 years of age.

LUNA is of no benefit.

Hysterectomy with bilateral salpingo-oophorectomy is the definitive management if the woman has completed the family. A woman must be informed prior to surgery that hysterectomy may not completely cure her disease [67].

CONCLUSION

To conclude, endometriosis is a debilitating disease affecting quality of life of the patient. Various risk factors for recurrence have been studied which include young age, advanced stage of disease, bilaterality of lesions, incomplete previous surgery, high revised American Fertility Society Score, deep endometriosis, and so on. Various biomarkers have been studied so far, but none has been validated independently as a biomarker for endometriosis. Management of recurrent endometriosis varies with symptomatology as well as previous history. As far as fertility is concerned, a second surgery is even more detrimental. Artificial reproductive techniques should be management of choice. Medical management in the form of combined oral contraceptives, progesterone, dienogest, and GnRH analogues can be used.

REFERENCES

1. Armstrong C. ACOG updates guidelines on diagnosis and treatment of endometriosis. *Am Fam Physician* 2011 Jan 1;83(1):84–5.
2. Guo SW. Recurrence of endometriosis and its control. *Hum Reprod Update* 2009 Jul-Aug;15(4):441–61.
3. Busacca M, Chiaffarino F, Candiani M. Determinants of long-term clinically detected recurrence rates of deep, ovarian, and pelvic endometriosis. *Am J Obstet Gynecol* 2006; 195(2):426–32.
4. Vignali M, Bianchi S, Candiani M, Spadaccini G, Oggioni G, Busacca M. Surgical treatment of deep endometriosis and risk of recurrence. *J Minim Invasive Gynecol* 2005;12(6):508–13.
5. Parazzini F, Bertulessi C, Pasini A. Determinants of short-term recurrence rate of endometriosis. *Eur J Obstet Gynecol Reprod Biol* 2005;121(2):216–9.
6. Li HJ, Leng JH, Lang JH, Wang HL, Liu ZF, Sun DW, Zhu L, Ding XM. Correlative factors analysis of recurrence of endometriosis after conservative surgery. *Zhonghua Fu Chan Ke Za Zhi* 2005;40:13–6.
7. Saleh A, Tulandi T. Reoperation after laparoscopic treatment of ovarian endometriomas by excision and by fenestration. *Fertil Steril* 1999;72:322–4.
8. Porpora MG, Pallante D, Ferro A, Crisafi B, Bellati F, Benedetti Panici P. Pain and ovarian endometrioma recurrence after laparoscopic treatment of endometriosis: A long-term prospective study. *Fertil Steril* 2010;93:716–21.
9. Koga K, Takemura Y, Osuga Y et al. Recurrence of ovarian endometrioma after laparoscopic excision. *Hum Reprod* 2006;21:2171–4.
10. Vercellini P, Frontino G, De Giorgi O, Aimi G, Zaina B, Crosignani PG. Comparison of a levonorgestrel-releasing intrauterine device versus expectant management after conservative surgery for symptomatic endometriosis: A pilot study. *Fertil Steril* 2003;80:305–9.
11. Shen F, Wang Y, Lu Y, Yuan L, Liu X, Guo SW. Immunoreactivity of progesterone receptor isoform B and nuclear factor kappa-B as biomarkers for recurrence of ovarian endometriomas. *Am J Obstet Gynecol* 2008 Nov;199(5):486.e1–486.e10.
12. Wessels JM, Kay VR, Leyland NA, Agarwal SK, Foster WG. Assessing brain-derived neurotrophic factor as a novel clinical marker of endometriosis. *Fertil Steril* 2016;105:119–28.e5.
13. Edwards AK, Ramesh S, Singh V, Tayade C. A peptide inhibitor of synuclein-g reduces neovascularization of human endometriotic lesions. *Mol Hum Reprod* 2014;20:1002–8.
14. Mol BWJ, Bayram N, Lijmer JG et al. The performance of CA-125 measurement in the detection of endometriosis: A meta-analysis, *Fertil Steril* 1998;70(6):1101–8.
15. Socolov R, Butureanu S, Angioni S et al. The value of serological markers in the diagnosis and prognosis of endometriosis: A prospective case-control study. *Eur J Obstet Gynecol Reprod Biol* 2011;154(2):215–7.
16. Tokmak A, Ugur M, Tonguc E, Var T, Moraloğlu O, Ozaksit G. The value of urocortin and Ca-125 in the diagnosis of endometrioma. *Arch Gynecol Obstet* 2011;283(5):1075–9.
17. Mabrouk M, Elmakky A, Caramelli E et al. Performance of peripheral (serum and molecular) blood markers for diagnosis of endometriosis. *Arch Gynecol Obstet* 2012;285(5):1307–12.

18. Agic A, Djalali S, Wolfler MM, Halis G, Diedrich K, Hornung D. Combination of CCR1 mRNA, MCP1, and CA125 measurements in peripheral blood as a diagnostic test for endometriosis. *Reprod Sci* 2008;15(9):906–11.

19. Mihalyi A, Gevaert O, Kyama CM et al. Noninvasive diagnosis of endometriosis based on a combined analysis of six plasma biomarkers. *Hum Reprod* 2010;25(3):654–64.

20. Ozhan E, Kokcu A, Yanik K, Gunaydin M. Investigation of diagnostic potentials of nine different biomarkers in endometriosis. *Eur J Obstet Gynecol Reprod Biol* 2014;178:128–33.

21. Tuten A, Kucur M, Imamgluetal M. Copeptin is associated with the severity of endometriosis. *Archf Gynecol Obstet* 2014;290(1):75–82.

22. Vodolazkaia A, El-Aalamat Y, Popovic D et al. Evaluation of a panel of 28 biomarkers for the non-invasive diagnosis of endometriosis. *Hum Reprod* 2012;27(9):2698–711.

23. Signorile PG, Baldi A. Serum biomarker for diagnosis of endometriosis. *J Cell Physiol* 2014;229(11):1731–5.

24. Kocbek V, Vouk K, Mueller MD, Rižner TL, Bersinger NA. Elevated glycodelin-A concentrations in serum and peritoneal fluid of women with ovarian endometriosis. *Gynecol Endocrinol* 2013;29(5):455–9.

25. Drosdzol-Cop A, Skrzypulec-Plinta V, Stojko R. Serum and peritoneal fluid immunological markers in adolescent girls with chronic pelvic pain. *Obstet Gynecol Surv* 2012;67(6):374–81.

26. Tuten A, Kucur M, Imamoglu M, Oncu IM, Acikgoz AS, Sofiyeva N, Ozturk Z, Kaya B, Oral E. Serum YKL-40 levels are altered in endometriosis. *Gynecol Endocrinol* 2014May;30(5):381–4. doi: 10.3109/09513590.2014.887671. [Epub 2014 Feb 17. PMID: 24533749]

27. Borrelli GM, Abrão MS, Mechsner S. Can chemokines be used as biomarkers for endometriosis? A systematic review. *Hum Reprod* 2014;29(2):253–66.

28. Verit FF, Erel O, Celik N. Serum paraoxonase-1 activity in women with endometriosis and its relationship with the stage of the disease. *Hum Reprod* 2008;23(1):100–4.

29. Prieto L, Quesada JF, Camberoetal O. Analysis of follicular fluid and serum markers of oxidative stress in women with infertility related to endometriosis. *Fertil Steril* 2012;98(1):126–30.

30. Lambrinoudaki IV, Augoulea A, Christodoulakos GE et al. Measurable serum markers of oxidative stress response in women with endometriosis. *Fertil Steril* 2009;9(1):46–50.

31. May KE, Conduit-Hulbert SA, Villar J, Kirtley S, Kennedy SH, Becker CM. Peripheral biomarkers of endometriosis: A systematic review. *Hum Reprod Update* 2010;16(6): 651–74.

32. Amico FD, Skarmoutsou E, Quaderno G et al. Expression and localisation of osteopontin and prominin-1 (CD133) in patients with endometriosis. *Int J Mol Med* 2013;31(5): 1011–6.

33. Matarese G, de Placido G, Nikas Y, Alviggi C. Pathogenesis of endometriosis: Natural immunity dysfunction or autoimmune disease? *Trends Mol Med* 2003;9(5):223–8.

34. Huang H-F, Hong L-H, Tan Y, Sheng J-Z. Matrix metalloproteinase 2 is associated with changes in steroid hormones in the sera and peritoneal fluid of patients with endometriosis. *Fertil Steril* 2004;81(5):1235–9.

35. Singh AK, Chattopadhyay R, Chakravarty B, Chaud-hury K. Altered circulating levels of matrix metalloproteinases 2 and 9 and their inhibitors and effect of progesterone supple- mentation in women with endometriosis undergoing *in vitro* fertilization. *Fertil Steril* 2013;100(1);127.e1–134.e1.

36. Kianpour M, Nematbakhsh M, Ahmadi SM et al. Serum and peritoneal fluid levels of vascular endothelial growth factor in women with endometriosis. *Int J Fertil Steril* 2013;7(2):96–9.

37. Chen L, Fan R, Huang X, Xu H, Zhang X. Reduced levels of serum pigment epithelium-derived factor in women with endometriosis. *Reprod Sci* 2012;19(1):64–9.

38. Nabeta M, Abe Y, Haraguchi R, Kito K, Kusanagi Y, Ito M. Serum anti-PDIK1L autoantibody as a novel marker for endometriosis. *Fertil Steril* 2010;94(7):2552–7.

39. Nabeta M, Abe Y, Takaoka Y, Kusanagi Y, Ito M. Identification of anti-syntaxin 5 autoantibody as a novel serum marker of endometriosis. *J Reprod Immunol* 2011;91(1–2):48–55.

40. Griffiths-Jones S, Saini HK, van Dongen S, Enright AJ. miRBase: Tools for microRNA genomics. *Nucleic Acids Res* 2008;36(1): D154–8.

41. Hoefig KP, Thorns C, Roehle A et al. Unlocking pathology archives for microRNA-profiling. *Anticancer Res* 2008;28(1):119–23.

42. Resnick KE, Alder H, Hagan JP, Richardson DL, Croce CM, Cohn DE. The detection of differentially expressed microRNAs from the serum of ovarian cancer patients using a novel real-time PCR platform, *Gynecol Oncol* 2009;112(1):55–9.

43. Fassbender A, Dorien O, de Moor B et al. Biomarkers of endometriosis. In Harada T, ed. *Pathogenesis and Treatment*. Berlin, Germany: Springer; 2014.

44. Suryawanshi S, Vlad AM, Lin H-M et al. Plasma MicroRNAs as novel biomarkers for endometriosis and endometriosis-associated ovarian cancer. *Clin Cancer Res* 2013;19(5):1213–24.

45. Jia S-Z, Yang Y, Lang J, Sun P, Leng J. Plasma miR-17- 5p, miR-20a and miR-22 are down-regulated in women with endometriosis. *Hum Reprod* 2013;28(2):322–30.

46. Khanaki K, Nouri M, Ardekani AM et al. Evaluation of the relationship between endometriosis and omega-3 and omega-6 polyunsaturated fatty acids. *Iran Biomed J* 2012;16(1):38–43.

47. Vouk K, Hevir N, Ribić-Pucelj M et al. Discovery of phosphatidylcholines and sphingomyelins as biomarkers for ovarian endometriosis. *Hum Reprod* 2012;27(10):2955–65.

48. Fassbender A, Burney RO, O DF, D'Hooghe T, Giudice L. Update on biomarkers for the detection of endometriosis. *BioMed Res Int* 2015:14. Article ID 130854. https://doi.org/10.1155/2015/130854.

49. Zachariah R, Schmid S, Radpour R et al. Circulating cell-free DNA as a potential biomarker for minimal and mild endometriosis, *Reprod BioMed Online* 2009;18(3):407–11.

50. Olkowska-Truchanowicz J, Bocian K, Maksym RB et al. CD4 CD25 FOXP3 regulatory T cells in peripheral blood and peritoneal fluid of patients with endometriosis. *Hum Reprod* 2013;28(1):119–24.

51. Cho SH, Oh YJ, Nam A et al. Evaluation of serum and urinary angiogenic factors in patients with endometriosis. *Am J Reprod Immunol* 2007;58(6):497–504.

52. Becker CM, Louis G, Exarhopoulos A et al. Matrix metalloproteinases are elevated in the urine of patients with endometriosis, *Fertil Steril* 2010;94(6):2343–6.

53. Cho S, Choi YS, Yim SY et al. Urinary vitamin D-binding protein is elevated in patients with endometriosis. *Hum Reprod* 2012;27(2):515–22.

54. May KE, Villar J, Kirtley S, Kennedy SH, Becker CM. Endometrial alterations in endometriosis: A systematic review of putative biomarkers. *Hum Reprod Update* 2011;17(5), Article ID dmr013:637–53.

55. Teague EMCO, van der Hoek KH, van der Hoek MB et al. MicroRNA-regulated pathways associated with endometriosis. *Mol Endocrinol* 2009;23(2):265–75.

56. Braza-Boïls A, Marí-Alexandre J, Gilabert J et al. MicroRNA expression profile in endometriosis: Its relation to angiogenesis and fibrinolytic factors. *Hum Reprod* 2014;29(5):978–88.

57. Burney RO, Hamilton AE, Aghajanova L et al. MicroRNA expression profiling of eutopic secretory endometrium in women with versus without endometriosis. *Mol Hum Reprod* 2009;15(10):625–31.

58. Aghajanova L, Giudice LC. Molecular evidence for differences in endometrium in severe versus mild endometriosis. *Reprod Sci* 2011;18(3):229–51.

59. Petracco R, Grechukhina O, Popkhadze S, Massasa E, Zhou Y, Taylor HS. MicroRNA 135 regulates HOXA10 expression in endometriosis. *J Clin Endocrinol Metab* 2011;96(12):E1925–33.

60. Fassbender A, Verbeeck N, Brnigen D et al. Combined mRNA microarray and proteomic analysis of eutopic endometrium of women with and without endometriosis. *Hum Reprod* 2012;27(7):2020–9.

61. Ding X, Wang L, Ren Y, Zheng W. Detection of mitochondrial biomarkers in eutopic endometria of endometriosis using surface-enhanced laser desorption/ionization time-of-flight mass spectrometry. *Fertil Steril* 2010;94(7):2528–30.

62. Kyama CM, Mihalyi A, Gevaert O et al. Evaluation of endometrial biomarkers for semi-invasive diagnosis of endometriosis. *Fertil Steril* 95;2011(4):1338.e3–43.e3.

63. Berkley KJ, Dmitrieva N, Curtis KS, Papka RE. Innervation of ectopic endometrium in a

rat model of endometriosis. *Proc Natl Acad Sci U S A* 2004;101(30):11094–8.

64. Bokor A, Kyama CM, Vercruysse L et al. Density of small diameter sensory nerve fibres in endometrium: A semi-invasive diagnostic test for minimal to mild endometriosis. *Hum Reprod* 2009;24(12):3025–32.

65. Meibody A, Mehdizadeh Kashi A, Zare Mirzaie A et al. Diagnosis of endometrial nerve fibers in women with endometriosis. *Arch Gynecol Obstet* 2011;284(5):1157–62.

66. Leslie C, Ma T, McElhinney B, Leake R, Stewart CJ. Is the detection of endometrial nerve fibers useful in the diagnosis of endometriosis? *Int J Gynecol Pathol* 2013;32(2):149–55.

67. Good clinical practice recommendations on endometriosis, FOGSI 2014–2016, Convener Kriplani A, Editorial grant-Jagsonpal, p. 1–38.

68. Wu B, Yang Z, Tobe RG, Wang Y. Medical therapy for preventing recurrent endometriosis after conservative surgery: A cost-effectiveness analysis. *BJOG* 2018 Mar;125(4):469–77.

69. Aizzi FJ. Recurrent endometrioma; outcome of medical management with dienogest. *Eur Exp Biol* 2017;7(6):39.

70. Lee JH, Song JY, Yi KW et al. Effectiveness of dienogest for treatment of recurrent endometriosis: Multicenter data. *Reprod Sci* 2018;25(10):1515–22.

71. Muzii L, Achilli C, Lecce F et al. Second surgery for recurrent endometriomas is more harmful to healthy ovarian tissue and ovarian reserve than first surgery. *Fertil Steril* 2015;103:738–43.

72. Hwang H, Chung YJ, Lee SR et al. Clinical evaluation and management of endometriosis: Guideline for Korean patients from Korean Society of Endometriosis. *Obstet Gynecol Sci* 2018;61(5):553–64.

18

Quality of life affected by endometriosis: Lifestyle modification for symptom alleviation

SEEMA CHOPRA AND ARSHI SYAL

Endometriosis is an estrogen-dependent, long-term condition that causes acute and chronic pain and fatigue. As a result, it has a significant impact on the woman's quality of life and day-to-day activities, including interpersonal relationships and sexuality and infertility, as well as the ability to carry out daily tasks, work, physical, and mental fitness. Chronic pain is the root cause of an adverse impact of endometriosis in the affected population, such as interruption of education and careers and curtailed social participation. In order to successfully self-manage the condition, women need evidence-based, easily accessible information about the condition and ways that support surgical and medical treatment [1,2].

Endometriosis affects an estimated 1 in 10 women, which is approximately 176 million women worldwide, during their reproductive years (15–49 years). However symptoms can start as early as menarche and continue until menopause, especially if there is scarring or adhesions from the disease or as a consequence of prior surgery [3].

Sometimes, endometriosis remains asymptomatic. However, most of the symptoms include painful menstruation (dysmenorrhea), painful intercourse (dyspareunia), painful micturition (dysuria), painful defecation (dyschezia), lower back or abdominal discomfort, chronic pelvic pain (noncyclic abdominal and pelvic pain of at least 6 months duration), and

cyclic rectal bleeding or hematuria (bowel or bladder invasion). Rarely, the woman can present with respiratory distress during menstruation in every cycle secondary to catamenial pneumothorax, long-term untreated disease leading to increased risk of development of adenocarcinoma, and, lastly, bleeding into the surrounding tissues, leading to inflammation, scarring, and adhesion formation. It is of concern that severity of symptoms does not actually correlate well with the extent or progression of the endometriotic lesions [4,5].

Endometriosis is a chronic disease, which is under-diagnosed, under-reported, and under-researched, and the average time between onset of pain and diagnosis is nearly 8 years in the United Kingdom and 12 years in the United States [6]. As of now, there is no permanent cure for endometriosis, and even if treated, more often than not, it will recur [7]. In addition to prolonged patient discomfort, the economic implications, similar to other chronic diseases such as diabetes, Crohn's disease, and rheumatoid arthritis, are high. A survey across 10 countries estimated that the average annual cost of endometriosis per affected woman was high, consisting of healthcare costs and for productivity losses (€9579, €3113 and €6298 respectively as per an estimate) [8]. The quality of life is affected by physical pain, while there is an emotional impact because of fertility-related issues, mood disorders related to disease recurrence, and uncertainty regarding need for repeated surgeries or long-term medical therapy in the future. Thus, endometriosis has negative impacts on different aspects of daily life and is multidimensional and more complex than just negatively affecting physical and psychological parameters [6–8].

The experience of living with endometriosis correlates with the symptomatology of chronic pelvic pain related to endometriosis, delayed diagnosis because of stigmatization and late referrals to specialists, and treatment of endometriosis that is delayed due to late diagnosis and lack of "one-treatment-fits-all" protocols. Women have unpleasant experiences with healthcare providers who may not be compassionate and consider the symptoms to be psychological issues and lack of information to the lay person regarding the pathogenesis and treatment options available.

There are a multitude of ways by which endometriosis has an impact on women's lives, such as (1) physical impact, (2) psychological impact, (3) marital/sexual relationship impact, (4) social life impact, (5) impact on education, (6) impact on employment, (7) financial impact, (8) impact on life opportunities, and (9) impact on lifestyle. Some women reported negative impacts on their lifestyle such as using more analgesic medication, consuming more alcohol, smoking more cigarettes (tobacco), and, in two cases, using illicit drugs to help them cope with pain or feelings and their condition [6].

In a young population, impact of disease on daily life poses certain challenges such as social isolation from friends due to unexpected bouts of physical pain, not being able to participate in sports or physical activities, and anxiety over impeded education because of missing classes. Learning to manage the stress in one's life is important when your health feels out of your control. One usually feels frustrated, but it is essential to manage your life even when you are living with chronic pain. Most of these young women with endometriosis feel overwhelmed as they have to manage their disease and consequent pain and the other social/emotional events that impact their lives. It usually is of help to have their own personalized list of things that give relief in such situations, such as having a bath or shower with warm water, fomentation with a heating pad, relaxation exercise with yoga, or de-stressing mentally with music, story books, or movies [9].

Plotkin, in his study, showed that once diagnosed with endometriosis, this entity had an adverse effect on all aspects of the lives of adolescents, such as missing out on school, avoiding social gatherings, and difficulties adjusting with the peers. Teenagers were mostly anxious and worried about future fertility, and, as a result, sometimes were encouraged to plan an early pregnancy by the treating physician [10].

Some foods boost our immune system, which in turn protect our bodies from some illnesses and diseases. It is recommended to eat foods rich in fiber and with less saturated fats and more omega-3 fats for overall health. Regular physical activity such as walking, swimming, or dancing (about 60 minutes each day) can help to maintain a healthy weight and may help symptoms as a result [11]. When we exercise, our brain releases "feel-good" chemicals called endorphins. These naturally occurring hormones work like pain relievers to lower pain. It only takes about 10 minutes of moderate exercise (any exercise that makes you sweat or breathe hard) for your body to start making these chemicals and to improve the blood flow to our organs. Regular exercise lowers the amount of estrogen in the body. Women who averaged 2.5 hours of high-intensity activity (jogging, bicycling, or aerobics) were 63% less likely to have endometriosis [12].

Regarding the role of diet in endometriosis, it is thought that dietary fat leads to production of prostaglandins, which stimulate uterine contractions and also affect ovarian functioning. Another mechanism of influence of diet on disease is that high levels of prostaglandins could lead to higher production of estrogens, thus leading to growth of ectopic endometrial tissue. This is seen in obese women who follow a diet high in red meat and low in fruits and vegetables [5]. Evidence has suggested that the symptoms associated with endometriosis result from a local inflammatory peritoneal reaction caused by ectopic endometrial tissue. In addition, regular physical exercise seems to have protective effects against diseases that involve inflammatory processes as there is an increase in the systemic levels of cytokines with anti-inflammatory and antioxidant properties with regular exercise and a decrease in estrogen levels in endometrial implants [14]. There is a cumulative effect of reduction of menstrual flow, of ovarian stimulation, and of the action of estrogen caused by regular physical exercise. It has been hypothesized that participation in recreational or occupational physical activity may decrease estrogen levels and, with extreme exercise, reduce the frequency of ovulation [15]. Further, physical activity may increase levels of sex hormone–binding globulin (SHBG), which would reduce bioavailable estrogens [16,17].

It is well known that hyperinsulinemia acts by decreasing concentrations of SHBG, thereby increasing concentrations of estrogens and of insulin-like growth factor-1 (IGF-1) through decreasing concentrations of insulin-like growth factor binding protein (IGFBP) that stimulates endometrial cell proliferation. With regular physical activity, insulin resistance and hyperinsulinemia are reduced [18].

Dhillon and Holt [19] conducted a case control study about the risk of endometrioma associated with recreational physical activity. Based on the intensity of physical activity as metabolic equivalent (MET), a significant 76% reduction of the risk to develop an endometrioma was observed in patients who exercised at high intensity (6.0 METs or more—running, bicycle riding, and playing tennis) three times a week or more, 30 minutes or more per episode, and 10 months or more per year for 2 years, which was not seen in exercise of low intensity (less than 4.0 METs—golf, bowling, and light walking). In a large prospective cohort (Nurse's Health Study), a small association between physical activity such as aerobic exercise and the rates of endometriosis was confirmed by laparoscopy, although the effect of the other activities was small. It was also shown that pain can have a negative influence on the practice of physical exercise in women with endometriosis [20].

For any disease per se, curative treatment alone is not enough to promote good health. The main goal of health promotion is to support healthy behavior through a multidimensional approach. Healthy behavior is not only physical activity, but also a combination of mental, educational, and environmental factors that enables us to lead a healthy life. Especially in the perception of pain because of endometriosis, social and environmental factors play an important role, emphasizing the role of the social and psychological support.

Exercise has been shown to activate endogenous analgesia in healthy individuals and thereby an increased pain threshold due to the release of endogenous opioid and activation of (supra) spinal nociceptive inhibitory mechanisms mediated by the brain. Release of beta-endorphins from the pituitary (peripherally) and the hypothalamus (centrally) is triggered by exercise which in turn enables analgesic effects by activating μ-opioid receptors peripherally and centrally. Through its projections on the periaqueductal gray matter, the hypothalamus has the capacity to activate descending nociceptive inhibitory mechanisms. Some patients with chronic pain show dysfunctional response of and aberrations in central pain modulation to exercise; therefore, exercise should be individually tailored for prevention of symptom flares [21]. As was demonstrated in this study, analgesics could be less effective for pain relief in women with endometriosis who exercise regularly [13].

Dyspareunia, an important debilitating symptom associated with endometriosis has been announced as a research priority by the World Endometriosis Society, which called it a neglected aspect of endometriosis [22]. It is well known that the experience of pain during physical relations limits sexual activity, which in turn leads to lower self-esteem and a negative effect on interpersonal relationships [23].

Still, the gray areas not previously studied in women with endometriosis are regarding concern about finding new partners, financial constraints because of losing a job or cost of treatment, pain attacks while in a public place, need for lots of drugs or painkillers, worry about unexpected heavy bleeding, and sometimes concern among single parents regarding losing eligibility for child custody because of being too sick or in too much pain and excessive intake of pain killers that may be harmful [6].

On the brighter side, few women, however, believed that there had been a positive impact of endometriosis on their lifestyle such as choosing a healthy diet or doing regular exercise and giving up smoking. A number of women believed that living with endometriosis has taught them to be more "determined" and "stronger," "dealing with disease instead of fighting," and listening to their body, and that their pain tolerance had increased and that now they can understand and help others with the same symptoms. Experiences of living with endometriosis were similar between the hospital-based and community-based study groups [6].

At the same time, there are no controlled and randomized studies to establish the role of physical exercise in preventing the occurrence or progression of the endometriosis and how and to what intensity of physical exercise would be beneficial for women with endometriosis. The observational existing studies, with little or no statistical significance, indicate an inverse relationship between the practice of physical exercise and the risk of endometriosis, possibly that the nonprotective effect of exercise can be due the discomfort during exercise, thus preventing the practice of exercise. In this respect, well-controlled studies, in experimental models of endometriosis, well-defined study groups using validated instruments for evaluation and follow-up, and well-established exercise protocols can elucidate whether or not physical exercise is indeed able to interfere with the development of the endometriosis and its sequel. In addition, it should be possible to determine the intensity of exercise to be used in a preventive and curative manner [14].

REFERENCES

1. *Endometriosis: Diagnosis and Management NICE Guideline*. Published: 6 September 2017. 1–24 http://nice.org.uk/guidance/ng73
2. Ghonemy GE, El Sharkawy NB. Impact of changing lifestyle on endometriosis related pain IOSR. *J Nurs Health* Mar–Apr. 2017;6(2):Ver. V, 120–9.
3. Adamson GD, Kennedy S, Hummelshoj L. Creating solutions in endometriosis: Global collaboration through the World Endometriosis Research Foundation. *J Endometriosis* 2010; 2(1):3–6.
4. Giudice LC. Clinical practice. Endometriosis. *N Engl J Med* 2010;362(25):2389–98.
5. Parazzini F, Viganò P, Candiani M, Fedele L. Diet and endometriosis risk: A literature review. *Reprod Bio-Med Online* 2013;26:323–36.
6. Moradi M et al. Impact of endometriosis on Women's health: A qualitative study. *BMC Women's Health* 2014;14:123.
7. Denny E, Mann CH. A clinical overview of endometriosis: A misunderstood disease. *Br J Nurs* 2007;16(18):1112–6.
8. Simoens S, Dunselman G, Dirksen C, Hummelshoj L, Bokor A, Brandes I, D'Hooghe T. The burden of endometriosis: Costs and quality of life of women with endometriosis and treated in referral centres. *Hum Reprod* 2012;27(5):1292–9.
9. Center for Young Women's Health. A Collection of Resources for Teens and Young women with endometriosis. Cener for young women's health Health https://youngwomenshealth.org/wp-content/.../Endometriosis-Teen.pdf
10. Plotkin KM. Stolen Adolescence: The Experience of Adolescent Girls with Endometriosis, *Electronic Doctoral thesis*. University of Massachusetts, Amherst; 2004. Paper AAI3136765.
11. Health Guides, Endometriosis: Nutrition and Exercise Posted under Health Guides. Updated 20 January 2017.
12. *Healthy Women, Lifestyle and Dietary Changes for Endometriosis*. National Women's Health Resource Center, 2017, Inc. http://www.healthywomen.org/sites/default/files/endometriosis-lifestyle.jpg
13. Koppan A, Hamori J, Vranics I, Garai J, Kriszbacher I, Bodis J, Rebek-Nagy G, Koppan M. Pelvic pain in endometriosis: Painkillers or sport to alleviate symptoms? *Acta Physiol Hung* 2010;97:234–9.
14. Bonocher CM, Montenegro ML, Rosa e Silva JC, Ferriani RA, Meola J. Endometriosis and physical exercises: A systematic review. *Reprod Biol Endocrinol* 2014;12:4.
15. Warren MP, Perlroth NE. The effects of intense exercise on the female reproductive system. *J Endocrinol* 2001;170:3–11.
16. Colditz GA, Cannuscio CC, Frazier AL. Physical activity and reduced risk of colon cancer: Implications for prevention. *Cancer Cause Control* 1997;8:649–67.
17. Wu MH, Shoji Y, Chuang PC et al. Endometriosis: Disease pathophysiology and the role of prostaglandins. *Expert Rev Mol Med* 2007;9:1–20.
18. Friberg E, Wallin A, Wolk A. Sucrose, high-sugar foods, and risk of endometrial cancer—a population-based cohort study. *Cancer Epidemiol Biomark Prev* 2011;20:1831–7.
19. Dhillon PK, Holt VL: Recreational physical activity and endometrioma risk. *Am J Epidemiol* 2003;158:156–64. [14].
20. Vitonis AF, Hankinson SE, Hornstein MD, Missmer SA. Adult physical activity and endometriosis risk. *Epidemiology* 2010;21:16–23.

21. Nijs J, Kosek E, Van Oosterwijck J, Meeus M. Dysfunctional endogenous analgesia during exercise in patients with chronic pain: To exercise or not to exercise? *Pain Physician* 2012 Jul;15(3 Suppl):ES205–13.

22. Vercellini P, Meana M, Hummelshoj L, Somigliana E, Vigano P, Fedele L. Priorities for endometriosis research: A proposed focus on deep dyspareunia. *Reprod Sci* 2011;18(2):114–8.

23. Culley L, Law C, Hudson N, Denny E, Mitchell H, Baumgarten M, RaineFenning N. The social and psychological impact of endometriosis on women's lives: A critical narrative review. *Hum Reprod Update* 2013;19(6):625–39.

19

Literature review: Guidelines for the management of endometriosis

RASHMI BAGGA AND JAPLEEN KAUR

INTRODUCTION

Endometriosis is a disease associated with significant financial, as well as psychological, burden. These guidelines aim to provide direction to treating physicians and are a compilation of recommendations, developed by a group of experts, which are based on the best-available scientific evidence [1]. Various international as well as national guidelines have been compiled for endometriosis. Some salient ones are enumerated below:

1. Management of Women with Endometriosis—European Society of Human Reproduction and Embryology (ESHRE) [2]
2. Management of Endometriosis—American College of Obstetricians and Gynecologists (ACOG) Practice Bulletin [3]
3. Endometriosis—Society of Obstetricians and Gynecologists of Canada (SOGC) [4]
4. World Endometriosis Society (WES) Consensus on Current Management of Endometriosis [5]
5. Endometriosis and Infertility—A consensus Management—Australasian Certificate of Reproductive Endocrinology and Infertility Consensus Expert Panel on Trial Evidence (ACCEPT) [6]

6. College National des Gynecologues et Obstetriciens Francais (CNGOF) Guidelines for the Management of Endometriosis [7]
7. Guideline for the diagnosis and treatment of endometriosis—National German Guideline (S2k) Diagnosis and Treatment of Endometriosis (NGG) [8]
8. Endometriosis: Diagnosis and Management—National Institute for Health and Care Excellence (NICE) Guidelines [9]

Guidelines can be developed and modified for region-wide, nationwide, or worldwide application, depending on the attributes of the target population, such as racial, socioeconomic, and cultural backgrounds. Thus, Good Clinical Practice Recommendations on Endometriosis have been put forth by the FOGSI (Federation of Obstetricians and Gynecologists of India) Endometriosis Committee of 2014–2016, under the aegis of FOGSI [10].

METHODOLOGICAL QUALITY OF THE GUIDELINES

A systematic review of national and international guidelines on diagnosis and management of endometriosis was published in 2017 [11]. Seven guidelines were included in the review for assessment of methodological quality and variation in recommendations [2–8]. They found significant variation in the recommendations, with only 10 out of 152 (7%) recommendations being comparable among the evaluated guidelines. It was also noted that almost one-third (28%) of recommendations were not evidence based. The ESHRE guideline was rated the highest on methodological quality, as assessed by the Appraisal of Guidelines for Research and Evaluation (AGREE II) instrument (methodological quality score of 88/100) [12]. Interestingly, none of the seven guidelines assessed were found to have followed the standardized guideline development methods according to the AGREE II instrument. These findings also reiterate the fact that guidelines should not be blindly translated into clinical practice. Rather they should be used only for "guidance," and decision making should be individualized on the basis of the patient's unique characteristics [13].

The highest-rated ESHRE guidelines are summarized below, with the grades of recommendation given in parenthesis. Salient features of NICE, ACOG, and FOGSI good clinical practice recommendations (GCRP) are also enumerated, where they differ from the ESHRE guidelines.

ESHRE GUIDELINES

Grading system adapted from SIGN (Scottish Intercollegiate Guidelines Network, 2010).

1. **Diagnosis of endometriosis**
   a. Symptoms that can be associated with endometriosis in reproductive aged women:
      - Gynecological: Infertility, dysmenorrhea, chronic pelvic pain, dyspareunia, fatigue in the presence of any of the above good practice point (GPP).
      - Nongynecological: Dysuria, hematuria, dyschezia, rectal bleeding, shoulder pain (GPP).
   b. Clinical examination, bimanual pelvic or per rectal examination (as appropriate), is recommended for diagnosis (GPP). Predictive signs include visible vaginal nodules in the posterior vaginal fornix or tender induration and nodules of the rectovaginal wall for deep infiltrating endometriosis,

adnexal mass for endometrioma (C). But normal examination also does not rule out endometriosis (C).
   c. Transvaginal ultrasonography is indicated for diagnosis of ovarian endometrioma and rectal endometriosis in suspected cases (A).
   d. Laparoscopy is the current gold standard for diagnosis, preferably with positive histology, although negative histology does not rule out the disease (GPP).
   e. Biomarkers like CA-125 are not recommended for diagnosis (A).
   f. Role of MRI in diagnosis of peritoneal endometriosis is not clear (D). However, if deep endometriosis is suspected, additional imaging like CT urography or MRI is recommended to map extent of disease with respect to bowel, bladder, or uretric involvement (GPP).

2. **Treatment of endometriosis:** This is divided into treatment of pain and treatment of subfertility as they are diametrically opposite.
   2.1 **Treatment of endometriosis-associated pain**
      a. Empirical treatment: Counseling, analgesics, combined oral contraceptives (COCs), and progestogens (GPP)
      b. Medical treatment: Analgesics (GPP), COCs (B), progestogens (medroxyprogesterone acetate [oral or depot], dienogest, cyproterone acetate, norethisterone acetate, danazol), antiprogestogens (gestrinone), and GnRH agonists preferably with add-back therapy[A], LNG-IUS (B); choice depending on availability, patient preference, expense, and side effect profile (GPP). GnRH agonists to be avoided in adolescents and young adults due to concerns about bone mineral density (GPP). In special circumstances, such as refractory pain in rectovaginal endometriosis, aromatase inhibitors may be added to COCs, progestogens, or GnRH analogues (B).
      c. Surgical treatment:
         i. Peritoneal endometriosis: "See-and-treat" approach (A), ablation equivalent to excision (C). Laparoscopic uterine nerve ablation (LUNA) is not recommended (A). Presacral neurectomy is effective,

but requires consideration of expertise and associated hazards (A).

ii. Ovarian endometrioma: Cystectomy is preferable to drainage and coagulation OR CO_2 laser vaporization (better pain relief [A] and lower recurrence rates [B]).

iii. Deep endometriosis: Consider excision (B), preferably at a center with multidisciplinary facility (GPP).

iv. Refractory cases: Can consider hysterectomy with bilateral oophorectomy if patient has completed child-bearing, with counseling regarding failure also (GPP).

v. Adhesion prevention: Oxidized regenerated cellulose recommended (B). Icodextrin not recommended (B), polytetrafluoroethylene surgical membrane, hyaluronic acid products, proven role in pelvic surgery, although not particularly for endometriosis (GPP).

vi. Role of preoperative hormonal therapy: No (A), Only role: For symptomatic relief during waiting period until surgery.

vii. Role of postoperative adjunctive hormonal therapy: Short term (within 6 months only); does not improve outcome of surgery for pain (A).

Long term (6–24 months): Postoperative LNG-IUS or oral contraceptives can be prescribed for the prevention of endometriosis-associated dysmenorrhea and for recurrence (continuous and cyclic have equal efficacy) (A).

viii. Extragenital disease: Surgical or medical management can be considered for symptomatic relief (D).

ix. Complementary or alternative medicine or nutritional supplements: Not recommended as benefits or harms are unclear (GPP).

2.2 Treatment of endometriosis-associated infertility

a. Hormonal treatments: Not recommended (A).

b. American Fertility Society/American Society for Assisted Reproduction (AFS/ASRM) stage I/II: Operative laparoscopy (A) including adhesiolysis and ablation (CO_2 laser vaporization better than monopolar coagulation [C]) is recommended.

c. Ovarian endometrioma: Excision (better than drainage and coagulation) improves spontaneous pregnancy rates (A). Preoperative counseling regarding effect of ovarian reserve is advised (GPP).

d. AFS/ASRM stage III/IV: Consider operative laparoscopy to increase spontaneous pregnancy rates (B).

e. Adjunctive hormonal therapy: Preoperative use is not known to improve spontaneous pregnancy rates (GPP). Postoperative use is definitely not recommended (A).

f. Nutritional supplements, complementary or alternative medicine: Not recommended (GPP).

g. Medically assisted reproduction (MAR): Includes controlled ovarian stimulation (COS), intrauterine insemination (IUI), and assisted reproductive techniques (ART)

  i. AFS/ASRM stage I/II: COS/IUI is recommended as first line or within 6 months after surgical treatment (C). ART can be considered if (GPP)
- Tubal function is compromised
- Associated male infertility
- Other treatments have failed

  ii. ART can be considered after surgery without increasing recurrence rate (C). Antibiotic prophylaxis can be considered at the time of ovum pickup (D).

  iii. Role of medical therapy prior to ART: GnRH (gonadotropin-releasing hormone) agonists for a period of 3–6 months prior to ART is beneficial (B).

  iv. Role of surgery prior to ART.
- AFS/ASRM stage I/II: May consider complete removal of lesions, in those already undergoing laparoscopy, although benefit is not well established (C).
- AFS/ASRM stage III/IV (without endometrioma): No Definite Recommendation for benefit.

- Ovarian endometrioma: Size >= 3 cm, surgery is not recommended for improving pregnancy rates (A). Exceptions: Significant endometriosis-associated pain or inaccessibility of follicles (GPP). Caution: Counseling regarding ovarian reserve, especially if undergone previous ovarian surgery (GPP).
- Data insufficient to make recommendations regarding surgery for smaller endometriomas (<3 cm) prior to ART.
- Deep nodular lesions: Role not well defined (C).

2.3 Menopause in endometriosis

a. For menopausal symptoms after surgically induced menopause, estrogen/progestogen therapy or tibolone is recommended (B).

2.4 Asymptomatic endometriosis

a. Routine surgical excision and ablation for an incidental finding of asymptomatic endometriosis at the time of surgery is not recommended, although woman should be informed and counseled regarding the finding (GPP). Differentiating it from incidentally detected endometrioma, clinicians are advised to follow national guidelines for the management of ovarian cysts detected incidentally on ultrasound scan.

2.5 Primary prevention of endometriosis

Usefulness of COCs or exercise for primary prevention is uncertain (C).

2.6 Endometriosis and cancer

Counsel women who ask that there is no evidence that endometriosis causes cancer. Some cancers are slightly more common in these women, such as non-Hodgkin's lymphoma and endometrioid and clear-cell ovarian carcinoma, but no change in clinical management is currently recommended, as there is paucity of data on how to lower this risk (GPP).

Salient features of other guidelines which are different from or in addition to the ESHRE guidelines are presented below:

A. **NICE Guidelines**
1. Lay emphasis on specialist endometriosis centers, patient information, and support groups.
2. Offer endometriosis treatment according to the woman's symptoms, preferences, and priorities, rather than the stage of the endometriosis.
3. Consider outpatient follow-up (with or without examination and pelvic imaging) for women with confirmed endometriosis, particularly women who choose not to have surgery, if they have
   - Deep endometriosis involving the bowel, bladder, or ureter or
   - 1 or more endometrioma that is larger than 3 cm
4. As an adjunct to surgery for deep endometriosis involving the bowel, bladder, or ureter, consider 3 months of gonadotropin-releasing hormone agonists before surgery.

B. **ACOG Guidelines**
1. Confirmed diagnosis of endometriosis can only be made on histology and imaging studies cannot be used for diagnosis.
2. ACOG guidelines separately mention recurrent endometriosis: Options of medical treatment, including analgesics, COCs, GnRH agonists, oral or injectable progestins, and LNG-IUS have been recommended. Any surgical intervention in recurrent cases should be individualized on a case-by-case basis.
3. After complete surgery for endometriosis, ACOG does not necessitate addition of progestin to the estrogen-only hormone replacement therapy.

C. **Good Clinical Practice Recommendation by FOGSI**
[Grading system in accordance to the AACE protocol]
1. Utility of 3D ultrasound for detection of rectovaginal endometriosis is not well established (D).
2. MRI may be helpful in detecting small lesions (but more than 1 cm) and distinguishing endometriomas from dermoids (A).
3. Types of lesions on laparoscopy have been described: Powder-burn or black lesions, glandular excrescences, flame-like red

lesions, peritoneal pockets or windows, white opacified peritoneum, clear vesicles, adherence of ovary to ovarian fossa, encysted collections of chocolate-colored fluids, and adhesions (A).

4. Although biomarkers are not recommended for routine clinical use, CA-125 is thought to have a role in ruling out ovarian malignancies and the presence of extensive peritoneal lesions. Also, it may be useful for treatment follow-up in selected cases (A).

5. Cabergolin (0.5 mg weekly twice for 3 months) reduced EAPP in early lesions and reduced the size of endometrioma with comparable effect to LHRH agonist.

6. Dietary modifications, exercise, psychotherapy, yoga, and meditation may have a role in symptom relief (GPP).

7. The management of asymptomatic endometriosis depends on the accuracy of diagnosis, size of the mass, age of the patient, desire to preserve fertility, and her psychological makeup (GPP). When ultrasound features are suggestive of benign disease, follow-up with imaging every 3–6 months can be opted for. If there is suspicion of malignancy any time, further investigation and referral to oncologist is advised (Evidence Level B).

8. Additionally, it includes guidelines on the management of scar endometriosis.
   a. Cyclical change of size or pain intensity over scar may indicate scar endometriosis. Requires high index of suspicion (A).
   b. Skin and subcutaneous tissue are usually involved (A).
   c. Preferred diagnostic modalities: Ultrasound and color Doppler, rarely CT/MRI. Trucut biopsy is definitive.
   d. First-line treatment: Wide local excision. Medical management: Temporary measure for very small lesions.
   e. Careful exclusion of decidua and use of different mops and needles for different layers during cesarean can be helpful in prevention.

In 2011, a consensus meeting was held in France, involving 56 representatives of 34 major stakeholding organizations (national, international, medical, lay organizations, and support groups) from five continents [5]. A set of 69 consensus statements on management of endometriosis, encompassing various treatment options for endometriosis, impact of endometriosis on quality of life, and the role of endometriosis organizations and support groups was compiled. In a similar manner, the World Endometriosis Society developed a set of 28 consensus statements on classification of endometriosis in a meeting held in 2014 [14]. It was agreed upon that until better systems are available, a classification toolbox including revised ASRM classification and, in addition, ENZIAN or Endometriosis Fertility Index (EFI), where indicated, should be used. Although the consensus process was different from formal guideline development, it was based on the same available scientific evidence. Another limitation of such consensus statements is that they may differ if a different set of experts are included.

It is evident from the above discussion that the various guidelines are heterogenous. Thus, the need of the hour is collaboration of various guideline development groups to formulate a comprehensive set of guidelines for endometriosis, in accordance with the highest methodological quality standards. Although this will require extensive resources, it is expected to be beneficial for the healthcare professionals and researchers as well as the women with endometriosis. The newer guidelines can also take into consideration the recent literature. There is no dearth of research on the subject of endometriosis. Multiple systematic reviews and meta-analyses have been published in recent years, exploring newer fields in the symptomatology, diagnosis, or management of endometriosis in an attempt to solve some riddles pertaining to this enigmatic disease.

RECENT SYSTEMATIC REVIEWS AND META-ANALYSES

A. **Depressive Symptoms among Women with Endometriosis**
Author: Gambadauro et al. [15]
Methodology: 24 eligible studies were included in the meta-analysis.
Results: Women with endometriosis showed higher levels of depression compared with controls (standardized mean difference [SMD] = 0.22%, 95% CI: 0.12–0.32). In the endometriosis group, patients with pelvic pain

had significantly higher levels of depression compared with those without pain. In patients with pelvic pain, levels of depression were not different between patients with or without endometriosis.

Conclusion: There is complex association between endometriosis and depressive symptoms, determined largely by chronic pain, but also may be affected by individual vulnerabilities.

B. **Quality of Life (QoL) in Women with Endometriosis**

Author: Chaman-Ara et al. [16]

Methodology: Seven studies which had used the Endometriosis Health Profile-30 (EHP-30) for evaluation of QoL in women with endometriosis were included.

Results: The QoL scores varied from 43.70 to 56.14 in the five dimensions of the core questionnaire.

Conclusion: Endometriosis significantly alters the quality of life of the affected women.

C. **Transvaginal Ultrasound versus Magnetic Resonance Imaging (MRI) for Diagnosing Deep Infiltrating Endometriosis (DIE)**

Author: Guerriero et al. [17]

Methodology: Literature search from January 1989 to October 2016, six studies reporting the use of both modalities for preoperative diagnosis of DIE in suspected cases and comparing with surgical were found eligible.

Results: In the detection of DIE in the rectosigmoid, MRI had a pooled sensitivity of 0.85 (95% CI, 0.78–0.90) and specificity was 0.95 (95% CI, 0.83–0.99). In the detection of DIE in the rectosigmoid, TVS had a pooled sensitivity of 0.85 (95% CI, 0.68–0.94) and specificity was 0.96 (95% CI, 0.85–0.99).

Conclusion: The diagnostic performance of TVS and MRI is similar for detecting DIE involving rectosigmoid, uterosacral ligaments, and rectovaginal septum.

D. **Systematic Review and Meta-Analysis of Complementary Treatments for Women with Symptomatic Endometriosis**

Author: Mira et al. [18]

Methodology: Two RCTS relating to complementary pelvic pain treatment and adverse effects using the search terms "physical therapy" OR "complementary treatment" AND "endometriosis" were included.

Results: Meta-analysis of acupuncture showed a significant benefit in pain reduction as compared with placebo (P = 0.007). Exercise, electrotherapy, and yoga were inconclusive, but demonstrated a positive trend in the treatment of symptoms of endometriosis.

Conclusion: Only acupuncture has demonstrated significant benefit as of now. But further studies should be designed to confirm benefit of other approaches considering that they have shown positive trends.

Thus, endometriosis seems to affect all aspects of a woman's health, including physical, mental, and psychological well-being. Therefore, other than allopathy and pharmacotherapy, online portals and support groups are becoming popular.

ROLE OF SUPPORT GROUPS, LAY ORGANIZATIONS, AND ONLINE PORTALS

Importance of support groups

First and foremost, being part of a support group gives the women psychological consolation that they are not alone. Interacting with other patients suffering from the same disease can help them to learn new coping mechanisms. By sharing their experiences, patients can offload their mental agony, which might prove beneficial in alleviating physical symptoms as well.

Limitations

Recently, an article titled, "Googling Endometriosis: A Systematic Review of Information Available on the Internet" has been published [19]. The researchers identified 750 World Wide Web pages on five search engines (i.e., Google.com, Yahoo.com, AOL.com, ASK.com, and BING.com). Out of them, 54 pages were assessed for credibility, quality, readability, and accuracy. None of the pages scored high on all four domains as noted above. Therefore, they concluded that patients should be wary of inaccurate and outdated, or even dangerous, information online.

Significant delay in diagnosis of endometriosis has been reported [20,21]. Possible reasons attributed to the diagnostic delay are delay in seeking medical care as young women are told dysmenorrhea is a natural process or delay in diagnosis on the part of healthcare professionals, who assume that endometriosis takes longer to develop and is unlikely in the adolescent [22]. Therefore, there is a need for increasing awareness about the disease. March has been designated as "Endometriosis Awareness Month." Endometriosis awareness has further picked up momentum with the "Yellow Ribbon" campaigns. There are numerous organizations involved in disseminating information, making sincere efforts in improving the lives of women with endometriosis as well as promoting research in the field. Some of the prominent ones are listed below:

- Endometriosis Association (oldest), https://endometriosisassn.org
- Endometriosis Foundation of America (EndoFound), https://www.endofound.org
- Endometriosis UK, https://www.endometriosis-uk.org
- Australian Coalition for Endometriosis (ACE), https://www.endometriosisaustralia.org
- #HerYellowRibbon, http://www.heryellowribbon.org
- Endo Warriors, http://endowarriorssupport.com
- The Endometriosis Coalition, https://theendo.co

CONCLUSION

Numerous national and international guidelines have been framed for endometriosis, with ESHRE guidelines scoring highest on methodological quality. Consensus statements, which have taken into account the opinions of women suffering from endometriosis, are also available. Online portals, support groups, and lay organizations are involved in spreading awareness about this enigmatic disease and mitigating the suffering of affected women. It must be mentioned that there is a need for conducting well-planned research studies on various aspects of diagnosis and management of endometriosis. In addition, development of a comprehensive set of recommendations, for ready reference by all the stakeholders involved, needs further attention.

REFERENCES

1. Grol R, Dalhuijsen J, Thomas S, Veld C, Rutten G, Mokkink H. Attributes of clinical guidelines that influence use of guidelines in general practice: Observational study. *BMJ* 1998;317:858.

2. Dunselman GA, Vermeulen N, Becker C et al. ESHRE guideline: Management of women with endometriosis. European Society of Human Reproduction and Embryology. *Hum Reprod* 2014;29:400–12.

3. Practice bulletin no. 114: Management of endometriosis. *Obstet Gynecol* 2010;116:223–36.

4. Leyland N, Casper R, Laberge P, Singh SS, SOGC. Endometriosis: Diagnosis and management. *J Obstet Gynaecol Can* 2010;7(Suppl 2):S1–32.

5. Johnson NP, Hummelshoj L. World Endometriosis Society Montpellier Consortium. Consensus on current management of endometriosis. *Hum Reprod* 2013;28:1552–68.

6. Koch J, Rowan K, Rombauts L, Yazdani A, Chapman M, Johnson N. Endometriosis and infertility—A consensus statement from ACCEPT (Australasian CREI Consensus Expert Panel on Trial evidence). *Aust N Z J Obstet Gynaecol* 2012;52:513–22.

7. www.cngof.fr/pratiques-cliniques/guidelines/apercu?path=RPC_endometriosis_en.pdf&i=227

8. Ulrich U, Buchweitz O, Greb R et al. National German Guideline (S2k): Guideline for the diagnosis and treatment of endometriosis: Long version – AWMF Registry No. 015–045. *Geburtshilfe Frauenheilkd* 2014;74:1104–18.

9. NICE guideline Endometriosis: Diagnosis and management. September 2017.

10. FOGSI Good Clinical Practice Recommendations on endometriosis 2017.

11. Hirsch M, Begum MR, Paniz E, Barker C, Davis CJ, Duffy JMN. Diagnosis and management of endometriosis: A systematic review of international and national guidelines. *BJOG* 2018;125:556–64.

12. AGREE Collaboration. Development and validation of an international appraisal instrument for assessing the quality of clinical practice guidelines: The AGREE project. *Qual Saf Health Care* 2003;12:18–23.

13. Cheong Y. How good are the current guidelines on endometriosis? *BJOG* 2018;125:565.

14. Johnson NP, Hummelshoj L, Adamson GD et al. World Endometriosis Society consensus on the classification of endometriosis. *Hum Reprod* 2017;32:315–24.

15. Gambadauro P, Carli V, Hadlaczky G. Depressive symptoms among women with endometriosis: A systematic review and meta-analysis. *Am J Obstet Gynecol* 2019 Mar 1;220(3):230–41.

16. Chaman-Ara K, Bahrami MA, Moosazadeh M, Bahrami E. Quality of life in women with endometriosis: A systematic review and meta-analysis. *World Cancer Res J (Accepted Article)* 2017;4(1):e839.

17. Guerriero S, Saba L, Pascual MA, Ajossa S, Rodriguez I, Mais V, Alcazar JL. Transvaginal ultrasound vs magnetic resonance imaging for diagnosing deep infiltrating endometriosis: Systematic review and meta-analysis. *Ultrasound Obstet Gynecol* 2018;51:586–95.

18. Mira TA, Buen MM, Borges MG, Yela DA, Benetti-Pinto CL. Systematic review and meta-analysis of complementary treatments for women with symptomatic endometriosis. *Int J Gynecol Obstet* 2018;143:2–9.

19. Hirsch M, Aggarwal S, Barker C, Davis CJ, Duffy JM. Googling endometriosis: A systematic review of information available on the Internet. *Am J Obstet Gynecol* 2017;216:451–8.

20. Hudelist G, Fritzer N, Thomas A et al. Diagnostic delay for endometriosis in Austria and Germany: Causes and possible consequences. *Hum Reprod* 2012;27:3412–6.

21. Husby GK, Haugen RS, Moen MH. Diagnostic delay in women with pain and endometriosis. *Acta Obstet Gynecol Scand* 2003;82:649–53.

22. Stratton P. The tangled web of reasons for the delay in diagnosis of endometriosis in women with chronic pelvic pain: Will the suffering end? *Fertil Steril* 2006;86:1302–4.

20

Hormone therapy after total surgery for endometriosis

BHARTI SHARMA

Endometriosis is a disease of the premenopausal phase of woman's life, and estrogen, the hormone produced by the ovaries, is the main culprit. The basis of most of the treatment modalities used for endometriosis is to suppress ovarian production of estrogen and to induce menopause. And it has been seen resolving with menopause either induced by medical therapy such as GnRH analogues or surgical menopause after total abdominal hysterectomy (TAH) with bilateral salpingo-oophorectomy (BSO) or suppression of ovarian functions by oral contraceptive pills. Total surgery—hysterectomy with or without bilateral salpingo-oophorectomy is considered the definitive option for women who have completed childbearing [1,2]. After total surgery, the patient is relieved from endometriosis-related symptoms, but climacteric symptoms such as hot flashes, vaginal dryness, sleep, and mood disturbances, which affect the quality of life, appear afterward. In endometriosis, although the total surgery is the last option, compared to all other indications, women at a younger age with endometriosis would definitely require hormone replacement therapy (HRT). In this particular group of women, there are issues on safety of HRT, risk of recurrence, and malignant transformation.

TOTAL SURGERY FOR ENDOMETRIOSIS

Total surgery is removal of the uterus with bilateral ovaries, along with all visible endometriosis, and is the only definite treatment for endometriosis. This is usually performed for intractable pain not responding to all available modalities, in women who have completed childbearing and, preferably, in advanced age [3]. In endometriosis, complete surgery is technically more demanding and, to keep the recurrence rate to a minimum, it is very crucial to eradicate the endometriotic lesions completely. A very high recurrence has been reported with deep infiltrating cases where ovaries were conserved [4].

NATURAL MENOPAUSE VERSUS SURGICAL (SUDDEN) MENOPAUSE

Surgical menopause is the induced menopause that develops after removal of both ovaries, which are the main producers of estrogen before normal menopause. The average age of natural menopause is around 51 years, but most women will start to notice menopausal symptoms from around 47 years [5]. Natural menopause takes years to achieve complete menopause from perimenopausal transition, whereas in surgical menopause, there is sudden hormonal interruption. The symptoms of surgical menopause are quite severe without any transition phase compared to natural menopause. The benefit of surgical menopause in cases of endometriosis is symptomatic pain relief but it has potential disadvantages, such as

- Sudden and more severe onset of menopausal symptoms (hot flushes, night sweats, and vaginal dryness)
- Loss of bone density and increased risk of osteoporosis and fracture
- Impaired sexual function due to reduced desire and due to discomfort from vaginal dryness
- Reduced sex drive (libido) associated with loss of ovarian testosterone production
- Increased risk of cardiovascular (heart) disease
- Increased risk of depression, dementia, Parkinson's disease

ENDOMETRIOSIS AND ESTROGEN DEPENDENCE

The pathophysiology of endometriosis is complex and multifactorial, but estrogen dependence and progesterone resistance is the hallmark of disease [6]. It has been demonstrated that endometriotic lesions have overexpression of estrogen receptor beta, high levels of steroidogenic acute regulatory protein, and reduced levels of 17 beta hydroxysteroid dehydrogenase type 2. This causes a very high level of a biologically active form of estrogen at local sites alleged to cause endometriosis [7,8].

HRT FOR SURGICAL MENOPAUSE FOLLOWING ENDOMETRIOSIS

Current international guidelines recommend HRT for all women who undergo menopause under the age of 45 years and should continue until the average age of menopause, provided no contraindication to it [9]. In cases of endometriosis, most of the women are young at the time of surgical menopause and get relief from their symptoms, but at the same time face severe menopausal symptoms

as well. HRT is known to improve the quality of life of these women with surgical menopause and helps them cope with the symptoms attributed to sudden cessation of hormones. It also plays a role to prevent urogenital atrophy, loss of libido, bone loss, and cardiovascular disease. But it is still controversial to prescribe HRT in cases of endometriosis and postsurgical menopause.

OPTIONS FOR HRT

There are no specific guidelines on the type of HRT to use, but estrogen only is advised following hysterectomy and women who retain their uterus should be given both estrogen and progesterone in combination preparation. As such, there is no consensus available on HRT regimen in this population of endometriosis, but considering low-dose estrogen preparation and discontinuing on recurrence of symptoms seems reasonable. In some cases, nonhormonal agents can be considered to treat the hot flushes and other vasomotor symptoms. In some circumstances, such as bowel involvement, progesterone may be added. But in cases of endometriosis, there are two important concerns for prescribing HRT: risk of reactivation of residual endometriosis and malignant transformation. These two factors were the main outcome reported in a systemic review on the management of menopause in women with a history of endometriosis in which 33 studies and 48 patients were included [10].

CONCERNS OF HRT IN ENDOMETRIOSIS

- Recurrence of extrauterine endometriosis
- Chances of malignant transformation of residual endometriosis tissue

Recurrence of extrauterine endometriosis after complete surgery

The risk of recurrence of endometriosis with HRT or without HRT is not clearly defined. Theoretically, recurrence is possible with exogenous estrogen therapy as endometriosis is estrogen dependent. Due to incomplete removal or adhesions and severity of disease, recurrence has been reported even after complete surgery and required reoperation as well. Only estrogen (unopposed) has been found to be associated with numerous cases of recurrence as compared to combined hormonal preparation (estrogen and progesterone) [11–16]. Different routes of administration (oral tablets, implants, and patches) and different doses have been prescribed and reported in the literature, which is associated with reactivation of residual endometriosis. The recurrence cases commonly present with pain in the abdomen, but cases of pelvic mass, vaginal bleeding, rectal bleeding, hematuria, and hemoptysis have also been reported [12,17,18]. The usual sites of recurrence are the genitourinary tract, bladder, ureter, and gastrointestinal organs. It has been hypothesized that spillage during surgery and reactivation with HRT is responsible for these presentations.

Malignant transformation of residual endometriosis tissue

Another important concern with HRT is that exogenous estrogen will promote malignant transformation of residual endometriotic tissue. Although the exact pathophysiology is not clear, in 1925, Sampson first described the malignant transformation of ovarian endometriosis [19]. Malignant transformation is a multistep pathway in which a normal endometriotic tissue progresses to atypical intermediate stage, finally to invasive carcinoma, and there are multiple contributory factors implicated such as oxidative stress, inflammation, and altered hormonal milieu [20]. In some cases, genetic alterations in PTEN, TP53, and ARIDIA have also been demonstrated in endometriosis-associated cancers [21]. Wang et al. also reported malignant transformation of endometriotic foci following unopposed estrogen in an animal model [22].

Unopposed estrogen, either oral or topical, was prescribed in the majority of cases where malignant transformation was reported and the duration of treatment ranges from 3 to 20 years with a median duration of 6.7 years as found during systemic review [10]. Most of these cases of malignant transformation present with vaginal bleeding, pain, or pelvic mass. Endometroid adenocarcinoma was found to the most common HRT associated malignancy in cases of endometriosis. Other histopathological types were adenosarcoma, clear-cell carcinoma, Müllerian carcinosarcoma, and endometrial stromal sarcoma [10].

CONCLUSION

At present, there are no clear guidelines; whether a woman should be denied for HRT on the basis of history of endometriosis, risk of recurrence or malignant transformation. As per available literature (systemic and Cochrane review), the suggested approach is

1. Women with history of endometriosis should be counseled carefully about the possibility of recurrence, especially those who had possible risk factors such as residual endometrial tissue, deep infiltrating endometriosis, or colorectal or rectovaginal disease.
2. Women should be aware of the risk of malignant transformation, although the risk is very low, but HRT may have effects even years after stopping the treatment.
3. Individualize each patient and discuss the benefits and risks of HRT in detail, which include family history, comorbidities, BMI, and grade of endometriosis.
4. Once the decision to start HRT is taken, consider combined (estrogen + progesterone) instead of only estrogen, keeping in mind the risk of breast cancer with combined HRT.
5. In cases where HRT does not seem feasible, consider alternative therapies like tibolone, aromatase inhibitors, or SERMs combined with estrogen.

REFERENCES

1. MacDonald SR, Klock SC, Milad MP. Long-term outcome of nonconservative surgery (hysterectomy) for endometriosis-associated pain in women <30 years old. *Am J Obstet Gynecol* 1999;180:1360–3. [PubMed]
2. Chalermchockchareonkit A, Tekasakul P, Chaisilwattana P et al. Laparoscopic hysterectomy versus abdominal hysterectomy for severe pelvic endometriosis. *Int J Gynecol Obstet* 2012;116:109–11. [PubMed]
3. MacDonald SR, Klock SC, Milad MP. Long-term outcome of nonconservative surgery (hysterectomy) for endometriosis-associated pain in women <30 years old. *Am J Obstet Gynecol* 1999 June 1;180(6):1360–3.
4. Rizk B, Fischer AS, Lotfy HA et al. Recurrence of endometriosis after hysterectomy. *Facts Views Vis Obgyn* 2014;6(4):219.

5. Harlow SD, Gass M, Hall JE, Lobo R, Maki P, Rebar RW, Sherman S, Sluss PM, de Villiers TJ, For the STRAW 10 Collaborative Group. Executive summary of the Stages of Reproductive Aging Workshop + 10: addressing the unfinished agenda of staging reproductive aging. *Menopause.* 2012;19(4):387–95.

6. Burney RO, Giudice LC. Pathogenesis and pathophysiology of endometriosis. *Fertil Steril* 2012 September 1;98(3):511–9.

7. Kitawaki J, Kado N, Ishihara H, Koshiba H, Kitaoka Y, Honjo H. Endometriosis: The pathophysiology as an estrogen-dependent disease. *J Steroid Biochem Mol Biol* 2002 December 1;83(1-5):149–55.

8. Bulun SE, Monsavais D, Pavone ME, Dyson M, Xue Q, Attar E, Tokunaga H, Su EJ. Role of estrogen receptor-β in endometriosis. *Semin in Reprod Med* 2012 January;30(01):39–45. Thieme Medical Publishers.

9. Hickey M, Davison S, Elliot J. Hormone Replacement Therapy. *BMJ* 2012 February 16;344:e763.

10. Gemmell LC, Webster KE, Kirtley S, Vincent K, Zondervan KT, Becker CM. The management of menopause in women with a history of endometriosis: A systematic review. *Hum Reprod Update* 2017 May 11;23(4):481–500.

11. Taylor AA, Kenny N, Edmonds S, Hole L, Norbrook M, English J. Postmenopausal endometriosis and malignant transformation of endometriosis: A case series. *Gynecol Surg* 2005;2:135–7.

12. Taylor M, Bowen-Simpkins P, Barrington J. Complications of unopposed oestrogen following radical surgery for endometriosis. *J Obstet Gynaecol* 1999;19:647–8.

13. Badawy SZA, Liberatore C, Farhat MA, Valente AL, Landas S. Cervical endometriosis stimulated by estrogen therapy following supracervical hysterectomy. *J Gynecol Surg* 2004;19:141–4.

14. Giarenis I, Giamougiannis P, Speakman CT, Nieto JJ, Crocker SG. Recurrent endometriosis following total hysterectomy with oophorectomy mimicking a malignant neoplastic lesion: A diagnostic and therapeutic challenge. *Arch Gynecol Obstet* 2009;279:419–21.

15. Chahine B, Malbranque G, Lelong J, Ramon P, Tillie-Leblond I. Catamenial hemoptysis during hormone replacement treatment. *Rev Mal Respir* 2007;24:339–42.

16. Mattar CN, Pang B, Fong YF. An unexpected presentation of endometriosis—a "parasitic" cyst of the bowel in a menopausal woman on hormone therapy. *Ann Acad Med Singapore* 2008;37:69–71

17. Manyonda IT, Neale EJ, Flynn JT, Osborn DE. Obstructive uropathy from endometriosis after hysterectomy and oophorectomy; two case reports. *Eur J Obstet Gynecol Reprod Biol* 1989;31:195–8.

18. Goh JT, Hall BA. Postmenopausal endometrioma and hormonal replacement therapy. *Aust N Z J Obstet Gynaecol* 1992;32:384–5.

19. Sampson JA. Endometrial carcinoma of the ovary, arising in endometrial tissue in that organ. *Arch Surg* 1925;10:1–72.

20. Gadducci A, Lanfredini N, Tana R. Novel insights on the malignant transformation of endometriosis into ovarian carcinoma. *Gynecol Endocrinol* 2014;30:612–7.

21. Munksgaard PS, Blaakaer J. The association between endometriosis and ovarian cancer: A review of histological, genetic and molecular alterations. *Gynecol Oncol* 2012;124:164–9.

22. Wang CT, Wang DB, Liu KR, Li Y, Sun CX, Guo CS, Ren F. Inducing malignant transformation of endometriosis in rats by long-term sustaining hyperestrogenemia and type II diabetes. *Cancer Sci* 2015;106:43–50.

21

Ethical dilemmas in the management of endometriosis

SEEMA CHOPRA

After 150 years of research and quite a number of proposed hypotheses, the etiology of endometriosis remains elusive. Because of varied presentation and no stringent diagnostic criteria, relevant epidemiological data regarding the incidence of endometriosis in the general population are lacking. Therefore, endometriosis often raises difficult ethical challenges in terms of establishing the diagnosis without delay and in a noninvasive manner in order to provide adequate advice and the best-available treatment options. The situation is further complicated by the associated infertility, which may be secondary to endometriosis or due to the diminished ovarian reserve subsequent to radical surgery for the disease. Endometriosis, along with infertility, affects the patient as well as the partner and the family [1].

Endometriosis is defined as the presence of ectopic endometrial tissue and stroma and is a hormone-dependent evolutionary disease as the pathogenesis is still unknown. The entity is responsible for symptoms such as nonmenstrual chronic pelvic pain, dysmenorrhea, dyspareunia, and infertility.

As the presentation is atypical and the symptoms nonspecific, the diagnosis of endometriosis from the onset of the symptoms is significantly delayed. Studies show the time gap of 11.7 years in the United States, 8 years in the United Kingdom, and 7.6 years in Norway [2,3]. Personal factors and medical factors are reasons for this delay, as shown in a study conducted by Ballard et al. [4]

An ethical dilemma faced by the treating physician while communicating the diagnosis of endometriosis as a cause in a patient with infertility is the conflict between the patient's right to confidentiality and the partner's right to have access to the information in order to make important decisions regarding the couple's life [5]. Still, it is for the patient herself to decide whether or not she wants to share the information with her life partner. Therefore the physician has the primary responsibility to share the information with the patient about the disease and consequent infertility as a possibility and to provide potential management options as the physician's main concern is the patient.

Since there is an overlap in symptoms, such as chronic pelvic pain and low backache, between the different underlying conditions, it is important from the perspective of the physician to consider alternative diagnoses before proceeding with invasive investigations and treatments for the presumptive diagnosis of endometriosis [6].

Chronic pelvic pain is a common and difficult condition, accounting for nearly one-fifth of all gynecology outpatient referrals. The affected woman also commonly presents to other specialties, including gastroenterology, as the symptomatology is same for in irritable bowel syndrome (IBS) and endometriosis [7].

Menstrual pain is both a normal part of many women's lives and also a principal symptom of women affected with endometriosis. It is a common experience among women with pelvic pain and endometriosis to be assessed or regarded in psychological terms by healthcare professionals [8]. During evaluation, patients are therefore at risk of being labeled as having difficult psyches, psychological conflicts, or ulterior motives, even with biopsy-proven disease. There were no particular differences between attitudes of attending nurses in managing such patients, expressed through speech and action, respectively. In some cases, they considered that women with endometriosis failed to meet their expectations of a woman and that they were undesirable as wives or girlfriends. However, they also recognized other patients for not allowing the disease to "rule their lives" [9]. It is not unusual to have the cause or validity of one's pain questioned and instead of gynecological assessment, be referred for psychiatric evaluation. Historically, other chronic pain patients have similar experiences and this also applied to pelvic pain in general. It becomes easy to "blame the victim" when the issues are personalized, when physical complaints are ignored or interpreted as being caused by psychological issues [10]. Furthermore, studies by Mik-Meyer and Werner have shown that it is more often than not, especially in the case of women, when the diagnostic choice is between biomedical disease and psychological problems, the latter is preferred over the organic cause [11].

Endometriosis, being a disease of heterogeneous etiopathogenesis, is not fully understood to date and its outcome not foreseen even by experienced clinicians. Therefore, in medical practice, many times it is difficult for the patients to properly comprehend the information provided to them by the physician and therefore to provide consent of being fully informed about the disease. Hence, there might be need of a more complex, or sometimes a more limited, treatment than the one anticipated when discussing therapeutic options with the patient. The intraoperative findings and the extension of pathology might not be the same as at the time of diagnosis that was established clinically and on imaging before starting the surgical procedure. If there is need for extensive surgery according to the intraoperative findings, the question arises that in the case that the surgeon cannot benefit the patient from an extensive procedure, whether or not it is ethical not to do adhesiolysis just to respect the principle of "do no harm," because then, at the same time, the surgeon is not complying with the principle of "doing good for the patient." Some other dilemmas in clinical practice are, first, failing to diagnose the extent of endometriosis preoperatively and the failure of surgical healing in the case of radical surgery undertaken at the time of surgery for unexpected findings [8].

One of the important lessons in surgical practice is that each generation must practice the art and science of surgery based on the principles of the moral and ethical foundations inherited from the preceding generation. Even with the same basic foundations, the applications of the knowledge thus acquired become more complex and the decisions more difficult as the advancing technology over a period of time enables us to have greater opportunities for pain relief and suffering and thus save lives [12].

The impact of these advancements in technologies has driven the ethical implications to the new dimensions of global health, population imperatives, and impact of the evolution of the human species. As a result, rather than revolving only around an individual patient or the conduct of medical practice, the ethical dilemmas have dramatically increased in scope.

In addition to having the clinical meaning of any medical measure in terms of statistical significance, the outcome of therapeutic intervention is also based on the complex relation between the effect size, the risk of harms, and the cost incurred. For example, the aim of destroying superficial peritoneal implants as minimum worthwhile effect size for a low-risk laparoscopy reasonably should be different from that of a technically demanding bowel procedure for deep colorectal endometriotic lesions with opening of the intestinal lumen to excise the disease. Therefore, it is worthwhile to have less focus on statistical p-values, and more emphasis should be placed on the effect size of intestinal surgery, which will benefit the patient. In order to have robust scientific evidence, it is suggested that submitted manuscripts should be evaluated by journal editors from the point of view that reporting the results of observational studies on bowel surgery for colorectal endometriosis performed with the sole intent of improving the chances of fertility include the step-by-step description of the shared decision-making process adopted, the text of the information leaflet/brochure for patients, and copies of the informed consent form for both the scheduled procedure and participation in the study. This supplemental material should be provided online to readers in case of eventual publication of the manuscript [13].

When necessary, it is justifiable that women with colorectal endometriosis should be referred to tertiary care centers of expertise in order to undergo in-depth evaluation to exclude pre-existing bowel stenosis or hydroureteronephrosis. When these conditions are reliably excluded, it is not likely to incur major lesion progression during hormonal treatment for IVF and pregnancy [14].

Treatment of colorectal endometriosis before IVF is promoted for the prevention of complications after ovarian stimulation or during pregnancy [15]. In fact, in women undergoing IVF without prior removal of colorectal endometriotic lesions, several cases of bowel occlusions, ureteral stenosis, and obstetrical problems have been reported [16]. It is urgently needed to have more data on these not-so-well-known aspects of endometriosis management in infertile women, with the study objective to compare the incidence and severity of complications during pregnancy and delivery in women with or without previous resection of bowel endometriotic lesions.

Many infertile patients would do almost anything to have a baby. This should induce physicians to raise the ethical bar even more than usual during information and counseling [17]. The information must be expressed quantitatively and in an easily comprehensible manner, using absolutes, and avoiding the use of estimates such as relative risks. The caring gynecologist must describe the uncertainties of treatment, the causal relation between different endometriotic lesions and outcome in terms of infertility, and the potential benefits versus harms of radical dissection versus conservative surgery for colorectal endometriotic lesions in diverse clinical conditions. It is crucial from a medico-legal perspective to understand that endometriosis is not a cancer even when severe, thus as long as there is no robust evidence of a benefit, should not be treated on the lines of malignancy. Furthermore, as the available data do not support this position, surgery is not indicated

to prevent disease aggravation or impending deep lesion progression [18]. The ethical obligation of describing the type of surgical activity performed in their division, including the number of major bowel procedures for colorectal endometriosis per year and the relative outcome, rests with the gynecologist if they are not specifically experienced in removal of bowel endometriotic lesions and is still unwilling to refer the patient to tertiary care centers of expertise.

One should develop patient decision aids according to the International Decision Aid Standards minimum qualifying and certifying criteria. For the benefit of the affected party, visual aids to help decision making regarding the risk of intra- and postoperative major complications, the likelihood of postoperative conception, and the pregnancy rate after IVF, with or without removal of deep bowel endometriotic lesions should be provided to the patients [19,20].

In order to prevent possible harm to the patient, the Endometriosis Treatment Italian Club (ETIC) [21] has developed a process to jointly identify those diagnostic and therapeutic measures which are supported by low-quality objective evidence and if these results are applied in women with endometriosis could lead to either an unjustified increase in the number of medical and surgical procedures, an untoward outcome and morbidity, a psychological impact on patients "life including wrong diagnostic labeling," and increased financial burden of treatment on individuals and their families. The objectives of the resulting position paper were twofold, the first objective being the selection of those 10 low-value medical interventions which should be discouraged owing to an unfavorable balance between potential benefits, potential harms, and costs. The second objective was with the aim of allowing them to make the decisions that most suits their priorities and references after defining the uncertainties and potential downstream consequences of the 10 considered measures to be discussed when counseling women for such interventions [21].

We all have the duty of providing a sufficiently robust demonstration toward patients, practicing clinicians, and the scientific community, that the incremental gain of this medical intervention is worth the risk of harm the women take to their health. This should apply also to IVF, given the complex nature of the intervention, the limited success rates, and the frequent need for repeated cycles [13].

It is well understood that the motto of any therapeutic intervention should be increasing the quality of life of the patient. But the tedious evolution of endometriosis-associated chronic pelvic pain and the high rate of recurrence despite various treatment modalities makes the patient choose radical surgery such as total hysterectomy with bilateral adnexectomy to be free of the disease symptomatology and a better quality of life. This radical choice is many times not acceptable to the surgeons because of iatrogenic menopause and its consequences and permanent infertility [8].

Because of the difficulties raised by diagnosing and treating endometriosis and the personal, family, and social implications of this disease, endometriosis remains an ethical challenge for gynecologists. The difficult dilemmas that arise by diagnosing and treating a patient suffering from endometriosis may be solved by efficient communication in the framework of a genuine therapeutic partnership between the patient and the gynecologist [21].

REFERENCES

1. Holicov M et al. Ethical challenges in the diagnosis and treatment of endometriosis. *Revista Română de Bioetică* 2015;13(2):338–48.
2. Hadfield R, Mardon H, Barlow D, Kennedy S. Delay in the diagnosis of endometriosis: A survey of women from the USA and the UK. *Hum Reprod* 1996;11(4):878–80.
3. Husby GK, Haugen RS, Moen MH. Diagnostic delay in women with pain and endometriosis. *Acta Obstet Gynecol Scand* 2003;82(7):649–53.
4. Ballard K, Lowton K, Wright J. What's the delay? A qualitative study of women's experiences of reaching a diagnosis of endometriosis. *Fertil Steril* 2006;86(5):296–301.
5. Ioan B, Gavrilovici C. Bioetica in lume? consiliul nuffield de bioetica. *Rev Rom Bioet* 2004;2(4).
6. Latthe P, Latthe M, Say L, Gülmezoglu M, Khan KS. WHO systematic review of prevalence of chronic pelvic pain: A neglected reproductive health morbidity. *BMC Public Health* 2006;6(177).
7. Issa B, Ormesher L, Whorwell PJ, Shah M, Hamdy S. Endometriosis and irritable bowel syndrome: A dilemma for the gynaecologist and gastroenterologist. *Obstet Gynaecol* 2016;18:9–16.
8. Bach AM, Risoer MB, Forman A, Seibaek L. Practices and attitudes concerning endometriosis among nurses specializing in gynecology. *Glob Qual Nurs Res* 2016;3: 2333393616651351. Published 2016 May 26.
9. Denny E. Women's experience of endometriosis. *J Adv Nurs* 2004 June;46(6):641–8. (1).
10. Ballweg ML. Blaming the victim. The psychologizing of endometriosis. *Obstet Gynecol Clin North Am* 1997 June;24(2):441–53.
11. Nanna Mik-Meyer. On being credibly ill: Class and gender in illness stories among welfare officers and clients with medically unexplained symptoms. *Health Sociol Rev* 2011;20:(1)28–40.
12. Satava RM. Laparoscopic surgery, robots, and surgical simulation: Moral and ethical issues. *Semin Laparosc Surg* 2002;9(4):230–8.
13. Vercellini P, Viganò P, Frattaruolo MP, Borghi A, Somigliana E. Bowel surgery as a fertility-enhancing procedure in patients with colorectal endometriosis: Methodological, pathogenic and ethical issues. *Hum Reprod* July 2018;33(7):1205–11.
14. Santulli P, Bourdon M, Presse M, Gayet V, Marcellin L, Prunet C, de Ziegler D, Chapron C. Endometriosis-related infertility: Assisted reproductive technology has no adverse impact on pain or quality-of-life scores. *Fertil Steril* 2016;105:978–87e4.
15. Darwish B, Chanavaz-Lacheray I, Roman H. Swimming against the stream: Is surgery worthwhile in women with deep infiltrating endometriosis and pregnancy intention? *J Minim Invasive Gynecol* 2018;25:1–3.
16. Touleimat S, Huet E, Sanguin S, Roman H. Differed surgery in patient with colorectal endometriosis and pregnancy intention: Is it reasonable? *J Gynecol Obstet Hum Reprod* 2018;47:29–31.
17. McCullough LB, Jones JW. Unravelling ethical challenges in surgery. *Lancet* 2009;374: 1058–59.
18. Fedele L, Bianchi S, Zanconato G, Raffaelli R, Berlanda N. Is rectovaginal endometriosis a progressive disease? *Am J Obstet Gynecol* 2004;191:1539–42.
19. Clinical Review (Drug and Therapeutics Bulletin). An introduction to patient decision aids. *BMJ* 2013;347. doi: https://doi.org/10.1136/bmj.f4147.

20. Joseph-Williams N, Elwyn G, Edwards A. Knowledge is not power for patients: A systematic review and thematic synthesis of patient-reported barriers and facilitators to shared decision making. *Patient Educ Couns* 2014 March;94(3):291–309.

21. ETIC Endometriosis Treatment Italian Club†. When more is not better: 10 "don'ts" in endometriosis management. An ETIC* position statement. *Hum Reprod Open* 2019;1–15. doi:10.1093/hropen/hoz009.

Conclusion

SEEMA CHOPRA

Endometriosis is a challenging medical condition with debilitating effects on the quality of life of women, as well as their mental and emotional health. More so, it remains a diagnostic dilemma as the symptoms are atypical or sometimes even asymptomatic. Endometriosis may have different clinical presentations depending on the primary location. Pelvic pain and infertility are two of the most common symptoms associated with it. Dysmenorrhea typically developing after years of pain-free menstrual cycle is suggestive of endometriosis. The pain most often begins 48 hours prior to the onset of menses and persists throughout the menstrual period. The pain may be unilateral or bilateral and is perceived as sensation of swelling of the internal organs or pelvic heaviness [1]. Cyclical pain soon progresses to noncyclical chronic pelvic pain severe enough to cause functional disability and to compromise day-to-day activities [2].

The average time taken to diagnose endometriosis from onset of clinical symptoms is 9 years, requiring an average of 4.2 physician visits, and is the longest in adolescent-aged patients [3]. This is mainly because the pelvic pain of endometriosis in adolescents may be noncyclic in comparison to adults who typically present with more specific complaints such as cyclical pain, dyspareunia, and infertility, making the diagnosis easier [4]. Also, dysmenorrhea in adolescents is more often considered "physiological" and hence rarely evaluated seriously.

Symptoms usually pertain to the anatomic site affected by the endometriosis. There could be involvement of pelvic organs alone or the gastrointestinal system or the urinary tract may be affected. Although clinical examination may have some pointers toward the diagnosis, on bimanual examination, there may be lateral displacement of the cervix due to unilateral involvement of the uterosacral ligaments. The uterus may be retroverted and exhibit tenderness, decreased mobility, or fixation. Ovarian endometrioma can present as a fixed, immobile, and tender adnexal mass. Ovarian endometriomas are bilateral in 30%–50% of cases [5]. Tender nodules can be palpated along the uterosacral ligaments or posterior cul-de-sac, especially if done before the onset of menses. Digital rectal examination reveals the nodularity and tenderness of the rectovaginal septum.

Advances in research have led to the identification of a number of noninvasive and/or minimally invasive biomarkers for early diagnosis of endometriosis. However, despite large number of biomarkers being available, promising results are sparse, and to date, no single biomarker is capable of accurately diagnosing endometriosis that can replace histopathological diagnosis. The major reason for this is the complex etiopathogenesis of the disease. Serum CA-125 may have a role in differentiating endometriomas from other benign cysts, especially when coupled with the transvaginal ultrasonography.

A recent study done by Othman and colleagues found elevated levels of IL-6 in the serum of patients with endometriosis when compared to infertile patients with no evidence of endometriosis [6].

The discovery of new biomarkers may be of particular advantage in diagnosing endometriosis.

Ultrasonography: Transvaginal ultrasonography (TVS) is a simple, widely available, and cost-effective method of imaging and, hence, is the first imaging modality in the evaluation of endometriosis. Ovaries are the most common site of endometriotic implants. The classical findings of an ovarian endometrioma on an ultrasound is the presence of a "chocolate cyst," owing to the presence of thick, degenerated blood products as a result of cyclical bleeding during the menses, a homogenous hypoechoic lesion with the ovary, with low to medium echoes (ground glass appearance), and no internal vascularity [7]. TVS has 88% sensitivity in differentiating endometriomas from other masses and a specificity of 90% [8]. The use of MRI comes into the play when the ultrasonography is inconclusive. MRI can be used as an adjunct to differentiate endometriomas from hemorrhagic cyst or dermoid.

Infertility is a challenging scenario in these patients. In reference to certain population-based studies, the estimated prevalence of endometriosis ranges from 0.8% to 6% in women in the reproductive age group; these figures rise drastically to as high as 20% to 50% in subfertile women, with variations according to age of patients and over time periods [9]. The possible mechanisms could be distortion of pelvic anatomy, endocrine and ovulatory abnormalities, fertilization and implantation defects, and early pregnancy loss.

The treatment objectives include the relief of pain and prevention of recurrence. These agents should suppress the synthesis of estrogen, reduce the bleeding, as well as induce atrophy of the endometriotic implants, thus creating a "pseudo pregnancy" or "pseudo menopause" status [10]. Although all agents are clinically effective, they differ in their mechanism of action, route of administration, length of therapy, and side effects. The first-line treatment includes oral contraceptive pills and progesterones, which have significant limitations. Thus it is essential to develop effective and well-tolerated therapies that are optimal for long-term use.

Despite medical/surgical/combined medical and surgical modalities, the recurrence of endometriosis is estimated to be 21.5% at 2 years and 40%–50% at 5 years [9]. Current hormonal therapies used to treat endometriosis have no role in improving endometriosis-related infertility, and

they aim only to alleviate pain symptoms. Thus, these therapies do not definitively "cure" the disease which may not only persist but may also progress. There are various pharmacological agents used for the treatment of endometriosis. These act by anti-inflammatory action, inhibiting ovulation, reducing estradiol levels, causing decidualization, and modulating immunological function and progesterone receptor activity [11]. Nonsteroidal anti-inflammatory drugs are invariably used for the relief of primary dysmenorrhea.

Surgery may be required as a primary modality when medical management fails or cannot be administered or as an adjunct to medical management. Various factors need to be taken into consideration while planning for surgery and choosing the mode of surgery, such as age, symptoms (pain, infertility, abnormal uterine bleeding [AUB]), aim of treatment (elimination of pain, improving fertility, ruling out malignancy), previous surgeries, and existing comorbidities of the patient. In women desiring fertility, risks associated with surgery, risk of laparoscopic procedure, reduction in ovarian reserve, risk of loss of ovary, reduction in future fertility, requirement of ART, and possibility of preoperative freezing of oocytes should be explained [12].

Deep infiltrating endometriosis is one of the most severe forms of endometriosis and is defined as endometriosis infiltration of more than 5 mm beneath the peritoneum. The symptomatology varies based upon the organ of involvement. The most commonly involved organ that a urologist encounters is the bladder followed by the ureter, the kidney, and the urethra. Traditionally, urinary tract endometriosis (UTE) is described as a rare entity with an incidence of 1% to 5.5% in patients with endometriosis. Its prevalence increases to 19%–53% among patients with DIE. Bladder involvement is the most frequent type of UTE, occurring in 70%–85% of cases, while ureteral involvement accounts for 9%–23% of UTE cases patients with DIE [13]. Ultrasonography remains the first line of investigations and MRI is regarded as second line. Medical management in the form of hormonal therapy alone is less effective in urinary tract endometriosis, and should be applied in selected groups of patients. The surgical approach and technique should be individualized based on the extent and severity of the disease and renal function status. A multimodality team including gynecologists, a urologist, and a gastrointestinal surgeon can improve the outcome in deep infiltrating endometriosis.

Bowel endometriosis is a complex problem for gynecologists and colorectal surgeons alike. The clinical presentation is varied and often deceptive. Symptoms include deep pelvic pain, dysmenorrhea, dyspareunia, dyschezia, tenesmus, and alteration of bowel habit. Severity of the bowel symptoms may vary according to the menstrual cycle. Up to 25% of patients also suffer from infertility. A high index of suspicion is necessary to suspect bowel endometriosis. Transvaginal or transrectal ultrasound, and magnetic resonance imaging remain the mainstays of diagnosis. Surgical resection is indicated when symptoms impair quality of life and activities of daily living.

The presence of endometrial glands outside the endometrium is defined as endometriosis, while occurrence of endometrial glands and stroma within the myometrium associated with myohyperplasia and hypertrophy is known as adenomyosis. Approximately 35% of women with adenomyosis are asymptomatic while 70% to 80% of women with adenomyosis present in the fourth and fifth decades of life. Furthermore, 5%–25% of adenomyosis cases may be seen in patients younger than 39 years and only 5% to 10% occur in elderly women more than 60 years of age. Diagnosis is usually made in symptomatic women in the forties and fifties age group; however, it may be found incidentally in younger women undergoing evaluation for infertility or who have abnormal uterine bleeding and dysmenorrhea. Partial or complete excision of adenomyoma can be planned. Hysterectomy is the mainstay of treatment for women who have completed their families; however, diagnosis of adenomyosis is rarely made with certainty before surgery and this invites many options of medical therapy.

Total surgery: Hysterectomy with or without bilateral salpingo-oophorectomy is considered the definitive option for women who have completed childbearing. After total surgery, the patient is relieved of endometriosis-related symptoms, but climacteric symptoms such as hot flashes, vaginal dryness, sleep, and mood disturbances which affect the quality of life appear. In endometriosis, although total surgery is the last option, compared to all other indications, women who with endometriosis are at younger ages would definitely require HRT. In this particular group of women there are issues on safety of HRT, risk of recurrence, and malignant transformation.

Experiences of living with endometriosis correlate with the symptomatology of chronic pelvic pain related to endometriosis, delayed diagnosis because of stigmatization, and late referrals to specialists. Treatment of endometriosis is often delayed due to late diagnosis and lack of "one-treatment-fits-all" protocols. For any disease per se, curative treatment alone is not enough to promote good health. The main goal of health promotion is to support healthy behavior through a multidimensional approach. Healthy behavior is not only physical activity, but also a combination of mental, educational, and environmental factors that enables us to lead a healthy life. Especially in the perception of pain because of endometriosis, social and environmental factors play an important role, emphasizing the role of the social and psychological support.

After 150 years of research and quite a number of proposed hypotheses, the etiology of endometriosis remains elusive. Therefore often endometriosis raises difficult ethical challenges in terms of establishing the diagnosis without delay and in a noninvasive manner in order to provide adequate advice and the best available treatment options. The situation is further complicated by the associated infertility, which may be secondary to endometriosis or due to the diminished ovarian reserve subsequent to radical surgery for the disease. In medical practice, many times it is difficult for patients to properly comprehend the information provided to them by the physician and therefore to provide consent of being fully informed about the disease. Hence, there might be a need for a more complex or sometimes a more limited treatment than the one anticipated when discussing therapeutic options with the patient. If there is a need for extensive surgery according to the intraoperative findings, it is ethical not to do adhesiolysis if the patient cannot benefit the patient from extensive procedure, just to respect the principle of "do no harm," because then, at the same time, the surgeon is not complying with the principle of "doing good for the patient?" Some other dilemmas in clinical practice are, first, failing to diagnose the extent of endometriosis preoperatively and the failure of surgical healing in the case of radical surgery undertaken at the time of surgery for unexpected findings.

Guidelines are essential to provide comprehensive recommendations on best course of action based on sound scientific evidence and expert opinion. Although a plethora of guidelines are available for management of endometriosis, it still remains a challenge for clinicians. Some of the prominent sets of guidelines are those given by ESHRE, ACOG, SOGC, FOGSI, and so on. Online portals, support groups, and lay organizations are involved in spreading awareness about this enigmatic disease and mitigating the suffering of affected women. It must be mentioned that there is a need for conducting well-planned research studies on various aspects of diagnosis and management of endometriosis. In addition, the development of a comprehensive set of recommendations, for ready reference by all the stakeholders involved, needs further attention.

REFERENCES

1. Bieber E. *Clinical Gynaecology*. 2nd ed. Cambridge: Cambridge university press; 2015.
2. Opoku-Anane J, Lau er MR. Prevalence of endometriosis in adolescent girls with chronic pelvic pain not responding to conventional therapy. Have we underestimated? *J Pediatr Adolesc Gynecol* 2012;25(2):e50.
3. Ballweg ML. Big picture of endometriosis helps provide guidance on approach to teens: Comparative historical data show endo starting younger, is more severe. *J Pediatr Adolesc Gynecol* 2003;16(3 Suppl):S21–6.
4. Laufer MR, Goietein L, Bush M, Cramer DW, Emans SJ. Prevalence of endometriosis in adolescent girls with chronic pelvic pain not responding to conventional therapy. *J Pediatr Adolesc Gynecol* 1997;10:199–202.
5. Carbognin G, Guarise A, Minelli L et al. Pelvic endometriosis: US and MRI features. *Abdom Imaging* 2004;29:609.
6. Othman EE, Hornung D, Salem HT et al. Serum cytokines as biomarkers for nonsurgical prediction of endometriosis. *Eur J Obstet Gynecol Reprod Biol* 2007;137:240–6.
7. Bennett GL, Slywotzky CM, Cantera M, Hecht EM. Unusual manifestations and complications of endometriosis—Spectrum of imaging findings: Pictorial review. *AJR Am J Roentgenol* 2010;194(6 Suppl):WS34–46.
8. Hudelist G, English J, Thomas AE, Tinelli A, Singer CF and Keckstein J. Diagnostic accuracy of transvaginal ultrasound for non-invasive diagnosis of bowel endometriosis: Systematic review and meta-analysis. *Ultrasound Obstet Gynecol* 2011;37:257–63.
9. Fuldeore MJ, Soliman AM. Prevalence and symptomatic burden of diagnosed endometriosis in the United States: National estimates from a cross-sectional survey of 59,411 women. *Gynecol Obstet Invest* 2017;82(5):453–61. doi: 10.1159/000452660. [Epub 2016 Nov 8.]
10. Mehedintu C, Plotogea MN, Ionescu S, Antonovici M. Endometriosis still a challenge. *J Med Life* 2014 September 15;7(3):349–57.
11. Han SJ, O'Malley BW. The dynamics of nuclear receptors and nuclear receptor coregulators in the pathogenesis of endometriosis. *Hum Reprod Update* 2014;20(4):467–84.
12. Somigliana E, Vigano P, Filippi F, Papaleo E, Benaglia L, Candiani M, Vercellini P. Fertility preservation in women with endometriosis: For all, for some, for none? *Hum Reprod* 2015;30:1280–6.
13. Knabben L, Imboden S, Fellmann B, Nirgianakis K, Kuhn A, Mueller MD. Urinary tract endometriosis in patients with deep infiltrating endometriosis: Prevalence, symptoms, management, and proposal for a new clinical classification. *Fertil Steril* 2015;103:147–52.

Index

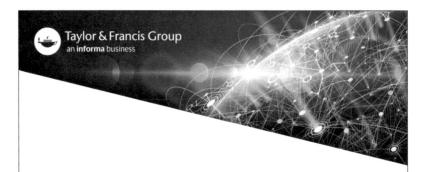